Clinical Infectious Diseases

Clinical Infectious Diseases

Edited by Cameron Harris

AMERICAN
MEDICAL PUBLISHERS
www.americanmedicalpublishers.com

American Medical Publishers,
41 Flatbush Avenue,
1st Floor, New York,
NY 11217, USA

Visit us on the World Wide Web at:
www.americanmedicalpublishers.com

ISBN: 978-1-63927-220-4

Cataloging-in-Publication Data

Clinical infectious diseases / edited by Cameron Harris.
p. cm.
Includes bibliographical references and index.
ISBN 978-1-63927-220-4
1. Communicable diseases. 2. Infection. 3. Epidemics. I. Harris, Cameron.
RC111 .C55 2022
616.9--dc23

Table of Contents

Preface

Infectious diseases, also known as transmissible diseases, are the illness caused by an infection. The invasion of an organism's body tissue by the biological pathogens such as viruses, bacteria, fungi, parasites, prions and anthropods causes infections. These pathogens enter the body of an organism and start multiplying. The immune system of the host tissues fights against them. The infections that show symptoms are categorized as clinical and the infections that do not show any apparent symptoms are known as subclinical infections. The symptoms of infectious diseases vary from one disease to another but the most common of them include fatigue, weight loss, fever, running nose, coughing, skin rashes, loss of appetite, night sweats, chills and body aches. The medications commonly used to treat the infectious diseases are antibiotics, antifungals, antiprotozoals, antivirals and antihelminthics. This book presents researches and studies performed by experts across the globe. It contains some path-breaking studies in the field of infectious diseases. It will provide comprehensive knowledge to the readers.

Significant researches are present in this book. Intensive efforts have been employed by authors to make this book an outstanding discourse. This book contains the enlightening chapters which have been written on the basis of significant researches done by the experts.

Finally, I would also like to thank all the members involved in this book for being a team and meeting all the deadlines for the submission of their respective works. I would also like to thank my friends and family for being supportive in my efforts.

Editor

1

Characteristics of ventilator-associated pneumonia due to hypervirulent *Klebsiella pneumoniae* genotype in genetic background for the elderly in two tertiary hospitals in China

Chao Liu[1] and Jun Guo[2,3*]

Abstract

Background: Aerobactin is a critical factor for the hypervirulent *Klebsiella pneumoniae* (hvKp), but data for the aerobactin-positive genotype of hvKp in elderly persons with ventilator-associated pneumonia (VAP) is limited. The purpose of this study is to understand the risk factors and characteristics of the hvKp genotype for elderly patients with VAP.

Methods: A retrospective study of 73 elderly patients with *Kp* was conducted from November 2008 to December 2017 in two tertiary hospitals. The clinical and microbiological data, including inflammatory reaction, nutritional status, antimicrobial susceptibility testing, string test, extended-spectrum-β-lactamase (ESBL) production, virulence-associated gene (capsular serotype-specific gene and rmpA/A2,magA,aerobaction) and multilocus sequence typing, of the hvKp group defined as aerobactin positive were compared with those of classic *Kp* strains.

Results: Of 73 *Kp* isolates, 46.6% were hvKp. ST23 is highly prevalent in two hospitals but is not highly associated with hvKp in different hospitals. Additionally, ST23, ST37 and ST2906 are more likely to induce lethal VAP. Most hvKp strains are sensitive to common antibiotics, but the number of multidrug-resistant (MDR) hvKp is increasing. Importantly, 38.2% of hvKp isolates produced ESBLs. Hypermucoviscosity and virulence-associated genes (K1,magA and rmpA/A2) were highly clustered in the hvKp group ($P < 0.001$). Cancer ($P = 0.004$), digestive disease ($P = 0.038$) and surgery ($P = 0.023$) within 1 month are strongly associated with the VAP-hvKp group. The incidence of septic shock ($P = 0.016$) and Sequential Organ Failure Assessment (SOFA) scores ($P < 0.001$) are significantly higher in the hvKp group. Multivariate analysis indicated that cancer (odds ratio [OR] = 5.365) is an independent risk factor for VAP-hvKp infection.

Conclusions: The morbidity for elderly patients with VAP due to hvKp is high. MDR-HvKp is emerging, which is a great challenge for clinical practice.

Keywords: *Klebsiella pneumoniae*, Hypervirulent, Aerobactin, Risk factor, ESBL-hvKp, Ventilator-associated pneumonia

* Correspondence: guojunhx301@163.com
[2]Department of Respiratory Medicine, School of Clinical Medicine, Beijing Tsinghua Changgung Hospital, Tsinghua University, Beijing, China
[3]Department of Geriatric Respiratory Medicine, Chinese PLA General Hospital, Beijing, China
Full list of author information is available at the end of the article

Background

Ventilator-associated pneumonia (VAP) is the most frequent life-threatening nosocomial infection in critically ill patients [1, 2]. *Klebsiella pneumoniae* (Kp) is one of the most common gram-negative bacteria causing hospital infections, especially various notoriously fatal infections. Kp includes two distinct groups: hypervirulent (hvKp) and classical (cKp). One of the characteristics of cKp is acquiring an antibiotic-resistant gene. The other type is hvKp, which is traditionally defined as hypermucoviscosity by string test, inducing aggressive invasive community infection, bloodstream infection, and pyogenic liver abscesses (PLA) for immunocompetent ambulatory younger adults with no underlying diseases [3–6]. However, the definition of hvKp by string test is controversial [7, 8]. Previous studies showed that certain hypermucoviscous *K. pneumonia* (hmvKp) strains are not closely related to high virulence in in vitro and in vivo models [7, 8]. Thus, to differentiate hvKp from cKp by the hypermucoviscosity phenotype alone may be inappropriate [9, 10]. Recently, aerobactin, a dominant component of the siderophore system, has been established as a critical virulence factor for the hvKp genotype [3, 10, 11]. A previous multi-centre study in China targeting middle-aged patients, illustrated the clinical and molecular characteristics of hvKp (defined as aerobactin positive) infection [10]. However, the data for the hospital infection in the elderly with hvKp VAP, who commonly suffer from various underlying disease and nutritional complications, is rare.

Although most previous studies demonstrated that hvKp is sensitive to most antibiotics, which is prominently different from cKp strains, the multi-drug resistance (MDR) and extended-spectrum-β-lactamase (ESBL)-producing hvKp, especially those resistant to colistin and carbapenems, are emerging in China [12–14]. However, there are not enough referable data for the elderly with VAP due to antimicrobial-resistant hvKp.

To date, no data about the clinical and microbiological characteristics of VAP caused by the hvKp genotype in the elderly have been demonstrated. The aim of this study was to further investigate the clinical characteristics of elderly patients with hvKp infection and microbiological features and the epidemiology of multi-centre hvKp. Therefore, we conducted a retrospective study in two tertiary hospitals focusing on the genotype of hvKp (defined as aerobactin positive) in China.

Methods

Patients

A retrospective study was conducted on 73 *Kp* culture-positive patients diagnosed from November 2008 to December 2017 at two tertiary hospitals: Beijing Tsinghua Changgung Hospital and Chinese PLA General Hospital. These two hospitals are located in Beijing, and the capacity of the hospitals is more than 800 beds. Patients currently receiving mechanical ventilation were included in this study. The definition of VAP is according to the 2016 ATS guideline [15]. Standard bronchoalveolar lavage and aspiration were achieved. The clinical characteristics, including underlying disease, infection type, nutritional status, mortality in 30 days, and sequential organ failure assessment (SOFA) were collected. The primary outcome of this study was to investigate the 30-day mortality of hvKp infection in the elderly with VAP compared with that of the cKp group. Additionally, the white blood cell count (WBC) and neutrophil percentage (NEU%) were applied as primary inflammatory factors. Total protein (TP) and albumin (ALB) were used to evaluate the nutrition status. The main inclusion criteria were 1) the definition of the elderly as 65 years old or older (≥65 year) and 2) at least one *K. pneumoniae*-positive culture. The exclusion criteria was 1) insufficient clinical data or bacterial strain sample storage and 2) cases of co-infection.

Clinical *Kp* strains

All isolates were stored at − 80 °C and identified by the API 20 NE system and the VITEK II system. Further species identification was confirmed by 16S rRNA gene sequencing. HvKp is defined as aerobactin positive. The hypermucoviscous phenotype was detected by the string test as described previously [16].

Antimicrobial susceptibility testing and phenotypic detection of ESBLs

Antimicrobial susceptibility testing was performed, and the results were interpreted according to 2017 Clinical and Laboratory Standards Institute (CLSI) guidelines. The antibiotics include amikacin, gentamicin, tobramycin, Sulbactam/sulbactam, aztreonam, cefazolin, cefepime, ceftriaxone, ceftazidime, ciprofloxacin, levofloxacin, piperacillin/tazobactam, and trimethoprim/sulfamethoxazole. ESBL was detected by an agar dilution test using ceftazidime and cefotaxime combined with clavulanate according to the CLSI guideline [10]. The definition of an MDR strain is resistance to three or more different antimicrobial categories, as described previously [17]. The carbapenem-resistant (CR) phenotype is defined as resistant to both imipenem and meropenem.

Detection of virulence-associated gene

Genomic DNA of all *Kp* isolates was extracted. *RmpA, rmpA2, magA, aerobactin* and the capsular serotype-specific (*cps*) genes (*K1, K2, K5, K20, K54,* and *K57*) were detected by polymerase chain reaction (PCR) as described previously [10, 18–20]. The primers are listed in Table 1.

Table 1 Primers

Name	sequence
rmpA	
Forward	5-ACTGGGCTACCTCTGCTTCA-3
Reverse	5-CTTGCATGAGCCATCTTTCA-3
rmpA2	
Forward	5-CTTTATGTGCAATAAG-GATGTT-3
Reverse	5-CCTCCTGGAGAGTAAGCATT-3
magA	
Forward	5-GGTGCTCTTTACATCATTGC-3
Reverse	5-GCAATGGCCATTTGCGTTAG-3
aerobactin	
Forward	5-GCATAGGCGGATACGAACAT-3
Reverse	5-CACAGGGCAATTGCTTACCT-3
K1	
Forward	5-GTAGGTATTGCAAGCCATGC-3
Reverse	5-GCCCAGGTTAATGAATCCGT-3
K2	
Forward	5-GGAGCCATTTGAATTCGGTG-3
Reverse	5-TCCCTAGCACTGGCTTAAGT-3
K5	
Forward	5-GCCACCTCTAAGCATATAGC-3
Reverse	5-CGCACCAGTAATTCCAACAG-3
K20	
Forward	5-CCGATTCGGTCAACTAGCTT-3
Reverse	5-GCACCTCTATGAACTTTCAG-3
K54	
Forward	5-CATTAGCTCAGTGGTTGGCT-3
Reverse	5-GCTTGACAAACACCATAGCAG-3
K57	
Forward	5-CGACAAATCTCTCCTGACGA-3
Reverse	5-CGCGACAAACATAACACTCG-3
rpoB	
Forward	5-GGCGAAATGGCWGAGAACCA-3
Reverse	5-GAGTCTTCGAAGTTGTAACC-3
gapA	
Forward	5-TGAAATATGACTCCACTCACGG-3
Reverse	5-CTTCAGAAGCGGCTTTGATGGCTT-3
mdh	
Forward	5-TGAAATATGACTCCACTCACGG-3
Reverse	5-CTTCAGAAGCGGCTTTGATGGCTT-3
pgi	
Forward	5-GAGAAAAACCTGCCTGTACTGCTGGC-3
Reverse	5-CGCGCCACGCTTTATAGCGGTTAAT-3
phoE	
Forward	5-ACCTACCGCAACACCGACTTCTTCGG-3
Reverse	5-TGATCAGAACTGGTAGGTGAT-3
infB	
Forward	5-CTCGCTGCTGGACTATATTCG-3
Reverse	5-CGCTTTCAGCTCAAGAACTTC-3
tonB	
Forward	5-CTTTATACCTCGGTACATCAGGTT-3
Reverse	5-ATTCGCCGGCTGRGCRGAGAG-3

Multilocus sequence typing (MLST) for Kp

Seven housekeeping genes (*gapA, mdh, phoE, tonB, infB, pgi and rpoB*) were detected by PCR according to the MLST website (*http://bigsdb.pasteur.fr/klebsiella/ klebsiella.html*) (Table 1). Allelic profiling and sequence types (STs) were also performed using the above website. Moreover, to further distinguish the relationship among different STs, phylogenetic analysis of the seven spliced housekeeping genes for these isolates that contributed to mortality was performed by the neighbour-joining method (MEGA 6.0). The common STs, including ST1, ST11, ST37, ST258 and ST412, were used as a reference.

Statistical analysis

SPSS software (version 20.0) was employed for data analysis. Measurement data was assessed as the means ± standard deviation (SD). The count data were analysed as percentages. Continuous variables were analysed by Student's *t*-tests and the Wilcoxon rank-sum tests. Categorical variables were analysed by the χ^2 or Fisher's exact tests. Univariate logistic regression analysis was performed for the risk factors. A multivariable logistic regression analysis was conducted for independent risk factors (the variables with $P<0.05$ were included). All tests were 2-tailed. A p-value<0.05 was considered significant.

Results

Clinical characteristics

Seventy-three *Kp* culture-positive patients were diagnosed at the two hospitals from November 2008 to December 2017 (Table 2). Thirty-four (46.6%) strains were hvKp, and 37 (50.7%) were hmvKp. Most of the patients (67, 91.8%) presented with sepsis, and 24 patients (32.9%) were diagnosed with septic shock. Sixty-six (90.4%) were males, and the mean age of patients in this study was 84.96 ± 8.33 years. Patients with cancer (38.2% versus 7.7%; $P = 0.004$), surgery history within 1 month (23.5% versus 5.1%; $P = 0.023$) and digestive diseases (29.4% versus 10.3%; $P = 0.046$) were more likely to be infected with hvKp. Although host responsibility (WBC and NEU%) and nutritional status (TP and ALB) were not significantly different at the primary endpoint (30-day mortality), the SOFA scores of the patients with hvKp were notably higher at 30-day mortality (8.94 ± 3.03 vs 6.62 ± 2.09, $P = 0.000$) (Table 2).

Genetic and phenotype characteristics: hvKp vs cKp

It is noted that hypermucoviscosity was strongly clustered in the hvKp group ($P < 0.001$). Our results showed that *K1, rmpA, rmpA2* and *magA* were highly clustered in hvKp ($P < 0.001$), but *K2, K5, K20, K54,* and *K57* were not associated with hvKp ($P = 0.073$, 0.213, 1.000, 0.096 and 0.849, respectively). Additionally, there is no isolate in the cKp group with K5 or K54 (Table 3).

Antimicrobial resistance analysis and detection rate of ESBL-producing *Kp* isolates

All Kp strains were resistant to Sulbactam. Most of the hvKp isolates represented a higher antimicrobial sensitivity rate to most of the antibiotics than cKp, except cefepime, ceftriaxone, ciprofloxacin, levofloxacin, imipenem, meropenem, and amikacin (Table 4). Although the detection rate of MDR (41.2% vs 74.4%, $P = 0.001$) and ESBLs (38.2% vs 69.2%, $P = 0.001$) was significantly lower than cKp, it is noted that 41.2% (14/34) of hvKp isolates were MDR and 38.2% (13/34) of hvKp isolates were ESBL-producing. Moreover, 8 isolates were identified as CR-hvKp.

Table 2 Clinical features of patients with VAP due to hvKp

Characteristic	HvKp(34)	cKp(39)	*P* value
Basic demographics			
Age	83.06 ± 8.55	86.62 ± .87	0.068
Male	31 (91.2%)	35 (89.7%)	1.000
Underlying diseases			
Pulmonary disease	31 (91.2%)	32 (82.1%)	0.321
Diabetes	19 (55.9%)	18 (46.2%)	0.407
Cardiovascular disease	12 (35.3%)	17 (43.6%)	0.470
Cerebrovascular disease	11 (32.4%)	15 (38.5%)	0.587
Cancer	**13 (38.2%)**	**3 (7.7%)**	**0.004**
Surgery within 1 mo	**8 (23.5%)**	**2 (5.1%)**	**0.023**
Digestive disease	**10 (29.4%)**	**4 (10.3%)**	**0.038**
Infection type			
Sepsis	30 (88.2%)	37 (94.9%)	0.408
Septic shock	**16 (47.1%)**	**8 (20.5%)**	**0.016**
Host responsibility			
WBC	12.57 ± 4.47	11.68 ± 4.36	0.397
NEU%	78.99 ± 9.54	77.13 ± 7.14	0.344
Nutrition status			
TP	63.38 ± 6.34	61.88 ± 6.02	0.304
ALB	33.33 ± 3.75	32.51 ± 3.39	0.326
SOFA score	**8.94 ± 3.03**	**6.62 ± 2.09**	**0.000**
Infection occurred in ICU	11 (32.4%)	10 (25.6%)	0.527
Mortality in 30 days	14 (41.2%)	14 (35.9%)	0.644

TP total protein, *ALB* albumin, *WBC* white blood cell count, *NEU%* neutrophils percentage

Table 3 Microbiological features of patients with VAP due to hvKp

Characteristic	HvKp(34)	cKp(39)	*P* value
K serotype			
K1	**17 (50.0%)**	**1 (2.6%)**	**0.000**
K2	7 (2.9%)	2 (5.1%)	0.073
K5	2 (5.9%)	0 (0%)	0.213
K20	2 (5.9%)	2 (5.1%)	1.000
K54	3 (8.8%)	0 (0%)	0.096
K57	4 (11.8%)	3 (7.7%)	0.849
rmpA	**27 (79.4%)**	**4 (10.3%)**	**0.000**
rmpA2	**28 (82.4%)**	**5 (12.8%)**	**0.000**
magA	**30 (88.2%)**	**17 (43.6%)**	**0.000**
Hypermucoviscosity	**29 (85.3%)**	**8 (20.5%)**	**0.000**

Risk factors for VAP-hvKp

Univariate regression analysis showed that cancer (odds ratio [OR] = 7.429), digestive diseases (OR = 3.646) and surgery history within 1 month (OR = 5.692) were risk factors for hvKp infection. Multivariate analysis revealed that cancer history (OR = 5.365) was an independent risk factor for hvKp infection (Table 5).

MLST genotypic analysis

New STs were not detected among the 73 Kp isolates. The most prevalent ST in this study was ST23 ($n = 15$; 20.5%), followed by ST412 ($n = 5$; 6.8%), ST17 ($n = 4$; 5.5%), ST37 ($n = 3$; 4.1%), and ST2906 ($n = 3$; 4.1%). The above STs accounted for 41.1% (30/73) of the total strains. Among the prevalent STs, 73.3% ST23 (11/15), 60.0% ST412 (3/5), and 100% ST17 (4/4) were hvKp. The detailed features of patients with prevalent hvKp are shown in Table 6. The CR-hvKp distributed in ST17 ($n = 2$), ST23 ($n = 1$), ST347 ($n = 1$), ST412 ($n = 1$), ST2874 ($n = 1$), and ST2905 ($n = 1$). The most common clone complex (CC) of the CR-hvKp was CC17 ($N = 2$). The phylogenetic tree demonstrated the relationship between the prevalent STs in our study and the common STs in the world (Fig. 1).

Discussion

To our knowledge, this is the largest multi-centre study focusing on elderly patients with VAP due to hvKp in China. Nearly half (46.6%, 34/73) of the hvKp-induced VAP in the elderly patients occurred among mechanically ventilated patients. The hvKp group showed a higher

Table 4 Antibiotics resistance: hvKp vs cKp

Antibiotic agent	HvKp(34)	cKp(39)	*P* value
MDR	**14 (41.2%)**	**29 (74.4%)**	**0.004**
ESBLs	**13 (38.2%)**	**27 (69.2%)**	**0.008**
Ampicillin	34 (100%)	39 (100%)	NA
Amikacin	6 (17.6%)	12 (30.8%)	0.194
Gentamicin	**8 (23.5%)**	**21 (53.8%)**	**0.008**
Ampicillin/Sulbactam	**13 (38.2%)**	**27 (69.2%)**	**0.008**
Aztreonam	**10 (29.4%)**	**21 (53.8%)**	**0.035**
Cefazolin	**14 (41.2%)**	**28 (71.8%)**	**0.008**
Cefotetan	**8 (23.5%)**	**16 (41.0%)**	**0.112**
Cefepime	9 (26.5%)	18 (46.2%)	0.082
Ceftriaxone	13 (38.2%)	23 (59.0%)	0.077
Ceftazidime	**10 (29.4%)**	**23 (59.0%)**	**0.011**
Ciprofloxacin	10 (29.4%)	20 (51.3%)	0.058
Levofloxacin	9 (26.5%)	19 (48.7%)	0.051
Trimethoprim/Sulfamethoxazole	**7 (20.6%)**	**22 (56.4%)**	**0.002**
Piperacillin/Tazobactam	**8 (23.5%)**	**18(46.2%)**	**0.044**
Imipenem	8 (23.5%)	10(25.6%)	0.835
Meropenem	9 (26.5%)	10(25.6%)	0.936
Tobramycin	**10 (29.4%)**	**21(53.8%)**	**0.027**

severity of disease than did the cKp group. The primary virulence factors, such as K1, rmpA/A2, and magA, were highly clustered in the hvKp group. ST23 was the most prevalent ST in two hospitals. However, the ST23 isolated in different hospitals was not highly associated with the aerobactin genetic background or hypermucoviscous phenotype, and it was concluded that just relying on STs to identify hvKp may be not appropriate. In our study, 50.7% of *K. pneumonia* isolates were identified as hypermucoviscous by the string test experiment, which is higher than that in a previous retrospective study conducted in a single centre in China, with a prevalence of 33% [16]. Thus, plasmid type, biofilm production, serotypes and the ability to induce inflammatory factors may be needed to further define hvKp. The prevalence of hvKp may be incorrectly estimated because of the lack of definite and objective diagnostic methods.

Aerobactin was considered a potential virulence trait for the hvKp genotype in in vitro and in vivo models [3]. Importantly, previous studies showed that the hvKp genotype (aerobactin-positive) often induced more serious invasive infection [10, 11, 21]. Previous studies reported that the detection rate of hvKp ranged from 4.5 to 37.8% in various clinical specimens [7, 10, 16, 19, 22]. In this study, 34 isolates (46.6%) were defined as hvKp due to aerobactin-positivity, which is the highest incidence for hospital-acquired infection (HAI) caused by the hvKp genotype. It is noted that the detection of the hvKp genotype in this study was also higher than that in previous multicentre studies(37.8%) based on adults [10] and a single centre retrospective study (28.6%) focusing on VAP [23]. It is concluded that hvKp may emerge as a major pathotype for elderly with VAP in the two hospitals.

Additionally, capsular serotype-specific genes are essential factors for *K. pneumoniae.* To date, various types of K-antigen have been reported [20, 24, 25]. In Asia, K1 and K2 are the most important elements, inducing severe infections. However, they are not the unique trait for hvKp [26–29]. Previous studies demonstrated that K1 distribution in hvKp ranged from 23 to 98% in various specimens in various populations [29–33]. The detection rate of K2 in hvKp ranged from 10 to 46% [16, 31, 33]. Moreover, a previous single centre study focusing on VAP showed that *K1* and *K2* among hvKp accounted for 42.9 and 21.4%, respectively [23]. The above data implied that K1 might be highly associated with hvKp compared with K2. In our study, half of the hvKp (50%) isolates were associated with *K1*, and *K2* was detected in 7 hvKp isolates (2.9%), which was consistent with previous studies. In addition to *K1* and *K2*, there were no significant difference between hvKp and cKp in *K5, K20, K54,* and *K57* due to small specimens. Moreover, *rmpA/rmpA2* and *magA* genes responsible for

Table 5 Risk factor for hvKp vs cKp

Variable	Univariate OR (95% CI)	*P* value	Multivariate OR (95% CI)	*P* value
Infection occurred in ICU	1.387 (0.502–3.832)	0.528		
Male	1.181 (0.245–5.694)	0.836		
Pulmonary diseases	2.260 (0.536–9.539)	0.267		
Diabetes	1.478 (0.586–3.725)	0.408		
Cardiovascular disease	0.706 (0.274–1.818)	0.471		
Cerebrovascular disease	0.765 (0.291–2.010)	0.587		
Cancer	**7.429 (1.895–29.114)**	**0.004**	**5.365 (1.199–24.007)**	**0.028**
Surgery within 1 mo	**5.692 (1.117–29.013)**	**0.036**		
Digestive diseases	**3.646 (1.023–12.990)**	**0.046**	3.713 (0.970–14.212)	0.055

Table 6 Features of patients with prevalent hvKp(n ≥ 3)

	ST2906(3)		ST37(3)		ST17(4)		ST412(5)		ST23(15)	
	$N^a = 0$	$N^b = 3$	$N^a = 2$	$N^b = 1$	$N^a = 2$	$N^b = 2$	$N^a = 2$	$N^b = 3$	$N^a = 10$	$N^b = 5$
K serotype										
K1	0	0	0	0	0	2	0	1	9	0
K2	0	1	1	1	0	2	0	1	0	0
K5	0	1	0	0	0	0	0	0	0	1
K20	0	1	0	0	0	0	0	0	0	1
K54	0	0	0	0	0	1	0	0	0	0
K57	0	0	1	0	2	1	1	0	0	0
rmpA	0	0	1	0	2	2	2	0	10	0
rmpA2	0	0	1	0	2	2	2	1	9	0
magA	0	0	2	0	2	2	2	1	9	1
Hmv	0	0	0	0	2	2	2	1	9	0
hvKp (aerobactin)	0	1	0	0	2	2	2	1	10	1
Sepsis Shock	0	3	0	1	2	1	0	1	8	1
Died in 30 Days	0	3	2	1	2	0	0	0	8	1

Hmv hypermucoviscosity, *a* and *b* different hospital

the hypermucoviscous phenotype were proposed as virulence factors in addition to major cps *K1/K2* [5, 19, 30, 34]. In our study, 2 hvKp isolates inserted *rmpA* did not show hypermucoviscosity. It is implied that there might exist other regulatory mechanisms for hypermucoviscosity. Importantly, our results are consistent with previous study: most of the dominant virulence-associated factors (*K1*, *rmpA/A2* and *magA*) and hypermucoviscosity are highly clustered in the hvKp group [10].

Although there was no significant difference in sepsis incidence and mortality between the two VAP groups, the incidence of sepsis shock and SOFA score was higher than those in the cKp group. Thus, to further understand the risk factors for hvKp, timely and appropriately prevention is essential. Our results showed that elderly patients with cancer, digestive disease and surgery history within 1 month were more likely to be infected with hvKp. Moreover, cancer history was an independent risk factor for VAP-hvKp infection in the elderly, and cancer patients should be monitored more intensively to prevent infection due to immunocompromise, which may also be a critical factor for VAP-hvKp [10]. Previous multi-centre study of the hvKp genotype based on adults in China concluded that diabetes and cancer were independent risk factors for hvKp [10]. However, the incidence of diabetes (50.7%, 37/73) in our study is far more than previous multi-centre study focused on adults (17.0%, 39/230) [10]. This may be the characteristics of the elderly who often suffer from various underlying diseases. Additionally, a previous study concluded that major histocompatibility complex (MHC) variants, nutritional status, and the gut microbiota might be potential host factors for improving the understanding of the hypervirulence phenomenon [9]. Although the incidence of septic shock and SOFA score in our study were higher than those of the cKp group, there was no significant difference in the nutritional status (TP and ALB) and inflammatory reaction (WBC and NEU%), which was consistent with a previous study [23]. Thus, other inflammatory factors may be needed to screen as a marker for elderly patients with VAP-hvKp.

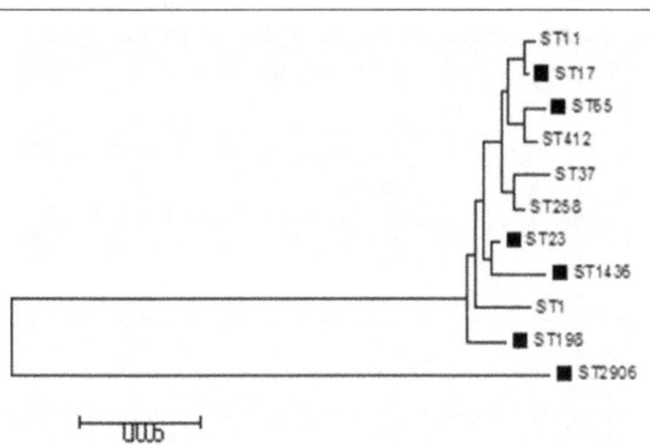

Fig. 1 Neighbour-joining dendrogram of concatenated sequences of seven housekeeping genes from the MLST database for prevalent STs in our study and the common STs in the world. (Black solid box represents death in our study)

Previous studies revealed that most cKp and antimicrobial-resistant patterns were overlapping, which is not frequent in hvKp [10, 16]. In this study, most of the hvKp isolates were sensitive to most of the above antibiotics. However, in the hvKp group, the number of ESBL-hvKp (41.2%) and MDR-hvKp (38.2%) is significantly higher than that in previous studies [10, 23]. It is alarming that MDR-hvKp may prefer to induce VAP in the elderly. Moreover, eight CR-hvKp isolates were identified as another "superbug". Taken together, these data revealed that MDR-hvKp is emerging among elderly patients with VAP, which needs to be confirmed by further investigations in larger populations. The CR-hvKp isolates were not detected in the nosocomial environment by routine nosocomial infection surveillance. Additionally, the composition of the gut microbiota was unclear because anal swabs were not applied for nosocomial infection surveillance. Previous study suggested that wards previously infected with CR-hvKp should be disinfected and left unoccupied for more than 2 weeks [12]. It may be a good choice to prevent fatal outbreaks of infection, especially in critically ill and immunocompromised elderly patients with mechanical ventilation.

The main limitation in our study is that it is a retrospective study from over 10 years. Although this study included two large tertiary hospitals, fewer patients with VAP-hvKp were included. However, this study is the largest cohort to investigate the clinical and microbiological characteristics of elderly patients with VAP-hvKp to now. Additionally, most of the key inflammatory factors, nutrition statue markers and environmental samples were not achieved. Moreover, the expression of aerobactin is unclear. Whole genome sequencing, transcriptomics and proteomics may be needed for further study to identify genetic expression.

Conclusions

HvKp is emerging as a common pathogen of VAP in the elderly in China. There is various epidemiology of VAP-hvKp in different hospitals. Although STs may not be associated with hvKp, ST23, ST37 and ST2906 are more likely to induce poor prognosis. Although the definition of hvKp is still controversial, the hvKp genotype is more likely to cause septic shock and a higher SOFA score. The emerging MDR-hvKp, especially CR-hvKp, will be a "superbug", which is a great challenge for clinicians. It is essential to enhance clinical awareness and infection surveillance for various hvKp infections, especially in immunocompromised elderly patients.

Acknowledgements
We thank the team of curators at the Institut Pasteur MLST and whole genome MLST databases for curating the data and making them publicly available at http://bigsdb.pasteur.fr.

Funding
This work was supported by the China postdoctoral science foundation (grant number 2014 M562610); the Excellent Young Program of the Organization Department of Beijing Municipal Party Committee (grant number 2016000057592G258).

Authors' contributions
JG and CL were responsible for study design and article writing. CL and JG collected clinical data and performed PCR and statistical analyses. JG performed critical data review. All authors read and approved the final version of the manuscript.

Consent for publication
Not applicable.

Competing interests
The authors declare that they have no competing interests.

Author details
[1]Department of Respiratory Medicine, Peking Union Medical College, Chinese Academy of Medical Sciences, China-Japan Friendship Hospital, Beijing, China. [2]Department of Respiratory Medicine, School of Clinical Medicine, Beijing Tsinghua Changgung Hospital, Tsinghua University, Beijing, China. [3]Department of Geriatric Respiratory Medicine, Chinese PLA General Hospital, Beijing, China.

References

1. Timsit JF, Esaied W, Neuville M, Bouadma L, Mourvllier B. Update on ventilator-associated pneumonia. F1000Res. 2017;6:2061.
2. Torres A, Niederman MS, Chastre J, Ewig S, Fernandez-Vandellos P, Hanberger H, Kollef M, Li Bassi G, Luna CM, Martin-Loeches I, et al. International ERS/ESICM/ESCMID/ALAT guidelines for the management of hospital-acquired pneumonia and ventilator-associated pneumonia: guidelines for the management of hospital-acquired pneumonia (HAP)/ ventilator-associated pneumonia (VAP) of the European Respiratory Society (ERS), European Society of Intensive Care Medicine (ESICM), European Society of Clinical Microbiology and Infectious Diseases (ESCMID) and Asociacion Latinoamericana del Torax (ALAT). Eur Respir J. 2017;50:1700582.
3. Russo TA, Olson R, MacDonald U, Beanan J, Davidson BA. Aerobactin, but not yersiniabactin, salmochelin, or enterobactin, enables the growth/ survival of hypervirulent (hypermucoviscous) Klebsiella pneumoniae ex vivo and in vivo. Infect Immun. 2015;83(8):3325–33.
4. Shon AS, Bajwa RP, Russo TA. Hypervirulent (hypermucoviscous) Klebsiella pneumoniae: a new and dangerous breed. Virulence. 2013; 4(2):107–18.
5. Siu LK, Yeh KM, Lin JC, Fung CP, Chang FY. Klebsiella pneumoniae liver abscess: a new invasive syndrome. Lancet Infect Dis. 2012;12(11):881–7.
6. Pomakova DK, Hsiao CB, Beanan JM, Olson R, MacDonald U, Keynan Y, Russo TA. Clinical and phenotypic differences between classic and hypervirulent Klebsiella pneumonia: an emerging and under-recognized pathogenic variant. Eur J Clin Microbiol Infect Dis. 2012;31(6):981–9.
7. Zhang Y, Zeng J, Liu W, Zhao F, Hu Z, Zhao C, Wang Q, Wang X, Chen H, Li H, et al. Emergence of a hypervirulent carbapenem-resistant Klebsiella pneumoniae isolate from clinical infections in China. J Infect. 2015;71(5):553–60.
8. Lin YC, Lu MC, Tang HL, Liu HC, Chen CH, Liu KS, Lin C, Chiou CS, Chiang MK, Chen CM, et al. Assessment of hypermucoviscosity as a virulence factor for experimental Klebsiella pneumoniae infections: comparative virulence analysis with hypermucoviscosity-negative strain. BMC Microbiol. 2011;11:50.
9. Catalan-Najera JC, Garza-Ramos U, Barrios-Camacho H. Hypervirulence and hypermucoviscosity: two different but complementary Klebsiella spp. phenotypes? Virulence. 2017:1–13.
10. Zhang Y, Zhao C, Wang Q, Wang X, Chen H, Li H, Zhang F, Li S, Wang R, Wang H. High prevalence of Hypervirulent Klebsiella pneumoniae infection in China: geographic distribution, clinical characteristics, and antimicrobial resistance. Antimicrob Agents Chemother. 2016;60(10): 6115–20.

11. Russo TA, Olson R, Macdonald U, Metzger D, Maltese LM, Drake EJ, Gulick AM. Aerobactin mediates virulence and accounts for increased siderophore production under iron-limiting conditions by hypervirulent (hypermucoviscous) Klebsiella pneumoniae. Infect Immun. 2014;82(6): 2356–67.
12. Gu D, Dong N, Zheng Z, Lin D, Huang M, Wang L, Chan EW, Shu L, Yu J, Zhang R, et al. A fatal outbreak of ST11 carbapenem-resistant hypervirulent Klebsiella pneumoniae in a Chinese hospital: a molecular epidemiological study. Lancet Infect Dis. 2018;18(1):37–46
13. Gu DX, Huang YL, Ma JH, Zhou HW, Fang Y, Cai JC, Hu YY, Zhang R. Detection of Colistin resistance gene mcr-1 in Hypervirulent Klebsiella pneumoniae and Escherichia coli isolates from an infant with diarrhea in China. Antimicrob Agents Chemother. 2016;60(8):5099–100.
14. Zhang R, Lin D, Chan EW, Gu D, Chen GX, Chen S. Emergence of Carbapenem-resistant serotype K1 Hypervirulent Klebsiella pneumoniae strains in China. Antimicrob Agents Chemother. 2015;60(1):709–11.
15. Kalil AC, Metersky ML, Klompas M, Muscedere J, Sweeney DA, Palmer LB, Napolitano LM, O'Grady NP, Bartlett JG, Carratala J, et al. Management of Adults with Hospital-acquired and Ventilator-associated Pneumonia: 2016 clinical practice guidelines by the Infectious Diseases Society of America and the American Thoracic Society. Clin Infect Dis. 2016;63(5):e61–e111.
16. Li W, Sun G, Yu Y, Li N, Chen M, Jin R, Jiao Y, Wu H. Increasing occurrence of antimicrobial-resistant hypervirulent (hypermucoviscous) Klebsiella pneumoniae isolates in China. Clin Infect Dis. 2014;58(2):225–32.
17. Magiorakos AP, Srinivasan A, Carey RB, Carmeli Y, Falagas ME, Giske CG, Harbarth S, Hindler JF, Kahlmeter G, Olsson-Liljequist B, et al. Multidrug-resistant, extensively drug-resistant and pandrug-resistant bacteria: an international expert proposal for interim standard definitions for acquired resistance. Clin Microbiol Infec. 2012;18(3):268–81.
18. Choi MJ, Ko KS. Loss of hypermucoviscosity and increased fitness cost in colistin-resistant Klebsiella pneumoniae sequence type 23 strains. Antimicrob Agents Chemother. 2015;59(11):6763–73.
19. Yu WL, Ko WC, Cheng KC, Lee HC, Ke DS, Lee CC, Fung CP, Chuang YC. Association between rmpA and magA genes and clinical syndromes caused by Klebsiella pneumoniae in Taiwan. Clin Infect Dis. 2006;42(10):1351–8.
20. Cheng NC, Yu YC, Tai HC, Hsueh PR, Chang SC, Lai SY, Yi WC, Fang CT. Recent trend of necrotizing fasciitis in Taiwan: focus on monomicrobial Klebsiella pneumoniae necrotizing fasciitis. Clin Infect Dis. 2012;55(7):930–9.
21. Nassif X, Sansonetti PJ. Correlation of the virulence of Klebsiella pneumoniae K1 and K2 with the presence of a plasmid encoding aerobactin. Infect Immun. 1986;54(3):603–8.
22. Lee HC, Chuang YC, Yu WL, Lee NY, Chang CM, Ko NY, Wang LR, Ko WC. Clinical implications of hypermucoviscosity phenotype in Klebsiella pneumoniae isolates: association with invasive syndrome in patients with community-acquired bacteraemia. J Intern Med. 2006;259(6):606–14.
23. Yan Q, Zhou M, Zou M, Liu WE. Hypervirulent Klebsiella pneumoniae induced ventilator-associated pneumonia in mechanically ventilated patients in China. Eur J Clin Microbiol Infect Dis. 2016;35(3):387–96.
24. Pan YJ, Fang HC, Yang HC, Lin TL, Hsieh PF, Tsai FC, Keynan Y, Wang JT. Capsular polysaccharide synthesis regions in Klebsiella pneumoniae serotype K57 and a new capsular serotype. J Clin Microbiol. 2008;46(7): 2231–40.
25. Chuang YP, Fang CT, Lai SY, Chang SC, Wang JT. Genetic determinants of capsular serotype K1 of Klebsiella pneumoniae causing primary pyogenic liver abscess. J Infect Dis. 2006;193(5):645–54.
26. Yeh KM, Kurup A, Siu LK, Koh YL, Fung CP, Lin JC, Chen TL, Chang FY, Koh TH. Capsular serotype K1 or K2, rather than magA and rmpA, is a major virulence determinant for Klebsiella pneumoniae liver abscess in Singapore and Taiwan. J Clin Microbiol. 2007;45(2):466–71.
27. Brisse S, Fevre C, Passet V, Issenhuth-Jeanjean S, Tournebize R, Diancourt L, Grimont P. Virulent clones of Klebsiella pneumoniae: identification and evolutionary scenario based on genomic and phenotypic characterization. PLoS One. 2009;4(3):e4982.
28. Fang CT, Lai SY, Yi WC, Hsueh PR, Liu KL, Chang SC. Klebsiella pneumoniae genotype K1: an emerging pathogen that causes septic ocular or central nervous system complications from pyogenic liver abscess. Clin Infect Dis. 2007;45(3):284–93.
29. Lin JC, Koh TH, Lee N, Fung CP, Chang FY, Tsai YK, Ip M, Siu LK. Genotypes and virulence in serotype K2 Klebsiella pneumoniae from liver abscess and non-infectious carriers in Hong Kong, Singapore and Taiwan. Gut Pathogens. 2014;6:21.
30. Fang CT, Chuang YP, Shun CT, Chang SC, Wang JT. A novel virulence gene in Klebsiella pneumoniae strains causing primary liver abscess and septic metastatic complications. J Exp Med. 2004;199(5):697–705.
31. Liu YM, Li BB, Zhang YY, Zhang W, Shen H, Li H, Cao B. Clinical and molecular characteristics of emerging hypervirulent Klebsiella pneumoniae bloodstream infections in mainland China. Antimicrob Agents Chemother. 2014;58(9):5379–85.
32. Compain F, Babosan A, Brisse S, Genel N, Audo J, Ailloud F, Kassis-Chikhani N, Arlet G, Decre D. Multiplex PCR for detection of seven virulence factors and K1/K2 capsular serotypes of Klebsiella pneumoniae. J Clin Microbiol. 2014;52(12):4377–80.
33. Lee SS, Chen YS, Tsai HC, Wann SR, Lin HH, Huang CK, Liu YC. Predictors of septic metastatic infection and mortality among patients with Klebsiella pneumoniae liver abscess. Clin Infect Dis. 2008;47(5):642–50.
34. Struve C, Bojer M, Nielsen EM, Hansen DS, Krogfelt KA. Investigation of the putative virulence gene magA in a worldwide collection of 495 Klebsiella isolates: magA is restricted to the gene cluster of Klebsiella pneumoniae capsule serotype K1. J Med Microbiol. 2005;54(Pt 11):1111–3.

2

Epidemic characterization and molecular genotyping of *Shigella flexneri* isolated from calves with diarrhea in Northwest China

Zhen Zhu†, Mingze Cao†, Xuzheng Zhou, Bing Li and Jiyu Zhang*

Abstract

Background: The widespread presence of antibiotics resistance genes in pathogenic bacteria can cause enormous problems. Food animals are one of the main reservoirs of intestinal pathogens that pose a potential risk to human. Analyzing the epidemiological characteristics and resistance patterns of *Shigella flexneri* in calves is necessary for animal and human health.

Methods and results: A total of 54 *Shigella flexneri* isolates, including six serotypes (1a, 2a, 2b, 4a, 6 and Xv), were collected from 837 fecal samples obtained from 2014 to 2016. We performed pulsed-field gel electrophoresis (PFGE) and applied the restriction enzyme *NotI* to analyze the genetic relatedness among the 54 isolates and to categorize them into 31 reproducible and unique PFGE patterns. According to the results of antimicrobial susceptibility tests, all 26 *Shigella flexneri* 2a serotypes were resistant to cephalosporin and/or fluoroquinolones. The genes bla_{TEM-1}, bla_{OXA-1}, and $bla_{CTX-M-14}$ were detected in 19 cephalosporin-resistant *S. flexneri* 2a isolates. Among 14 fluoroquinolone-resistant isolates, the *aac(6')-Ib-cr* gene was largely present in each strain, followed by *qnrS* (5). Only one ciprofloxacin-resistant isolate harbored the *qepA* gene. Sequencing the quinolone resistance determining regions (QRDRs) of the fluoroquinolone-resistant isolates revealed two point mutations in *gyrA* (S83 L, D87N/Y) and a single point mutation in *parC* (S80I). Interestingly, two *gyrA* (D87N/Y) strains were resistant to ciprofloxacin.

Conclusions: The current study enhances our knowledge of *Shigella* in cattle, although continual surveillance is necessary for the control of shigellosis. The high level of cephalosporin and/or fluoroquinolone resistance in *Shigella* warns us of a potential risk to human and animal health.

Keywords: *Shigella flexneri*, Antimicrobial susceptibility, Resistant

Background

The majority of Enterobactericeae family bacteria, including *Salmonella*, *E. coli* and *Shigella* spp., the major etiological agent of diarrheal disease, are a global public health burden, particularly in low-income countries [1–3]. *Shigella* is phylogenetically distinct from several independent *E. coli* strains and has evolved through convergent evolution [4]. The genus *Shigella* consists of four subgroups differentiated according to their biochemical and serological properties: A (*S. dysenteriae*), B (*S. flexneri*), C (*S. boydii*), and D (*S. sonnei*). All four species of *Shigella* cause shigellosis, but *S. flexneri* is the predominant subgroup found in developing countries, whereas *S. sonnei* is found in industrialized countries [5]. The first *Shigella* species identified was *S. dysenteriae*, followed by *S. flexneri* at the end of the 19th century. Shigellosis became a notorious and widespread epidemic during World War 1 with the transmission of *S. flexneri* strain NCTC1, a 2a lineage [6, 7]. Based on the differing structural characteristics of the antigenic determinants of the O antigen, *S. flexneri* is divided into no fewer than 20 serotypes: 1a, 1b, 1c, 1d, 2a, 2b, 2v, 3a, 3b, 4a, 4av, 4b, 4c, 5a, 5b, X, Xv, Y, Yv, 6, and 7b [8, 9].

Given that shigellosis is a global public health burden, previous studies have focused on the human gastrointestinal pathogens but have ignored animal groups. *Shigella* spp. infect and also cause corresponding clinical

* Correspondence: infzjy@sina.com
†Equal contributors
Key Laboratory of New Animal Drug Project of Gansu Province, Key Laboratory of Veterinary Pharmaceutical Development of Ministry of Agriculture, Lanzhou Institute of Husbandry and Pharmaceutical Sciences of CAAS, Jiangouyan, Qilihe District, Lanzhou, People's Republic of China

symptoms in monkeys, cows, pigs, chickens and other animals [10–13]. Indeed, animals that live in environments characterized by poor sanitary hygiene, restricted access to clean drinking water and long-term exposure to contaminated food are prone to dysentery [14, 15]. Many antibiotics are used to control disease and promote growth during the breeding process, leading to the widespread dissemination of antibiotic resistance genes (ARGs). The spread of drug resistance among pathogenic bacteria in humans and animals may be disastrous.

The present study investigated the *Shigella* epidemic in cows in the northwest region of China. *S. flexneri* 2a was first isolated from a yak with diarrhea in Tibet in 2014. In this study, we used pulsed-field gel electrophoresis (PFGE) to analyze the relationships among *S. flexneri* isolates and tested for antimicrobial susceptibility patterns. Our results will help prevent diarrhea in calves and will assist in the selection of effective antibiotics against *Shigella*.

Methods

Bacterial isolation and identification

Fresh stool samples were isolated from 2014 to 2016 in Northwest China (Gansun, Shanxi, Qinghai, Xinjiang and Tibet) from calves (3 to 20 days) with diarrhea. Samples were stored in transport medium, cultured directly on *Salmonella-Shigella* (SS) agar and incubated at 37 °C for 24 h to select for *Shigella*. Resultant colonies (colorless, semitransparent, smooth, and moist circular) [16] were picked and grown at 37 °C for 24 h on MacConkey (MAC) Agar to verify identity. Colonies were selected and cultured in brain heart infusion broth at 37 °C for 5 h with shaking at 250 rpm. All isolates were confirmed using API20E test strips (bioMerieux Vitek, Marcy-l' Etoile, France) according to the manufacturer's recommendations. *Shigella* was serotyped using a commercially available kit (Denka Seiken, Tokyo, Japan) and confirmed by PCR [17].

Antimicrobial susceptibility testing

The antimicrobial susceptibility of *S. flexneri* isolates was determined via the Kirby–Bauer disc-diffusion method in accordance with the guidelines of the Clinical and Laboratory Standards Institute (CLSI) [18].

The antibiotic discs (OXOID, UK) included penicillin G (P, 10 μg), ampicillin (AMP, 10 μg), amoxicillin/clavulanic acid (AMC, 30 μg), cephalothin (KF, 30 μg), cephazolin (KZ, 30 μg), cefamandole (MA, 30 μg), cefoxitin (FOX, 30 μg), ceftriaxone (CRO, 30 μg), cefotaxime (CTX, 30 μg), cefoperazone (CFP, 75 μg), cefepime (FEP, 30 μg), meropenem (MEM, 10 μg), imipenem (IPM, 10 μg), norfloxacin (NOR, 10 μg), enrofloxacin (ENR, 5 μg), levofloxacin (LEV, 5 μg), ciprofloxacin (CIP, 5 μg), erythromycin (E, 15 μg), chloramphenicol (C, 30 μg), tetracycline (TE, 30 μg), streptomycin (S, 10 μg), gentamicin (CN, 10 μg), and amikacin (AK, 30 μg). *E. coli* strain ATCC25922 was used as a quality control strain in each test batch.

PCR amplification of ARGs

We performed PCR assays that targeted 24 different ARGs using the primers described in Table 1. To determine the underlying resistance mechanism of β-lactam antibiotics, we amplified extended-spectrum β-lactamase (ESBL) genes, specifically $bla_{CTX\text{-}M}$, bla_{SHV}, bla_{TEM}, and bla_{OXA}, as well as *ampC* genes, specifically bla_{MOX}, bla_{FOX}, bla_{DHA}, bla_{CIT}, bla_{ACC}, and bla_{MIR} [19–21]. Plasmid-mediated quinolone resistance (PMQR) determinant genes, including *qnrA*, *qnrB*, *qnrD*, *qnrS*, *qepA* and *aac(6')-Ib-cr* and four quinolone resistance determining region (QRDR) genes as well as DNA gyrase (*gyrA,gyrB*) and topoisomerase IV (*parC,parE*) were amplified to determine the underlying mechanism of quinolone resistance [16, 21–23]. The PCR fragments were sequenced after purification and compared to sequences in GenBank.

PFGE

Genotypes and transmission patterns were determined by performing PFGE according to the method described in a previous study [19]. *S. flexneri* isolates were digested with the restriction enzyme *Not*I (TaKaRa, Japan) at 37 °C for 3 h to generate a DNA fingerprinting profile. *Salmonella enterica* serotype Braenderup strain H9812 was digested with *Xba*I (TaKaRa, Japan) and used as a molecular size standard. Electrophoresis was performed on the CHEF Mapper XA system (Bio-Rad) with a 1% agarose SeaKem Gold gel (Lonza, USA). Electrophoretic parameters were determined by performing multiple screening runs and included switching times of 2.16 to 54.17 s, a voltage of 6 v/cm, a 120° angle and a run time of 21 h. PFGE images were obtained using a Universal Hood II (Bio-RAD, USA) and analyzed using BioNumerics software version 7.1 (Applied Maths, Sint-Martens-Latem, Belgium). A clustering tree that indicated relative genetic similarity was constructed using UPGMA (Unweighted Pair Group Method with Arithmetic Mean) and the Dice-predicted similarity value with a 1.0% pattern optimization and 1.5% band position tolerance.

Results

Bacterial isolation and identification

During our epidemiological survey of *Shigella*, we collected 873 fecal samples from calves with diarrhea and obtained 54 *S. flexneri* isolates from five provinces in northwest China from 2014 to 2016. Isolate information is shown in detail in Table 2. Among the 54 *S. flexneri* isolates, there were six serotypes: five (9.26%) isolates were 1a, twenty-six (48.15%) isolates were 2a, four (7.41%) isolates were 2b, six (11.11%) isolates were 4a,

Table 1 Primers for the detection of antibiotic resistance genes

Target	Primer sequence (5′ to 3′)	Amplicon size (bp)	Reference
β-lactamase			
$bla_{CTX-M-1}$	F: GGTTAAAAAATCACTGCGTC	873	Cui et al., 2015 [16]
	R: TTACAAACCGTCGGTGACGA		
$bla_{CTX-M-2}$	F: CGACGCTACCCCTGCTATT	552	Zong et al., 2008 [17]
	R: CCAGCGTCAGATTTTTCAGG		
$bla_{CTX-M-8}$	F: TCGCGTTAAGCGGATGATGC	689	Zong et al., 2008 [17]
	R: AACCCACGATGTGGGTAGC		
$bla_{CTX-M-9}$	F: AGAGTGCAACGGATGATG	868	Cui et al., 2015 [16]
	R: CCAGTTACAGCCCTTCGG		
$bla_{CTX-M-25}$	F: TTGTTGAGTCAGCGGGTTGA	497	Liu et al., 2015 [18]
	R: GCGCGACCTTCCGGCCAAAT		
bla_{SHV}	F: CGCCGGGTTATTCTTATTTGTCGC	1015	Zong et al., 2008 [17]
	R: TCTTTCCGATGCCGCCGCCAGTCA		
bla_{TEM}	F: ATGAGTATTCAACTTTCCG	876	This study
	R: CCAATGCTTAATCAGTGAG		
bla_{OXA}	F: ATTAAGCCCTTTACCAAACCA	890	Cui et al., 2015 [16]
	R: AAGGGTTGGGCGATTTTGCCA		
bla_{MOX}	F: GCTGCTCAAGGAGCACAGGAT	520	Cui et al., 2015 [16]
	R: CACATTGACATAGGTGTGGTGC		
bla_{FOX}	F: AACATGGGGTATCAGGGAGATG	190	Cui et al., 2015 [16]
	R: CAAAGCGCGTAACCGGATTGG		
bla_{DHA}	F: AACTTTCACAGGTGTGCTGGGT	405	Cui et al., 2015 [16]
	R: CCGTACGCATACTGGCTTTGC		
bla_{CIT}	F: TGGCCAGAACTGACAGGCAAA	462	Cui et al., 2015 [16]
	R: TTTCTCCTGAACGTGGCTGGC		
bla_{ACC}	F: AACAGCCTCAGCAGCCGGTTA	346	Cui et al., 2015 [16]
	R: TTCGCCGCAATCATCCCTAGC		
bla_{MIR}	F: TCGGTAAAGCCGATGTTGCGG	302	Cui et al., 2015 [16]
	R: CTTCCACTGCGGCTGCCAGTT		
PMQRs			
qnrA	F: ATTTCTCACGCCAGGATTTG	516	Colobatiu et al.,2015 [19]
	R: GATCGGCAAAGGTTAGGTCA		
qnrB	F: GATCGTGAAAGCCAGAAAGG	476	Colobatiu et al.,2015 [19]
	R: ACGATGCCTGGTAGTTGTCC		
qnrD	F: CGAGATCAATTTACGGGGAATA	656	Cui et al.,2015 [13]
	R: AACAAGCTGAAGCGCCTG		
qnrS	F: ACGACATTCGTCAACTGCAA	417	Colobatiu et al.,2015 [19]
	R: TAAATTGGCACCCTGTAGGC		
aac(6′)-Ib-cr	F: CCCGCTTTCTCGTAGCA	544	Colobatiu et al.,2015 [19]
	R: TTAGGCATCACTGCGTCTTC		
qepA	F: CGTGTTGCTGGAGTTCTTC	403	Colobatiu et al.,2015 [19]
	R: CTGCAGGTACTGCGTCATG		
QRDR			
gyrA	F: TACACCGGTCAACATTGAGG	648	Hu et al.,2007 [20]

Table 1 Primers for the detection of antibiotic resistance genes *(Continued)*

	R: TTAATGATTGCCGCCGTCGG		
gyrB	F: TGAAATGACCCGCCGTAAAGG	309	Hu et al.,2007 [20]
	R: GCTGTGATAACGCAGTTTGTCCGGG		
parC	F: GTACGTGATCATGGACCGTG	531	Hu et al.,2007 [20]
	R: TTCGGCTGGTCGATTAATGC		
parE	F: ATGCGTGCGGCTAAAAAAGTG	290	Hu et al.,2007 [20]
	R: TCGTCGCTGTCAGGATCGATAC		

eight (14.81%) isolates were 6, and five (9.26%) isolates were Xv (Fig. 1). Our surveillance of the Gansu isolates identified all of the serotypes, except 4a. All 4a serotypes were isolated from Shanxi, while all Xv and 1a serotypes were from Gansu. Additionally, serotype 2a was widely isolated from each province, with the exception of Xinjiang, and serotype 6 was found only in yaks. Interestingly, *Shigella* was primarily isolated in the first quarter and fourth quarter, accounting for 54% (29/54) and 30% (16/54), respectively (Fig. 2).

Antimicrobial susceptibility testing

The 54 *S. flexneri* isolates were examined for susceptibility to 23 antibiotics. More than 50% of isolates were resistant to 8 antibiotics. Among them, resistance to P (54/54, 100%), AMP (51/54, 94.44%) and TE (49/54, 90.74) was most common, followed by E (46/54, 85.19%), S (38/54, 70.37%), KZ (34/54, 62.96%), KF (29/54, 53.70%) and CN (29/54, 53.70%). None of the isolates were resistant to IMP, MEM and the fourth-generation cephalosporin FEP. In addition, although a certain number of isolates were resistant to second- and third-generation cephalosporins (MA, FOX, CRO, CTX and CFP) and fluoroquinolones (CIP, NOR, ENR and LEV), these comprised no more than 30% of the total number of isolates, and the resistance rate was lower than those of other antibiotics (Table 3, Fig. 3).

Remarkably, all 26 *S. flexneri* 2a isolates demonstrated varying degrees of resistance to cephalosporins and/or fluoroquinolones and exhibited multidrug resistance (MDR). The *S. flexneri* 2a isolates were resistant to 14 diverse cephalosporins/fluoroquinolones. Among them, 73.06% (19/26) of isolates were resistant to cephalosporin, 53.85% (14/26) of isolates were resistant to fluoroquinolones, and 26.92% (7/26) of isolates were resistant to both cephalosporin and fluoroquinolones. Furthermore, isolate GBSF1512433 was resistant to all cephalosporins (with the exception of FEP) and fluoroquinolones (with the exception of CIP). Compared with the *S. flexneri* 2a isolates collected from beef calves, the 4 yak isolates were sensitive to most cephalosporins and fluoroquinolones but resistant to KF, KZ and MA (Table 4).

ARGs analysis of cephalosporin- and/or fluoroquinolone-resistant *S. flexneri* 2a isolates

In this study, only three β-lactamase gene types (bla_{OXA-1}, bla_{TEM-1} and $bla_{CTX-M-14}$) were identified among the 19 cephalosporin-resistant *S. flexneri* 2a isolates (Table 5). All isolates harbored bla_{TEM-1} type ARGs (100%), 15 isolates harbored bla_{OXA-1} (15/19, 78.95%), and 14 harbored $bla_{CTX-M-14}$ (14/19, 73.68%). In total, 63.16% (12/19) of isolates harbored three β-lactamase gene types. All *S. flexneri* 2a isolates from yaks were negative for bla_{CTX-M} type ARGs.

Both PMQR genes and SNPs in QRDRs were identified for 14 quinolone-resistant isolates (Table 6). According to the PCR results, all quinolone-resistant isolates were positive for *aac(6')-Ib-cr* but negative for *qepA*, except strain GBSF1602098. Only five (5/14, 35.71%) strains isolated from Gansu harbored *qnrS*, and no isolate harbored all three ARGs simultaneously. The point mutations in the QRDR genes play important roles in determining quinolone and/or fluoroquinolone resistance [24]. In the present study, we successfully amplified all four QRDR genes and compared them to reference sequences. We found two point mutations in *gyrA* and one point mutation each in *gyrA* and *parC* (Table 6). All quinolone-resistant strains carried mutations that altered the amino acid sequences of *gyrA* (S83 L) and *parC* (S80I). In addition, each strain carried the mutation 87 (D → N or Y) in *gyrA*, with the exception of GBSF1510390. Interestingly, GBSF1505314 and GBSF1602098 harbored the *gyrA* D87Y mutation, which confers resistance to ciprofloxacin.

PFGE pattern analysis

PFGE was performed to determine the genetic relatedness among the isolates and to study the molecular epidemiology in specific geographical regions [25]. The PFGE patterns of the 54 *Not*I-digested *S. flexneri* isolates were heterogeneous, and multiple PFGE patterns were present among the strains. Thus, diverse factors such as geography and environment may affect PFGE patterns. At an 80% similarity level, *S. flexneri* isolates generated 31 reproducible and unique PFGE patterns, including 11 common types (CT) and 20 single types (ST) (Fig. 3).

Table 2 Strain information of *S. flexneri* isolates from diarrheal calves, 2014 to 2016

Strain name	Serotype	Isolation year	Origin	Province
TYSF1412001	2a	2014	Yak	Tibet
GBSF1412056	2a	2014	Beef cattle	Gansu
GBSF1501026	2a	2015	Beef cattle	Gansu
GBSF1501071	Xv	2015	Beef cattle	Gansu
GYSF1501076	6	2015	Yak	Gansu
QYSF1501088	6	2015	Yak	Qinghai
XBSF1501093	2b	2015	Beef cattle	Xinjiang
GBSF1501105	2a	2015	Beef cattle	Gansu
SBSF1501123	4a	2015	Beef cattle	Shanxi
QYSF1502130	6	2015	Yak	Qinghai
GBSF1502176	2a	2015	Beef cattle	Gansu
GYSF1502197	6	2015	Yak	Gansu
SBSF1502219	4a	2015	Beef cattle	Shanxi
XBSF1502236	2b	2015	Beef cattle	Xinjiang
GBSF1503241	2a	2015	Beef cattle	Gansu
GYSF1503270	1a	2015	Yak	Gansu
GBSF1503288	1a	2015	Beef cattle	Gansu
GBSF1505314	2a	2015	Beef cattle	Gansu
SBSF1505331	2a	2015	Beef cattle	Shanxi
GBSF1506340	Xv	2015	Beef cattle	Gansu
GBSF1507358	1a	2015	Beef cattle	Gansu
GBSF1509369	2a	2015	Beef cattle	Gansu
GBSF1510375	2a	2015	Beef cattle	Gansu
GBSF1510390	2a	2015	Beef cattle	Gansu
QYSF1511395	2a	2015	Yak	Qinghai
GBSF1511401	2a	2015	Beef cattle	Gansu
GYSF1511409	2a	2015	Yak	Gansu
SBSF1512413	4a	2015	Beef cattle	Shanxi
GBSF1512419	2b	2015	Beef cattle	Gansu
GBSF1512425	2a	2015	Beef cattle	Gansu
GBSF1512433	2a	2015	Beef cattle	Gansu
GBSF1601015	Xv	2016	Beef cattle	Gansu
GBSF1601024	Xv	2016	Beef cattle	Gansu
TYSF1601031	2b	2016	Yak	Tibet
GBSF1601064	2a	2016	Beef cattle	Gansu
GYSF1601073	6	2016	Yak	Gansu
GBSF1602082	2a	2016	Beef cattle	Gansu
QYSF1602094	6	2016	Yak	Qinghai
GBSF1602098	2a	2016	Beef cattle	Gansu
GBSF1602103	2a	2016	Beef cattle	Gansu
SBSF1603115	4a	2016	Beef cattle	Shanxi
SBSF1603121	4a	2016	Beef cattle	Shanxi
GBSF1603138	2a	2016	Beef cattle	Gansu
GBSF1603149	2a	2016	Beef cattle	Gansu
QYSF1603158	6	2016	Yak	Qinghai
SBSF1604173	2a	2016	Beef cattle	Shanxi
SBSF1604195	4a	2016	Beef cattle	Shanxi
GBSF1605203	Xv	2016	Beef cattle	Gansu
GBSF1608241	2a	2016	Beef cattle	Gansu
GYSF1610256	2a	2016	Yak	Gansu
GYSF1610266	6	2016	Yak	Gansu
GBSF1610275	1a	2016	Beef cattle	Gansu
GBSF1611283	1a	2016	Beef cattle	Gansu
GBSF1611290	2a	2016	Beef cattle	Gansu

Among all isolates, the majority of *S. flexneri* 2a (26/54, 48.15%) isolates were classified into 11 PFGE patterns (4 CT and 7 ST). These PFGE patterns were closely related to each other, except the Tibet (TYSF1412001) and Qinghai (QYSF1511395) isolates, suggesting the strains isolated from different geographical locations exhibit diverse PFGE patterns and a capricious genetic diversity.

Discussion

ARGs are widespread and cause problems when present in pathogens [26]. Over the past decade, MDR *Shigella* has been reported in many countries [27]. However, only a few studies have described the prevalence of *Shigella* in animals worldwide. In the present study, we investigated the epidemiology of *S. flexneri* in cows in northwest

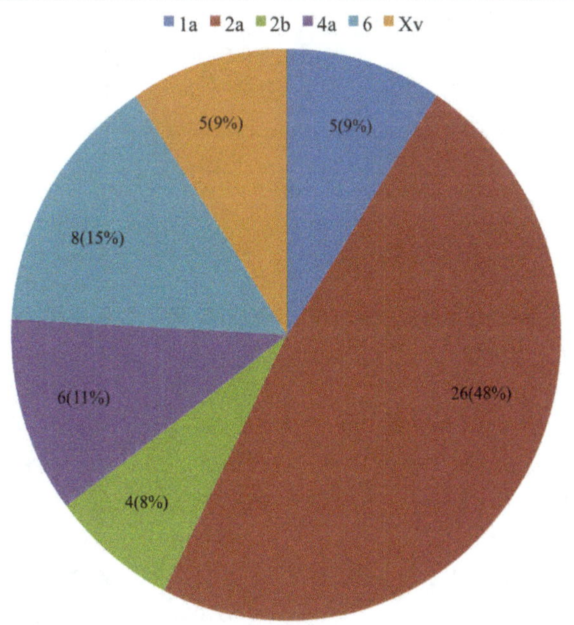

Fig. 1 *S. flexneri* serotypes collected from 2014 to 2016

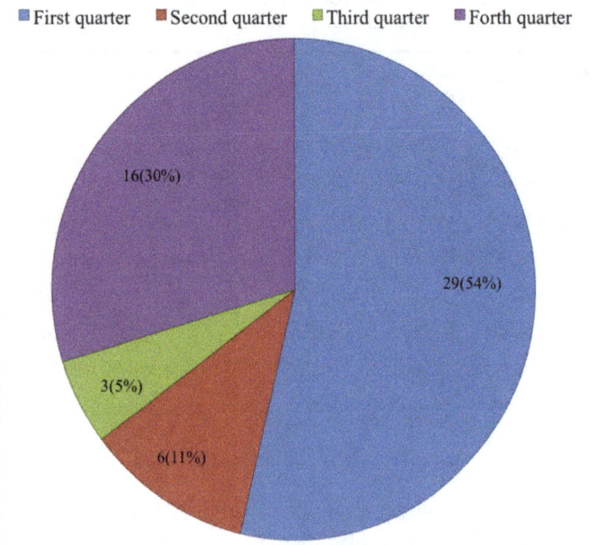

Fig. 2 Number of *S. flexneri* isolated from different quarters

China. During a 2-year survey, 54 *S. flexneri* isolates were obtained. Unfortunately, 16S rRNA gene sequence analysis does not effectively distinguish between closely related strains in a superfamily, such as *Shigella* and *E. coli* [28], and conventional biochemical and serological techniques are also insufficient. Therefore, PFGE was utilized to analyze the molecular characteristics of these isolates, to determine the relatedness among isolates and to study the molecular epidemiology in specific geographical regions. The clustering results allowed us to analyze the epidemiological trends of *S. flexneri*. Characterization of these isolates will be helpful for clinical diagnosis, treatment, prevention and the control of shigellosis [15].

Antimicrobial resistance has emerged as a serious problem [29], particularly for conventional, older-generation antibiotics such as P, AMP, TE, and E. According to the results of our antimicrobial susceptibility tests, cephalosporin and fluoroquinolone resistance rates in our isolates were higher than those in human isolates [19, 26]. Notably, the predominant *S. flexneri* 2a isolates were all resistant to cephalosporins, fluoroquinolones and multiple antibiotics. Two isolates (GBSF1505314 and GBSF1602098) were also resistant to ciprofloxacin, which is the first-line antibiotic

Table 3 Statistical analysis of the results of antimicrobial susceptibility to 23 antibiotics for 54 *S. flexneri*

Antibiotic	Antimicrobial resistance rate No. (%)					
	Total (*n* = 54)	Gansu (*n* = 37)	Shanxi (*n* = 8)	Xinjiang (*n* = 2)	Qinghai (*n* = 5)	Tibet (*n* = 2)
Penicillin G (P)	54 (100%)	37 (100%)	8 (100%)	2 (100%)	5 (100%)	2 (100%)
Ampicillin (AMP)	51 (94.44%)	37 (100%)	8 (100%)	2 (100%)	3 (60%)	1 (50%)
Amoxycillin/Clavulanic acid (AMC)	5 (9.62%)	3 (8.11%)	1 (12.5%)	1 (50%)	0	0
Cephalothin (KF)	29 (53.70%)	19 (51.35%)	5 (62.5%)	2 (100%)	2 (40%)	1 (50%)
Cephazolin (KZ)	34 (62.96%)	21 (56.76%)	7 (87.5%)	2 (100%)	3 (60%)	1 (50%)
Cefamandole (MA)	16 (29.63%)	12 (32.43%)	2 (25%)	1 (50%)	1 (20%)	0
Cefoxitin (FOX)	3 (5.56%)	2 (5.41%)	1 (12.5%)	0	0	0
Ceftriaxone (CRO)	12 (22.22%)	9 (24.32%)	2 (25%)	1 (50%)	0	0
Cefotaxime (CTX)	14 (25.93%)	10 (27.03%)	2 (25%)	1 (50%)	1 (20%)	0
Cefoperazone (CFP)	6 (11.11%)	6 (16.22%)	0	0	0	0
Cefepime (FEP)	0	0	0	0	0	0
Meropenem (MEM)	0	0	0	0	0	0
Imipenem (IPM)	0	0	0	0	0	0
Norfloxacin (NOR)	16 (29.63%)	12 (32.43%)	3 (37.5%)	1 (50%)	0	0
Enrofloxacin (ENR)	13(24.07%)	11 (29.73%)	2 (25%)	0	0	0
Levofloxacin (LEV)	14 (25.93%)	11 (29.73%)	2 (25%)	1 (50%)	0	0
Ciprofloxacin (CIP)	2 (3.70%)	2 (5.41%)	0	0	0	0
Erythromycin (E)	46 (85.19%)	35 (94.59%)	6 (75%)	2 (100%)	3 (60%)	0
Tetracycline (TE)	49 (90.74%)	35 (94.59%)	8 (100%)	2 (100%)	3 (60%)	1 (50%)
Chloramphenicol (C)	17 (31.48%)	10 (27.03%)	6 (75%)	1 (50%)	0	0
Streptomycin (S)	38 (70.37%)	30 (81.08%)	4 (50%)	2 (100%)	2 (40%)	0
Gentamicin (CN)	29 (53.70%)	23 (62.16%)	4 (50%)	2 (100%)	0	0
Amikacin (AK)	3 (5.56%)	3 (8.11%)	0	0	0	0

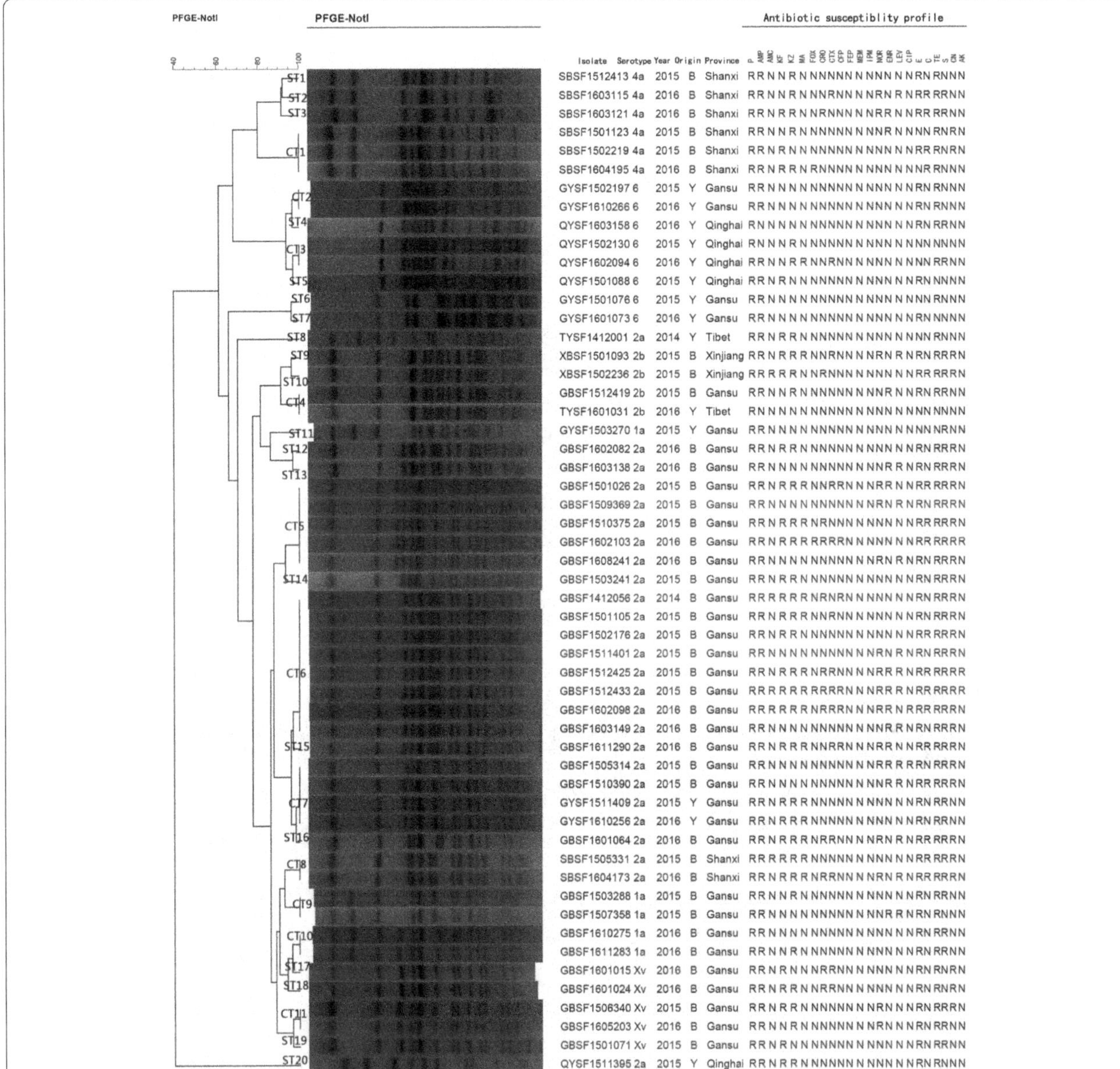

Fig. 3 PFGE dendrogram and antibiotic susceptibility profile of 54 *NotI*-digested *S. flexneri*. B = Beef cattle; Y = Yak. R = Resistance; N = Sensitive and Intermediary

treatment for shigellosis. The universal emergence of resistant and MDR strains in animals may be attributable to the unrestricted and excessive use of antibiotics in veterinary clinics. The widespread presence of MDR strains has reduced the selectivity of clinical medications to treat shigellosis [30]. Notably, our PFGE dendrogram showed various genetic patterns for *S. flexneri*, and there were diverse resistance profiles associated with each pattern. Based on these results, *S. flexneri* has the ability to adapt to the selective pressures of different antibiotics.

The high levels of resistance of S. *flexneri* 2a to cephalosporin/fluorquinolones, which are the most effective treatments for severe gastrointestinal infections caused by pathogenic bacteria, prompted us to study potential molecular resistance mechanisms. The emergence of ESBL-producing *Shigella* spp. has been observed in many countries [31]. In the current study, only 3 ARG genotypes (bla_{OXA-1}, bla_{TEM-1} and $bla_{CTX-M-14}$) were detected. Among them, the bla_{TEM-1} gene was detected in all 19 cephalosporin-resistant isolates. In total, 174 bla_{TEM} variants resistant to penicillin and other ß-lactamase antibiotics have been recorded. *TEM-1* confers resistance to ampicillin and cephalothin [32]. bla_{OXA}-type ARGs are class D β-lactamases, which were named for their ability to hydrolyze oxacillin [32]. Initially, bla_{OXA}-beta-lactamases were reported in *P. aeruginosa*,

Table 4 Statistical analysis of the cephalosporin and/or fluoroquinolone susceptibility for 26 *S. flexneri* 2a

Cephalosporin and/or Fluorquinolones resistance spectrum	Cephalosporin and/or Fluorquinolones resistance rate No. (%)				
	Total (n = 26)	Gansu (n = 22[a])	Shanxi (n = 2)	Qinghai (n = 1[a])	Tibet (n = 1[a])
KF/KZ	5 (19.23%)	3 (13.64%)	0	1[a] (100%)	1[a] (100%)
KF/KZ/MA	3 (11.54%)	2[a] (9.09%)	1 (50%)	0	0
KF/KZ/MA/CRO	1 (3.85%)	1 (4.55%)	0	0	0
KF/KZ/MA/CTX	1 (3.85%)	1 (4.55%)	0	0	0
KF/KZ/MA/CRO/CFP	1 (3.85%)	1 (4.55%)	0	0	0
KF/KZ/MA/FOX/CRO/CTX/CFP	1 (3.85%)	1 (4.55%)	0	0	0
NOR/LEV	3 (11.54%)	3 (13.64%)	0	0	0
ENR/LEV	3 (11.54%)	3 (13.64%)	0	0	0
NOR/ENR/LEV/CIP	1 (3.85%)	1 (4.55%)	0	0	0
KF/KZ/MA/CRO/CTX/NOR/LEV	2 (7.69%)	1 (4.55%)	1 (50%)	0	0
KF/KZ/MA/CRO/CTX/NOR/ENR/LEV	1 (3.85%)	1 (4.55%)	0	0	0
KF/KZ/MA/CTX/CFP/CIP/NOR/ENR	2 (7.69%)	2 (9.09%)	0	0	0
KF/KZ/MA/CRO/CTX/CFP/NOR/ENR/CIP	1 (3.85%)	1 (4.55%)	0	0	0
KF/KZ/MA/FOX/CRO/CTX/CFP/NOR/ENR/LEV	1 (3.85%)	1 (4.55%)	0	0	0

[a]a yak origin *S. flexneri* 2a isolate

although now the bla_{OXA} gene has been detected in plasmids and integrons in many Gram-negative organisms [32, 33]. According to some studies, the probable host preference for bla_{OXA}-type β-lactamase is *S. flexneri* [34]. In the present study, 15/19 (78.95%) isolates harbored bla_{OXA}- type genes, and sequencing results indicated that all the bla_{OXA} genes were $bla_{OXA\text{-}1}$. Additionally, $bla_{CTX\text{-}M}$ has become one of the most prevalent extended-spectrum-β-lactamases (ESBLs) [35]. This gene was widely harbored by S. *flexneri* 2a isolated

Table 5 Antimicrobial spectrum and ARGs analysis of *S. flexneri* 2a with resistance to cephalosporin

Strain name	Antimicrobial spectrum	ARGs in plasmid		
		TEM	*OXA*	*CTX-M-9*
TYSF1412001	KF/KZ	*TEM-1*	*OXA-1*	——
QYSF1511395	KF/KZ	*TEM-1*	——	——
GBSF1503241	KF/KZ	*TEM-1*	*OXA-1*	*CTX-M-14*
GBSF1502176	KF/KZ	*TEM-1*	*OXA-1*	*CTX-M-14*
GBSF1602082	KF/KZ	*TEM-1*	——	*CTX-M-14*
SBSF1505331	KF/KZ/MA	*TEM-1*	*OXA-1*	*CTX-M-14*
GYSF1511409	KF/KZ/MA	*TEM-1*	——	——
GYSF1610256	KF/KZ/MA	*TEM-1*	*OXA-1*	——
GBSF1510375	KF/KZ/MA/CRO	*TEM-1*	*OXA-1*	*CTX-M-14*
GBSF1501105	KF/KZ/MA/CTX	*TEM-1*	*OXA-1*	*CTX-M-14*
GBSF1412056	KF/KZ/MA/CRO/CFP	*TEM-1*	*OXA-1*	*CTX-M-14*
GBSF1602103	KF/KZ/MA/FOX/CRO/CTX/CFP	*TEM-1*	*OXA-1*	*CTX-M-14*
GBSF1601064	KF/KZ/MA/CRO/CTX/NOR/LEV	*TEM-1*	——	*CTX-M-14*
SBSF1604173	KF/KZ/MA/CRO/CTX/NOR/LEV	*TEM-1*	*OXA-1*	*CTX-M-14*
GBSF1611290	KF/KZ/MA/CTX/CFP/NOR/ENR	*TEM-1*	*OXA-1*	*CTX-M-14*
GBSF1501026	KF/KZ/MA/CTX/CFP/NOR/ENR	*TEM-1*	*OXA-1*	*CTX-M-14*
GBSF1512425	KF/KZ/MA/CRO/CTX/NOR/ENR/LEV	*TEM-1*	*OXA-1*	——
GBSF1602098	KF/KZ/MA/CRO/CTX/CFP/NOR/ENR/CIP	*TEM-1*	*OXA-1*	*CTX-M-14*
GBSF1512433	KF/KZ/MA/FOX/CRO/CTX/CFP/NOR/ENR/LEV	*TEM-1*	*OXA-1*	*CTX-M-14*

Table 6 Antimicrobial spectrum and amino acid types in QRDR and PMQRs genes analysis of *S. flexneri* 2a with resistance to fluoroquinolones

Strain name	Antimicrobial spectrum	QRDR			ARGs in plasmid		
		gyrA		*parC*	*aac(6')-Ib-cr*	*qnrS*	*qepA*
		83	87	80			
GBSF1509369	NOR/LEV	S83 L	D87N	S80I	+	−	−
GBSF1511401	NOR/LEV	S83 L	D87N	S80I	+	−	−
GBSF1608241	NOR/LEV	S83 L	D87N	S80I	+	−	−
GBSF1510390	ENR/LEV	S83 L	D87D	S80I	+	+	−
GBSF1603138	ENR/LEV	S83 L	D87N	S80I	+	−	−
GBSF1603149	ENR/LEV	S83 L	D87N	S80I	+	−	−
GBSF1505314	NOR/ENR/LEV/CIP	S83 L	D87Y	S80I	+	+	−
GBSF1601064	KF/KZ/MA/CRO/CTX/NOR/LEV	S83 L	D87N	S80I	+	−	−
SBSF1604173	KF/KZ/MA/CRO/CTX/NOR/LEV	S83 L	D87N	S80I	+	−	−
GBSF1611290	KF/KZ/MA/CTX/CFP/NOR/ENR	S83 L	D87N	S80I	+	−	−
GBSF1501026	KF/KZ/MA/CTX/CFP/NOR/ENR	S83 L	D87N	S80I	+	+	−
GBSF1512425	KF/KZ/MA/CRO/CTX/NOR/ENR/LEV	S83 L	D87N	S80I	+	+	−
GBSF1602098	KF/KZ/MA/CRO/CTX/CFP/NOR/ENR/CIP	S83 L	D87Y	S80I	+	−	+
GBSF1512433	KF/KZ/MA/FOX/CRO/CTX/CFP/NOR/ENR/LEV	S83 L	D87N	S80I	+	+	−

+: Presence corresponding genes
-: Absence corresponding genes

from beef cattle. Interestingly, all *S. flexneri* 2a isolated from yaks were negative for bla_{CTX-M} type ARGs.

Fluoroquinolones are highly effective for the treatment of shigellosis worldwide [36]. The primary mechanism of quinolone resistance involves the accumulation of sequential mutations in QRDRs that encode DNA gyrase and topoisomerase IV [37]. The most prevalent mutations in *Shigella* spp. are the point mutations in *gyrA* codons 83, 87 and 211, and *parC* codon 80 [38, 39]. Novel mutations in QRDRs are also being discovered [39]. In the present study, three mutations in *gyrA* codon 83 (S → L) and/or 87 (D → N or Y) and *parC* codon 80 (S → I) were detected in each fluoroquinolone-resistant isolate. All substitutions are responsible for reduced affinity. In addition, the amino acid diversity at the same position may lead to different levels of quinolone resistance [40, 41]. *GyrA* D87Y mutations were detected in only two ciprofloxacin-resistant isolates. However, the role of this mutation in ciprofloxacin resistance is unclear and requires further investigation.

Over the past few years, PMQR determinants have been deemed the most common ARGs in Enterobacteriaceae worldwide [42]. PMQR determinants mediate only low-level quinolone resistance. However, these resistance genes are usually associated with mobile or transposable elements that allow for dissemination among Enterobacteriaceae. In addition, the presence of PMQR genes may facilitate the selection of QRDR mutations that result in higher levels of quinolone resistance [37, 43, 44]. The *aac(6')-Ib-cr* gene encodes an acetyltransferase that is known to reduce quinolone activity. In the present study, all 14 isolates resistant to fluoroquinolones were positive for *aac(6')-Ib-cr,* indicating the *aac(6')-Ib-cr* gene is widespread in *S. flexneri* 2a. Compared with the *aac(6')-Ib-cr* gene, the transmembrane segment efflux pump *qepA* gene was scarcely detected in *Shigella,* and we found only one ciprofloxacin-resistant isolate that was *qepA*-positive. The qnr family (which includes the first PMQR genes) contains a variety of subtypes, including *qnrA*, *qnrB*, *qnrC*, *qnrD* and *qnrS* and several *qnr* family genes that have been reported in *Shigella* [39, 45]. The *Qnr* proteins protect DNA gyrase against quinolones and facilitate the selection of QRDR mutations that improve resistance to these antimicrobials.

Conclusion

In conclusion, cephalosporin and/or fluoroquinolone resistance in *Shigella* has been widely reported. To increase our understanding of *Shigella* in cattle, we investigated *Shigella* in calves with diarrhea and analyzed the genetic relatedness, antimicrobial susceptibility, QRDR mutations, and prevalence of PMQR and ß-lactamase in *S. flexneri* 2a isolates from five provinces in northwest China. However, this study also had limitations, including the lack of a systematic surveillance system to prospectively or retrospectively detect and analyze shigellosis in veterinary clinics. Furthermore, we are unable to effectively monitor and control antibiotic abuse and the resulting spread of ARGs. Therefore, it is essential to continually monitor rates of shigellosis and the development of resistance patterns.

Acknowledgements
The authors thank all the farms for providing the samples in this study.

Funding
This work was supported by funds from the National Natural Science Foundation of China (31,272,603, 31,101,836).

Authors' contributions
Conceived and designed the experiments: JYZ and ZZ. Performed the experiments: ZZ and MZC. Analyzed the data: ZZ, BL, and XZZ. Contributed reagents/materials/analysis tools: MZC and FSC. Wrote the paper: ZZ. All authors read and approved the final manuscript.

Consent for publication
All authors agreed on the publication of the paper.

Competing interests
The authors declare that they have no competing interests.

References

1. Nandre R, Matsuda K, Lee JH. Efficacy for a new live attenuated Salmonella Enteritidis vaccine candidate to reduce internal egg contamination. Zoonoses Public Health. 2014;61:55–63.
2. Nandre RM, Ruan X, Duan Q, Sack DA, Zhang W. Antibodies derived from an enterotoxigenic Escherichia coli (ETEC) adhesin tip MEFA (multiepitope fusion antigen) against adherence of nine ETEC adhesins: CFA/I, CS1, CS2, CS3, CS4, CS5, CS6, CS21 and EtpA. Vaccine. 2016;34:3620–5.
3. Rausch D, Ruan X, Nandre R, Duan Q, Hashish E, Casey TA, et al. Antibodies derived from a toxoid MEFA (multiepitope fusion antigen) show neutralizing activities against heat-labile toxin (LT), heat-stable toxins (STa, STb), and Shiga toxin 2e (Stx2e) of porcine enterotoxigenic Escherichia coli (ETEC). Vet Microbiol. 2017;202:79–89.
4. Pupo GM, Lan R, Reeves PR. Multiple independent origins of Shigella clones of Escherichia coli and convergent evolution of many of their characteristics. Proc Natl Acad Sci U S A. 2000;97:10567–72.
5. Livio S, Strockbine NA, Panchalingam S, Tennant SM, Barry EM, Marohn ME, et al. Shigella isolates from the global enteric multicenter study inform vaccine development. Clin Infect Dis. 2014;59:933–41.
6. Linton DS. "War dysentery" and the limitations of German military hygiene during world war I. Bull Hist Med. 2010;84:607–39.
7. Baker KS, Mather AE, McGregor H, Coupland P, Langridge GC, Day M, et al. The extant world war 1 dysentery bacillus NCTC1: a genomic analysis. Lancet. 2014;384:1691–7.
8. Sun Q, Lan R, Wang J, Xia S, Wang Y, Wang Y, et al. Identification and characterization of a novel Shigella flexneri serotype Yv in China. PLoS One. 2013;8:e70238.
9. Qiu S, Xu X, Yang C, Wang J, Liang B, Li P, et al. Shift in serotype distribution of Shigella species in China, 2003–2013. Clin Microbiol Infect. 2015;21:252. e5–8
10. Priamukhina NS, Kilesso VA, Tikhomirov ED. Animal carriers of Shigella and their possible epidemiological importance. Zh Mikrobiol Epidemiol Immunobiol. 1984;11:20–4.
11. Fang H, Wang H, Cai L, Yu Y. Prevalence of antibiotic resistance genes and bacterial pathogens in long-term manured greenhouse soils as revealed by metagenomic survey. Environ Sci Technol. 2015;49:1095–104.
12. Wang Q, Qian L, Jiang S, Cai C, Ma D, Gao P, et al. Safety evaluation of neo transgenic pigs by studying changes in gut microbiota using high-throughput sequencing technology. PLoS One. 2016;11:e0150937.
13. Mohammed AN, Abdel-Latef GK, Abdel-Azeem NM, El-Dakhly KM. Ecological study on antimicrobial-resistant zoonotic bacteria transmitted by flies in cattle farms. Parasitol Res. 2016;115:3889–96.
14. Qu F, Bao C, Chen S, Cui E, Guo T, Wang H, et al. Genotypes and antimicrobial profiles of Shigella sonnei isolates from diarrheal patients circulating in Beijing between 2002 and 2007. Diagn Microbiol Infect Dis. 2012;74:166–70.
15. Li S, Sun Q, Wei X, Klena JD, Wang J, Liu Y, et al. Genetic characterization of Shigella flexneri isolates in Guizhou Province, China. PLoS One. 2015;10: e0116708.
16. Cui X, Wang J, Yang C, Liang B, Ma Q, Yi S, et al. Prevalence and antimicrobial resistance of Shigella flexneri serotype 2 variant in China. Front Microbiol. 2015;6:435.
17. Sun Q, Lan R, Wang Y, Zhao A, Zhang S, Wang J, et al. Development of a multiplex PCR assay targeting O-antigen modification genes for molecular serotyping of Shigella flexneri. J Clin Microbiol. 2011;49:3766–70.
18. Clinical Laboratory Standards Institute. Performance standards for antimicrobial disk susceptibility testing; twenty-second informational supplement. Wayne: Clinical and Laboratory Standards Institute; 2013. p. m100–s23.
19. Cui X, Yang C, Wang J, Liang B, Yi S, Li H, et al. Antimicrobial resistance of Shigella flexneri serotype 1b isolates in China. PLoS One. 2015;10:e0129009.
20. Zong Z, Partridge SR, Thomas L, Iredell JR. Dominance of blaCTX-M within an Australian extended-spectrum beta-lactamase gene pool. Antimicrob Agents Chemother. 2008;52:4198–202.
21. Liu J, Zeng T, Su G, Lin LY, Zhao Y, Yang WQ, et al. The dissemination mode of drug-resistant genes in Enterobacter Cloacae. Indian J Med Microbiol. 2015;33:87–92.
22. Colobatiu L, Tabaran A, Flonta M, Oniga O, Mirel S, Mihaiu M. First description of plasmid-mediated quinolone resistance determinants and β-lactamase encoding genes in non-typhoidal *Salmonella* isolated from humans, one companion animal and food in Romania. Gut Pathog. 2015;7:16.
23. Hu LF, Li JB, Ye Y, Li X. Mutations in the GyrA subunit of DNA gyrase and the ParC subunit of topoisomerase IV in clinical strains of fluoroquinolone-resistant Shigella in Anhui, China. J Microbiol. 2007;45:168–70.
24. Komp Lindgren PD, Karlsson A, Hughes D. Mutation rate and evolution of fluoroquinolone resistance in Escherichia coli isolates from patients with urinary tract infections. Antimicrob Agents Chemother. 2003;47:3222–32.
25. Dutta S, Jain P, Nandy S, Matsushita S, Yoshida S. Molecular characterization of serologically atypical provisional serovars of Shigella isolates from Kolkata, India. J Med Microbiol. 2014;63:1696–703.
26. Pal C, Bengtsson-Palme J, Kristiansson E, Larsson DGJ. The structure and diversity of human, animal and environmental resistomes. Microbiome. 2016;4:54.
27. Ahmed AM, Furuta K, Shimomura K, Kasama Y, Shimamoto T. Genetic characterization of multidrug resistance in Shigella spp. from japan. J Med Microbiol. 2006;55:1685–91.
28. Demarta A, De Respinis S, Dolina M, Peduzzi R. Molecular typing of Yersinia frederiksenii strains by means of 16s rDNA and gyrB genes sequence analyses. FEMS Microbiol Lett. 2004;238:423–8.
29. Ud-Din AI, Wahid SU, Latif HA, Shahnaij M, Akter M, Azmi IJ, et al. Changing trends in the prevalence of Shigella species: emergence of multi-drug resistant Shigella sonnei biotype g in Bangladesh. PLoS One. 2013;8:e82601.
30. Wright DJ, Drasar BS. Dysentery in world war 1: Shigella a century on. Lancet. 2014;384:1651–3.
31. Tajbakhsh M, García Migura LM, Rahbar M, Svendsen CA, Mohammadzadeh M, Zali MR, et al. Antimicrobial-resistant Shigella infections from Iran: an overlooked problem? J Antimicrob Chemother. 2012;67:1128–33.
32. Pfeifer Y, Cullik A, Witte W. Resistance to cephalosporins and carbapenems in gram-negative bacterial pathogens. Int J Med Microbiol. 2010;300:371–9.
33. Sugumar M, Kumar KM, Manoharan A, Anbarasu A, Ramaiah S. Detection of OXA-1 β-lactamase gene of Klebsiella pneumoniae from blood stream infections (BSI) by conventional PCR and in-silico analysis to understand the mechanism of OXA mediated resistance. PLoS One. 2014;9:e91800.
34. Navia MM, Capitano L, Ruiz J, Vargas M, Urassa H, Schellemberg D, et al. Typing and characterization of mechanisms of resistance of Shigella spp. isolated from feces of children under 5 years of age from Ifakara, Tanzania. J Clin Microbiol. 1999;37:3113–7.
35. Robin F, Beyrouthy R, Bonacorsi S, Aissa N, Bret L, Brieu N, et al. Inventory of extended-spectrum-beta-lactamase-producing enterobacteriaceae in France as assessed by a multicenter study. Antimicrob Agents Chemother. 2017;61
36. Taneja N, Kumar A, Appannanavar S, Verma G, Sharma M. Plasmid-mediated quinolone resistance in Shigella isolates over a decade in India. J Glob Antimicrob Resist. 2014;2:59–60.
37. Yang H, Duan G, Zhu J, Zhang W, Xi Y, Fan Q. Prevalence and characterisation of plasmid-mediated quinolone resistance and mutations in the gyrase and topoisomerase IV genes among Shigella isolates from Henan, China, between 2001 and 2008. Int J Antimicrob Agents. 2013;42:173–7.

38. Kamonporn P, Ladaporn B, Sivhour C, Wilawan O, Sirigade R, Panida N, et al. Multidrug-resistant infections in patients with diarrhea, Cambodia, 2014–2015. Emerg Infect Dis. 2016;22:1640–3.
39. Gu B, Qin TT, Fan WT, Bi RR, Chen Y, Li Y, et al. Novel mutations in gyrA and parC among Shigella sonnei strains from Jiangsu Province of China, 2002–2011. Int J Infect Dis. 2017;59:44–9.
40. Ruiz J. Mechanisms of resistance to quinolones: target alterations, decreased accumulation and DNA gyrase protection. J Antimicrob Chemother. 2003; 51:1109–17.
41. Tamanna RJ, Ramana J. Structural insights into the fluoroquinolone resistance mechanism of Shigella flexneri DNA gyrase and topoisomerase IV. Microb Drug Resist. 2016;22:404–11.
42. Pu XY, Pan JC, Gu YM, Zheng W, Li J, Yu H. Complete sequences and characterization of two novel plasmids carrying aac(6')-Ib-cr and qnrS gene in Shigella flexneri. Microb Drug Resist. 2016;22:115–22.
43. Folster JP, Pecic G, Bowen A, Rickert R, Carattoli A, Whichard JM. Decreased susceptibility to ciprofloxacin among Shigella isolates in the United States, 2006 to 2009. Antimicrob Agents Chemother. 2011;55:1758–60.
44. Rodríguez-Martínez JM, Machuca J, Cano ME, Calvo J, Martínez-Martínez L, Pascual A. Plasmid-mediated quinolone resistance: two decades on. Drug Resist Updat. 2016;29:13–29.
45. Zaidi MB, Estrada-García T, Campos FD, Chim R, Arjona F, Leon M, et al. Incidence, clinical presentation, and antimicrobial resistance trends in Salmonella and Shigella infections from children in Yucatan, Mexico. Front Microbiol. 2013;4:288.

3

Effectiveness of surface coatings containing silver ions in bacterial decontamination in a recovery unit

Rafael Manuel Ortí-Lucas[1,2*] and Julio Muñoz-Miguel[1,2]

Abstract

Background: HAIs remain a frequent complication for hospitalised patients and pose a challenge that must be tackled by our health systems.

Methods: Quasi-experimental study. In order to determine the antimicrobial effectiveness of surface coating agents containing silver ions (BactiBlock®) the degree of contamination of several surfaces in two ICU wards was compared. The association between application of Bactiblock® and surface contamination was analysed using a relative risk (RR). Multivariate logistic regressions were performed for each product applied and each sampling location to adjust for the RR of the contamination of surfaces treated with Bactiblock® for the independent variables.

Results: Surface contamination was observed in 31.5% of treated samples and 27.4 of untreated samples. Contamination was equally prominent on bedside Tables (38.7%), bed rails (38.4%) and sinks (38.3%), while the walls showed minimum contamination (2.6%). For beds under isolation protocols, contamination was higher (32.6%) than when no protocol was followed (26.5%) but the difference was not significant ($p = 0.148$). After stratification for application method and adjusting the multivariate models for period of the study and presence of isolated patients, the risk of contamination after the intervention increased when the coating agent was applied using a spray (OR = 1. 79; 95% CI: 1.08-2.95, particularly in a dry and rugged surface such as that of bedside Tables (OR = 2.59; 95% CI: 1.22-5. 52); and decreased when the product was applied using a roller on a smooth and continuously cleaned (or wet) Surface (OR = 0.42; 95% CI: 0.19-0.92).

Conclusion: Coating of hospital surfaces with substances containing silver ions may reduce bacterial growth. However, the effectiveness of the coating agent is affected by application method and environmental conditions and the type and cleanness of the surface.

Keywords: Antimicrobial activity, Silver ions, Risk assessment, Environmental contamination, Surface coating, Healthcare-associated infection

Background

Despite efforts to promote infection control and prevention protocols [1], healthcare associated infections (HAIs) remain a frequent complication for hospitalized patients and a challenge for healthcare systems, not only because they result in high morbi-mortality rates, but also because of the additional associated costs. For over 20 years, the microbiome has been considered the main source of nosocomial infection, followed by horizontal transmission between patients and healthcare workers (20-40%), and the environment (20%) [2]. However, the role of environmental contamination may be more relevant than previously thought. The importance of surface contamination in patient settings is one of the most controversial aspects of HAI control. Microorganisms can survive in the environment for different amounts of time. Certain pathogens such as Meticillin-resistant *Staphylococcus aureus* (MRSA), *Acinetobacter spp.* or *Pseudomonas aeruginosa* are capable of surviving for up to several months [3]. Besides the microorganism itself,

* Correspondence: rm.orti@ucv.es
[1]Social Medicine and Public Health Department, Universidad Católica de Valencia San Vicente Mártir, C/ Espartero,7, Valencia 46007, Spain
[2]Preventive Medicine Department, Hospital Clínico Universitario de Valencia, Valencia, Spain

the variability of their survival times on inanimate surfaces is conditioned by the nature of the surface, humidity, temperature, the cleaning procedure used, and the use of disinfectants as well as their intensity [4]. However, the lack of surface cleanness-control standards for nosocomial pathogens and the scarcity of experimental studies in this area limit the scientific evidence for a link between environmental contamination and the incidence of HAIs. Thus, surface colonisation studies are only recommended in outbreak scenarios [5].

Healthcare environment decontamination is not limited to the use of water, detergents, and disinfectants because conventional cleaning practices are not sufficient to guarantee decontamination [4, 6]. Although a surface may look clean, further testing often reveals the presence of organic remains and nosocomial pathogens [7]. Moreover, the efficacy of an agent depends on its correct use and the thoroughness of the cleaning and decontamination process [8, 9]. Recently, healthcare professionals have pointed out a direct relationship between healthcare budget cuts and the prevalence of HAIs [10]. In the context of preventive medicine, this means that the application of hygiene protocols has become more limited and, as a result, high-touch surfaces can become a reservoir for microorganisms [6, 7] thus facilitating the proliferation of infection and colonisation through indirect contact between healthcare workers, patients, and family members [11, 12]. Besides questioning the quality of traditional cleaning and disinfection methods, healthcare practitioners are now also becoming increasingly concerned about multi-drug resistant organisms related to HAIs, which are on the rise [13]. This has renewed interest in the prevention of these infections and strategies for their control in healthcare facilities [14]. New approaches have been proposed, such as employing novel disinfectants, steam, automated aerosol dispensers, or the use of surfaces with antimicrobial properties. However, these techniques must be properly evaluated before their implementation as means to prevent infection during the provision of healthcare services [12].

The development of antimicrobial surface coatings may play an important role in HAI reduction. These active surfaces are capable of reducing microbial counts compared to regular, untreated surfaces, and could reinforce hygiene in clinical environments [15]. Metals with biocidal properties have been used successfully to treat surfaces in the healthcare context [16]. Several different antimicrobial technologies are now available for the control of pathogenic microorganisms. For example, both in vivo [17] and in vitro [18] studies have proven the effectiveness of metallic copper as an antimicrobial which can reduce bacterial count. Similarly, the antimicrobial effect of silver is also well known and has been scientifically demonstrated [19]. A pilot study carried out by the Heart of England NHS Foundation Trust in the U.K. revealed that treating surfaces with ionic silver can reduce the levels of contaminant bacteria in healthcare environments by up to 95.8% [12, 20]. The innovation in the surface coating agent used in this study is its incorporation into ionic laminar clays before these are added to a polymer matrix [15]. These nanoclays distribute the silver ions evenly through the matrix, thus conferring the material consistent antimicrobial activity throughout the entire surface [21], as well as assuring uniform liberation of the product over time. Given both the demonstrable value of the minimum inhibitory concentration of nanosilver particle additives in vitro, and their antimicrobial capacity as polymer-based products [15], this pilot study aimed to determine its effectiveness in a clinical practice context.

Methods

Study design

In this study of quasi-experimental design, the level of contamination of different surfaces treated with laminar nanoclay-based antimicrobial additives containing silver ions was compared to that of untreated control surfaces in a recovery unit (PACU).

The intervention consisted in the application of BB635A1 (Antimicrobial acrylic coating. 0.3% BactiBlock® 101 R4.47 and 0.3% Zinc Pyrithione) on bedside tables (melamine), walls (paint) and beds (metal railings). BB655A0 (Monolayer polyurethane coating. 0.3% BactiBlock® 101 R4.47) was applied on floors and sinks (metal) using a monolayer roll. Both product and application method were chosen depending on the surface that was to be treated. Since monitors have tactile surfaces they could not be included in this study. The PACU comprises two wards with similar design: si rooms per nurse control-unit which are both in daily transit. The study had a duration of 3 months, corresponding to the minimum time period the coating agent is expected to remain active, and was divided into two periods. In order to analyse the effectiveness of the intervention in the prevention of pathogen growth, one of the wards was treated with the coating agent while the other remained untreated as a control. There are no differences between the occupancy rate or type of patient in the different wards, as patients are checked in after surgery into any available bed. At the beginning of this study the unit had just been renovated. The whole unit was subjected to the same cleaning routine. Both wards were cleaned and disinfected following the standard protocols used at the hospital: the floor was cleaned following the 'double bucket' system with a disinfectant containing 15.05% alkyl dimethyl ammonium and 1.5% bis-(3-aminopropyl)-dodecylamine; surfaces were cleaned with a cloth and a quaternary ammonium-based disinfectant. All products were used according to their instructions and were applied consistently.

The variables "isolated patient" and "period" refer to infected or colonised patients and the endemic level of the PACU respectively. The floor surface was also treated with the coating agent, but no samples were taken due to its minimal role in HAI transmission. The recovery unit continued in normal operation at standard activity levels throughout the study.

Application quality control

In order to evaluate the effectiveness of the product through time, 5 × 5 cm aluminum squares were placed on the walls and floors of the treated wards before applying the antimicrobial products according to the international standard JIS Z 2801 test (ISO 22196) for antimicrobial activity of plastics [22]. These were placed in the same locations in both symmetrical wards in surfaces of different intensity of use such as the floor at the entrance of the ward, cabinets and walls. Once the product was applied on the surfaces, these strips were collected and analyzed every 15 days.

Microbiological sampling

Samples were taken from the surfaces weekly, on Tuesdays at 11 am, on 25 cm^2 plate count agar (PCA), replicate organisms detection and counting (RODAC) dishes in order to detect the total aerobic bacteria count. To sample a surface, the dish was opened and the side with exposed agar was rubbed along the surface being studied while applying constant and uniform pressure and avoiding abrupt movements. Once the sampling process was completed, the dish was closed and labelled with a detailed identifier before being sealed in Parafilm. The surface was then cleaned with isopropyl alcohol so as to eliminate any agar residue. The sealed dishes were transported in a portable fridge, in aseptic conditions, from the Hospital to the microbiology lab. The researchers at this lab were blinded to the sample's origin during the entirety of the study. After incubation for 48 h at 37 °C and 100% RH, the samples were analyzed and the results were expressed in terms of CFU/cm2, considering the area of the sample.

Statistical analysis

Firstly, the mean contamination results for all sampled surfaces expressed in CFU/cm2 were compared. The frequency of contamination was estimated for the different surfaces surrounding the patient. A surface was considered to be contaminated when the CFU count exceeded 0.03 CFU/cm2, a conservative threshold when compared to other approaches to the evaluation of surface hygiene [23]. A simple analysis was carried out using JI-2 estimation (or Fisher test) and relative risk (RR) analysis in order to compare the contamination of surfaces in terms of their treatment (with or without intervention) and other explicative variables: product application method (spray or roller), surface type (rough or smooth), patient isolation-status, and the observation period (weeks 1-7 or first period vs. weeks 8-13 or final period). To adjust the RR of contamination for treated surfaces to these variables, multivariate logistic regression analyzes were carried out for the product application at every sample point (ENTER method). The odds ratio (OR) values were estimated with a confidence interval of 95%; a *p*-value of less than 0.05 was considered significant, and a *p*-value of less than 0.20 was required for inclusion of a variable in the multivariate model. SPSS 15.0 was the statistical package of choice.

Results

A total of 155 samples were taken from tables, 154 from sinks, 151 from the beds, and 155 from the walls; 31.5% of the samples in the treated areas were contaminated, whereas 27.4% of samples from non-treated areas were contaminated, equivalent to a RR of 1.15 (95% CI: 0.90-1.47; $p = 0.261$). Contamination was higher on smooth surfaces (38.4%) such as the metal on the bed rails, than on rough areas (20.6%) including the wood on the tables and the walls ($p = 0.000$), giving a smooth/rough RR of 1.86 (95% CI: 1.43-2.41). Contamination was also higher when the product was applied with a roll compared to a spray (38.3% and 26.5%, respectively; $p = 0.005$), resulting in a roll/spray RR of 1.45 (95% CI: 1.13-1.86). It is noteworthy that samples from the first 7 weeks were more likely to be contaminated than samples from the second period of study (36.5% and 21.3%, respectively; $p = 0.000$), giving a RR of 1.71 (1.31-2.23). If the patient was isolated in the sampled room, contamination (32.6%) was slightly higher than if there had been no isolation (26.5%), but this difference was not significant ($p = 0.148$).

When comparing the mean results of contamination for the different sample points (See Fig. 1), higher contamination was observed on treated beside tables than on untreated ones ($p = 0.005$). This effect was inverted in the sampled sinks, were treated sinks had lower mean contamination results. However these results were statistically non-significant ($p = 0.13$).

Similar results were obtained when the frequency of contamination as a dichotomous variable was analysed (Table 1). Interestingly, contamination was higher on bedside Tables (38.7%), sinks (38.3%), and beds (38.4%), than on the walls (2.6%; $p = 0.000$). The proportion of contaminated samples was higher from treated bedside tables, whereas there were no differences between treated and untreated bed rails; contamination was lower for treated sinks, although these differences were not statistically significant. There were statistically significant differences in the contamination of bedside tables both when isolated patients had been present in the room and during the first 7 weeks of study. Higher levels of contamination

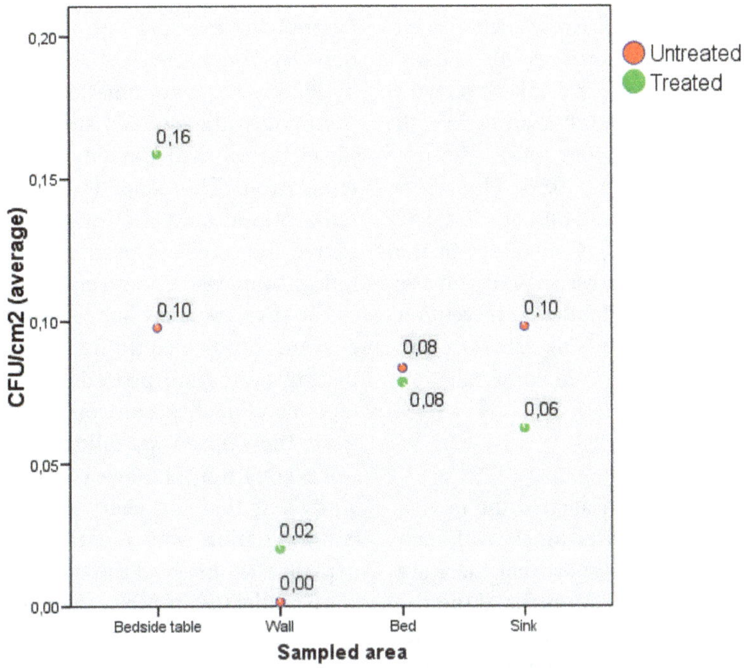

Fig. 1 Level of microbial contamination on environmental surfaces (cfu/cm^2), stratified according to intervention

were also observed during the first half of the study for beds and sinks.

Any of the determining factors described in Table 1 could have confounded our results, which resulted in a lower relative risk for the application of the product on dry, rough surfaces. Thus we prepared a logistic regression model for each type of sampled surface, adjusting for patient isolation and the study period as confounding factors. We explored the other possible explanatory variables mentioned above, but found that these resulted in no significant differences in the outcome.

The OR for the multivariate model considering the global risk associated with spray application of the coating agent, was 1.79 (95% CI: 1.08-2.95). In specific models,

Table 1 Contamination frequency and simple analysis according to the sampling point and determining factors

Risk factor	Global		Bedside table		Bed		Wall		Sink	
	n (%)	*p*	n (%)	*p*	n (%)	*p*	n (%)	P_f	n (%)	*p*
Intervention										
Yes	97 (31,5)	0.261	40 (51.3)*	0.001	29 (38.2)	0.949	3 (3.8)	0.317	25 (32.9)	0.172
No	84 (27,4)		20 (26.0)		29 (38.7)		1 (1.3)		34 (43.6)	
Surface type										
Rough (Wood or paint)	64 (20.6)*	0.000	60 (38.7)	-	-	-	4 (2.6)	-	-	-
Smooth (metal)	117 (38.4)		-		58 (38.4)		-		59 (38.3)	
Application Method										
Spray	122 (26.5)*	0.005	60 (38.7)	-	58 (38.4)	-	4 (2.6)	-	-	-
Monolayer roll	59 (38.3)		-		-		-		59 (38.3)	
Isolated patient										
Yes	56 (32.6)	0.148	23 (53.5)*	0.009	16 (37.2)	0.889	1 (2.3)	0.963	16 (37.2)	0.853
No	96 (26.5)		27 (30.0)		35 (38.5)		2 (2.2)		35 (35.6)	
Period										
Weeks 1-7	120 (36.5)*	0.000	40 (48.2)*	0.009	38 (46.9)*	0.021	0 (0.0)*	0.044	42 (51.2)*	0.000
Weeks 8-13	61 (21.3)		20 (7.8)		20 (28.6)		4 (5.6)		17 (23.6)	

* $P < 0.05$
f Denotes use of the Fisher test

according to the application method and sample point (Fig. 2), the intervention carries a relatively high risk of contamination for rough and dry surfaces like tables, which presented 2.6 times more risk ($p < 0.05$). This result also applies to the walls, although due to the low overall contamination incidence for this site, our model did not reach statistical significance and so $p > 0.05$. The result was also similar for the bed rails (smooth and dry surface), although the risk was lower ($p > 0.05$). Conversely, in the model that considered the global risk associated with the intervention using monolayer rolls, the intervention clearly had a protective effect for the sink (smooth and wet surface), with a nearly 60% decrease in contamination (OR = 0.42; 95% CI: 0.19-0.92).

Discussion

Here, as a preventive alternative, we evaluated the in vivo effectiveness of BactiBlock® silver ion coatings. Although our results are coherent, because they show that there are higher contamination levels in the environment of the patient (bedside table, bed, sink), the effect of the silver coatings contradicted the beneficial effects previously reported in vitro [15]. However, before refuting the effectiveness of the coating agent, we must first evaluate any other factors that could explain this pattern. Our results suggest that the antibacterial effect of these products depends on the characteristics of the treated surface, especially its roughness and if it is generally wet or dry.

In vitro studies did not reveal any relevant differences in the efficacy of the coating agent applied as a spray or from a roll. Therefore, it is surprising that intervening by applying the spray on a wooden table (a dry and inherently rough surface) has a counterproductive effect by increasing contamination, whereas applying the same protocol to the sinks (a smooth and wet surface) by applying a roll, had the intended effect by reducing contamination. The same interventions on the metal bed rails (smooth and dry) or the wall (rough and dry) presented intermediate results, without any evidence of significant differences between these application methods.

The discrepancies between our results and those from previous studies could not be explained by the contamination evaluation procedure, the bacterial culture contact plate quality controls, or by differences resulting from the chosen sampling points because our results were consistent in every case. One limitation of our study was that not every microorganism that produced contamination was identified, however this does not explain the observed differences because all the samples were collected in the same environment using both an appropriate threshold to discriminate differential growth and an appropriate sample size. The fact that the occupancy rate was equally high in both wards and that no epidemical clusters were observed during the study lead us to believe that these factors played no significant role in the changes in contamination. Similarly, it does not appear that the differences we observed between surfaces are due to the development of natural resistance. It remains unclear if ionic silver can generate bacterial resistance [24, 25].

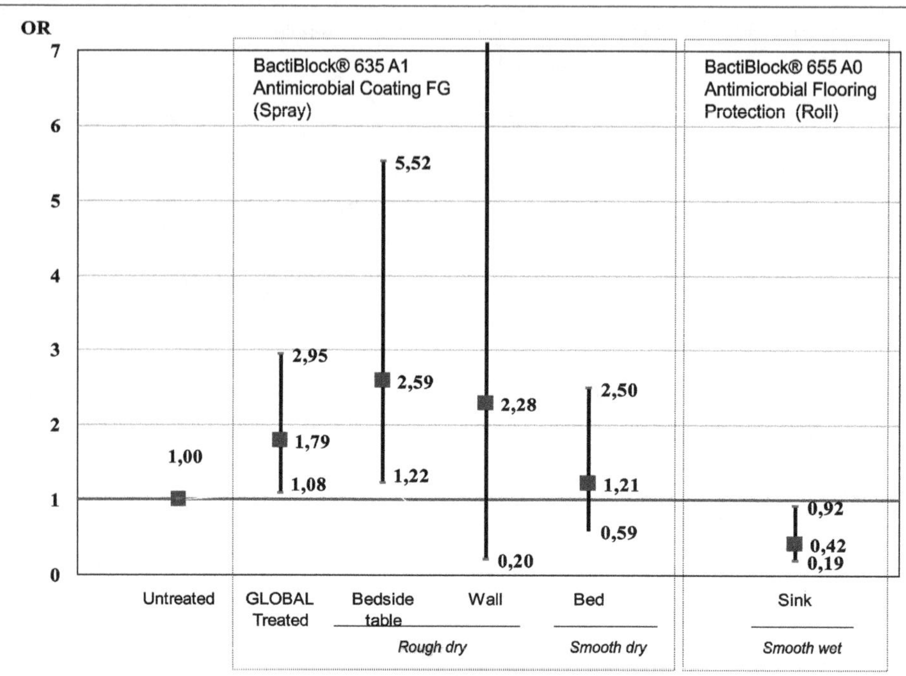

Fig. 2 ORintervention for surfaces treated with spray / roll. (Logistic Regression: Sample point models adjusted for period and presence of isolated patients)

In contrast, it does appear that surface texture affects outcome. Surfaces like that of wooden tables or the plaster walls are rough, and their roughness is increased by the application of the spray. Corresponding with the decreased RR trend we observed for these materials, the metal surfaces of the bed rails and sinks are relatively smoother but their roughness is also enhanced by application of the spray, although the rails are dryer than the sinks, thus increasing their relative smoothness. Therefore, perhaps our results could be explained if the roughness of some surfaces prevents effective cleaning and limits the decontaminant effect of surface coatings. According to this hypothesis any dirt deposited on top of the antibacterial covering would inhibit the action of the silver ions present by creating a layer which blocks their direct contact with the deposited microorganisms. This phenomenon is not new; it is comparable with the effect observed in water pipelines when biofilms develop which favour the resistance of bacteria like *Legionella pneumophila* or *P. aeruginosa* to antimicrobials such as chlorine and other disinfectants [26].

It could be argued that contamination was lower in the sinks because they are continuously washed with tap water, however, it is well known that sinks can act as potential reservoirs for particular Gram-negative bacteria [24, 26–28] such as *Escherichia coli, Klebsiella spp.*, or *Pseudomonas* spp. which are favoured in wet conditions, increasing their life expectancy to more than 1 year [3]. Nonetheless, if the dirt deposited on top of the antibacterial coatings is sufficient to render the antimicrobial action of the silver ions ineffective on rough 'dirty' (difficult to clean) surfaces, the near-continuous washing with water of the smooth (easy to clean) surface of the sinks would probably keep the coating 'clean', allowing it to be effective.

Although these products show in vitro biocidal activity against some microorganisms, it is important to assess their in vivo efficacy, because their effectiveness in real conditions depends on their proper application. This study suggests that the antimicrobial coating's application method should avoid increasing the roughness of the treated surfaces, and that for the effective action of BactiBlock® (especially for rough surfaces), they should be wet-cleaned using a rubbing action in order to improve the liberation of silver ions from the product. This explanation is not novel in the context of medicine aimed at preventing HAIs. It is similar to the need to wash dirty hands so as to maximize the effects of hydroalcoholic solutions [29]. However, if confirmed, this information would be important in decision making, since it would help those controlling infections to better understand and manage the risks related to environmental contamination of health centres. Thus, the availability and proper application of new technologies is crucial when cleaning services and practices are insufficient or unable to reduce infection risks.

Conclusions

Covering the surfaces of the hospital with silver ions may help to stop the increase in microorganisms, but further studies will first be required to confirm if the effect seen in previous studies is due to the product or to other concurrent factors present in these different environmental conditions such as the product type, application method, or whether the tested surface is dry or wet.

Abbreviations

CFU: Colony forming units; HAI: Healthcare associated infections; ICU: Intensive care unit; MRSA: Meticillin-resistant *Staphylococcus aureus*; OR: Odds ratio; PCA: Plate count agar; RODAC: Replicate organisms detection and counting; RR: Relative risk

Acknowledgements

The authors thank Nanobiomatters Bactiblock LTD for providing funding for the sampling and analysis of microbiological samples and INCLIVA for the translation and revision services provided.

Funding

The fieldwork was financially supported by Nanobiomatters Bactiblock LTD. The supporter had a role in data collection and analysis of microbiological samples; but no role in the study design, analysis, interpretation, writing of this manuscript, or the decision to submit the manuscript for publication.

Authors' contributions

RMOL carried out the design and coordination of the study, statistical analysis, interpretation and writing of the manuscript. JMM participated in the statistical analysis, interpretation and writing of the manuscript. Both authors read and approved the final manuscript.

Competing interests

The authors declare that they have no competing interests.

Consent for publication

Not applicable.

References

1. Schabrun S, Chipchase L. Healthcare equipment as a source of nosocomial infection: a systematic review. J Hosp Infect. 2006;63(3):239–45. doi:10.1016/j.jhin.2005.10.013.
2. Weinstein RA. Epidemiology and control of nosocomial infections in adult intensive care units. Am J Med. 1991;91(3B):179S–84S.
3. Kramer A, Schwebke I, Kampf G. How long do nosocomial pathogens persist on inanimate surfaces? A systematic review. BMC Infect Dis. 2006; 6(1):130. doi:10.1186/1471-2334-6-130.
4. Dancer SJ, White LF, Lamb J, Girvan EK, Robertson C. Measuring the effect of enhanced cleaning in a UK hospital: a prospective cross-over study. BMC Med. 2009;7(1):28. doi:10.1186/1741-7015-7-28.
5. Sehulster L, Chinn RYW. Guidelines for environmental infection control in health-care facilities. Morb Mortal Wkly Rep. 2003;52(RR10):1–42.
6. French G, Otter J, Shannon K, Adams NM, Watling D, Parks M. Tackling contamination of the hospital environment by methicillin-resistant *Staphylococcus aureus* (MRSA): a comparison between conventional terminal cleaning and hydrogen peroxide vapour decontamination. J Hosp Infect. 2004;57(1):31–7. doi:10.1016/j.jhin.2004.03.006.

7. Denton M, Wilcox M, Parnell P, et al. Role of environmental cleaning in controlling an outbreak of Acinetobacter Baumannii on a neurosurgical intensive care unit. J Hosp Infect. 2004;56(2):106–10. doi:10.1016/j.jhin.2003.10.017.
8. Griffith CJ, Cooper RA, Gilmore J, Davies C, Lewis M. An evaluation of hospital cleaning regimes and standards. J Hosp Infect. 2000;45(1):19–28. doi:10.1053/jhin.1999.0717.
9. Carling PC, Bartley JM. Evaluating hygienic cleaning in health care settings: what you do not know can harm your patients. Am J Infect Control. 2010; 38(5):S41–50. doi:10.1016/j.ajic.2010.03.004.
10. Humphreys H. Self-disinfecting and Microbiocide-impregnated surfaces and fabrics: what potential in interrupting the spread of healthcare-associated infection? Clin Infect Dis. 2014;58(6):848–53. doi:10.1093/cid/cit765.
11. Jiménez-Martín S., Andrea-Viola A. El sistema de salud en España en perspectiva comparada 2014.
12. Page K, Wilson M, Parkin IP. Antimicrobial surfaces and their potential in reducing the role of the inanimate environment in the incidence of hospital-acquired infections. J Mater Chem. 2009;19(23):3819. doi:10.1039/b818698g.
13. Sanborn WR. The relation of surface contamination to the transmission of disease. Am J Public health nations health. Am J Public Health. 1963;53(8):1278–83.
14. Dancer SJ. Importance of the environment in meticillin-resistant *Staphylococcus aureus* acquisition: the case for hospital cleaning. Lancet Infect Dis. 2008;8(2):101–13. doi:10.1016/S1473-3099(07)70241-4.
15. Monte-Serrano M, Fernandez-Saiz P, Ortí-Lucas RM. Effective Antimicrobial Coatings Containing Silver-Based Nanoclays and Zinc Pyrithione. J Microb Biochem Technol 2015;7(6). doi:10.4172/1948-5948.1000245.
16. Haggstrom JA, Klabunde KJ, Marchin GL. Biocidal properties of metal oxidenanoparticles and their halogenadducts. Nano. 2010;2(3):399–405. doi:10.1039/B9NR00245F.
17. Casey AL, Adams D, Karpanen TJ, et al. Role of copper in reducing hospital environment contamination. J Hosp Infect. 2010;74(1):72–7. doi:10.1016/j.jhin.2009.08.018.
18. Paul M, Shani V, Muchtar E, Kariv G, Robenshtok E, Leibovici L. Systematic review and meta-analysis of the efficacy of appropriate empiric antibiotic therapy for sepsis. Antimicrob Agents Chemother. 2010;54(11):4851–63. doi:10.1128/AAC.00627-10.
19. Dancer SJ. Controlling hospital-acquired infection: focus on the role of the environment and new technologies for decontamination. Clin Microbiol Rev. 2014;27(4):665–90. doi:10.1128/CMR.00020-14.
20. Taylor L, Phillips P, Hastings R. Reduction of bacterial contamination in a healthcare environment by silver antimicrobial technology. J Infect Prev. 2009;10(1):6–12. doi:10.1177/1757177408099083.
21. Chopra I. The increasing use of silver-based products as antimicrobial agents: a useful development or a cause for concern? J Antimicrob Chemother. 2007;59(4):587–90. doi:10.1093/jac/dkm006.
22. Percival SL, Bowler PG, Russell D. Bacterial resistance to silver in wound care. J Hosp Infect. 2005;60(1):1–7. doi:10.1016/j.jhin.2004.11.014.
23. Malik RE, Cooper RA, Griffith CJ. Use of audit tools to evaluate the efficacy of cleaning systems in hospitals. Am J Infect Control. 2003;31(3):181–7.
24. Hartemann P, Hoet P, Proykova A, et al. "Nanosilver: Safety, Health and Environmental Effects and Role in Antimicrobial Resistance." Materials Today 18.3. 2015:122-23.
25. Morgan DJ, Liang SY, Smith CL, et al. Frequent multidrug-resistant Acinetobacter Baumannii contamination of gloves, gowns, and hands of healthcare workers. Infect Control Hosp Epidemiol. 2010;31(7):716–21. doi:10.1086/653201.
26. Li L, Mendis N, Trigui H, Oliver JD, Faucher SP. The importance of the viable but non-culturable state in human bacterial pathogens. Front Microbiol. 2014;5 doi:10.3389/fmicb.2014.00258.
27. Shiomori T, Miyamoto H, Makishima K, et al. Evaluation of bedmaking-related airborne and surface methicillin-resistant *Staphylococcus aureus* contamination. J Hosp Infect. 2002;50(1):30–5. doi:10.1053/jhin.2001.1136.
28. Best EL, Fawley WN, Parnell P, Wilcox MH. The potential for airborne dispersal of Clostridium Difficile from symptomatic patients. Clin Infect Dis. 2010;50(11):1450–7. doi:10.1086/652648.
29. Who. Guidelines on hand hygiene in health care. First global patient safety challenge clean care is safer care. World Health. 2009;30(1):270. doi:10.1086/600379.

4

Incidence, clinical characteristics, and outcomes of nosocomial *Enterococcus* spp. bloodstream infections in a tertiary-care hospital in Beijing, China

Yangyang Zhang[1,2†], Mingmei Du[3†], Yan Chang[4], Liang-an Chen[1*] and Qing Zhang[2*]

Abstract

Background: *Enterococcus* spp. are the common cause of nosocomial bloodstream infections (BSIs) with high morbidity and mortality. The purpose of this study was to characterize the incidence, clinical and microbiological features, and mortality of nosocomial enterococcal BSIs at a large Chinese tertiary-care hospital in Beijing, China.

Methods: A retrospective cohort study on adult patients with nosocomial BSIs due to *Enterococcus* spp. was performed between January 1, 2012, and December 31, 2015 at the Chinese People's Liberation Army General Hospital. Patients' data were gathered by reviewing electronic medical records.

Results: A total of 233 episodes of BSI due to *Enterococcus* spp. occurred among 224 patients during these 4 years. The overall incidence was 3.9 episodes per 10,000 admissions. *Enterococcus faecium* (*E. faecium*) was the major pathogen (74%, 95% CI 68–80%), followed by *Enterococcus faecalis* (*E. faecalis*) (20%, 95% CI 15–25%). *E. faecium* showed higher antimicrobial resistance than *E. faecalis*. The 30-day mortality of nosocomial enterococcal BSI was 24% (95% CI 18–29%). Predictors for mortality included the Acute Physiology and Chronic Health Evaluation II (APACHE II) score, Charlson comorbidity index (CCI), impaired renal function, prior use of immunosuppressive agents, and appropriate empirical antimicrobial treatment.

Conclusions: This study emphasizes that *Enterococcus* spp. were major pathogens for nosocomial BSIs and associated with high mortality. Appropriate empirical antimicrobial treatment can improve outcomes. Vancomycin is the best choice for patients with *E. faecium* BSIs. Penicillins, aminoglycosides, fluoroquinolones, and vancomycin can be considered for patients with *E. faecalis* BSIs.

Keywords: *Enterococcus*, Nosocomial bloodstream infection, Bacteraemia, Epidemiology, Mortality

* Correspondence: chenliangan301@163.com; zhangqing_cyfy@163.com
[†]Equal contributors
[1]Department of Respiratory Medicine, Chinese PLA General Hospital, Fuxing Road No. 28, Beijing 100853, China
[2]Department of Respiratory Medicine, Affiliated Hospital of Chengde Medical University, Nanyingzi Street No. 36, Chengde, Hebei Province 067000, China
Full list of author information is available at the end of the article

Background

BSIs can cause high mortality and result in heavy social and economic burdens. As one of the common gram-positive pathogens, *Enterococcus* spp. are the fourth leading cause of BSIs in North America [1], and are rated as the third most prevalent pathogens of nosocomial BSIs in the United States [2], accounting for >9.0% of the BSIs. Several multicentre studies from China and Japan also reported that *Enterococcus* spp. were the fourth most common BSI pathogens [3–5]. And a systematic review focused on community-acquired BSIs in south and southeast Asia showed that *Enterococcus* spp. were the third most prevalent gram positive bacteria [6]. The crude mortality rates of enterococcal BSIs ranged between 21.4% and 64.2% [7–11]. Risk factors for developing enterococcal BSIs include the presence of comorbidities such as malignancy, diabetes; more severe illness; invasive devices, such as a central intravenous catheter; complicated surgery; solid organ transplantation; and hematopoietic stem cell transplantation [2, 12–16].

Enterococci are innately resistant to cephalosporins, and the commonly used antimicrobial agents such as fluoroquinolones and carbapenems are not recommended. The increasing prevalence of acquired resistance to penicillins and aminoglycosides has been observed in many countries [17, 18]. Vancomycin-resistant enterococci (VRE) are a great challenge in clinical treatment because there are limited bactericidal options to choose [19].

E. faecalis and *E. faecium* are the most frequently isolated species, and incidences of both have shown a rising trend, especially for *E. faecium* [11, 20]. *E. faecium* has significantly higher antibiotic resistance rates than *E. faecalis* and may lead to more serious disease and worse outcome [11, 21, 22].

Although there has been much research on enterococcal BSI, the incidence, species distribution, clinical features, and prognosis vary in different periods and different regions. In addition, nosocomial BSI is different from community-acquired BSI in several aspects, including a poor prognosis [11]. Little data exists regarding nosocomial enterococcal BSIs in China. The purpose of the present study was to characterise the incidence, clinical, and microbiological features, and to identify the predictors of crude mortality in patients with enterococcal BSIs at our hospital. The clinical and microbiological characteristics of *E. faecalis* and *E. faecium* were also compared.

Methods

Study design, hospital setting, and patients

We performed a retrospective cohort study on adult patients with nosocomial BSIs due to *Enterococcus* spp. between January 1, 2012, and December 31, 2015, at the Chinese People's Liberation Army General Hospital (PLAGH), a 2200-bed tertiary-level healthcare hospital in Beijing, China. It is one of the biggest comprehensive hospitals in China, with medical, health care, teaching, and scientific research that serves national military and nonmilitary personnel from across the country.

Eligible patients included all patients aged ≥18 years with at least 1 positive blood culture for *Enterococcus* spp. In patients with persistent BSIs caused by the same organism, only the first episode was included. If the patients had 2 or more separate BSIs, each infection was considered individually. All patients were identified by searching the real-time nosocomial infection surveillance system (RT-NISS) [23]. This platform utilises data from electronic medical record systems, such as hospital stay, temperature changes, and microbiology results with the application of clinically validated algorithms to identify and classify all of the patients' infections. RT-NISS was developed by the Infection Management and Disease Control Department of PLAGH.

Data collection

The patients' data were gathered by reviewing electronic medical records. We recorded the demographic data including age and gender. The clinical data collected included: body mass index (BMI), underlying diseases, the CCI score, the APACHE II score in the first 24 h following the onset of BSIs, the hospitalisation wards, previous exposures (prior hospital stay, previous treatment such as surgical procedures, immunosuppressive agents, chemotherapeutic agents, total parenteral nutrition, mechanical ventilation, renal replacement therapy, antibiotics, or invasive devices within 30 days prior to BSIs), treatment (antibiotic choice), and outcomes (length of hospital stay, and all-cause mortality at 7 days and 30 days). The microbiological data collected included: species of *Enterococcus*, likely source of BSIs (identified by treating doctors and/or physicians of the Infection Management and Disease Control Department), whether cultures were polymicrobial, and antimicrobial susceptibility results. We collected the annual admission data to calculate incidence rates, which are expressed as the number of BSI episodes per 10,000 hospital admissions.

Definitions

The diagnosis of enterococcal BSI should meet the following criteria: 1)isolation of *Enterococcus* spp. from one or more blood cultures; and one of the following 2) fever (>38 °C), chills, or hypotension; and 3) eliminated the possibility of contamination during the collection and cultivation of blood samples [24]. Nosocomial BSI was defined as the first positive blood culture obtained ≥48 h after hospital admission and with no evidence of infection at admission [15, 24]. An episode was defined as the positive isolation of enterococcus from at least one blood culture sample from a patient and without the prior blood culture isolating the same bacteria within the previous 30 days [2, 25]. Onset of BSIs was defined as the date when the blood culture was collected. Polymicrobial BSIs were defined as 2 or more clinically important organisms isolated from 1 single blood culture sample or different blood culture samples within 48 h. Appropriate antimicrobial treatment was defined as an active antimicrobial choice and an adequate dosage within 5 days from the onset. Empirical antimicrobial therapy was defined as the antimicrobial agents given within 24 h after the onset of BSIs. Active agents were confirmed according to the antimicrobial susceptibility test.

Identification and antibiotic susceptibility testing

Blood was cultured using BacT/ALERT 3D system (Becton-Dickinson, Sparks, MD, USA) in the microbiology laboratory. Species identification was performed using the VITEK 2 system (BioMérieux, Marcy 1'Étoile, France). Antibiotic susceptibility testing was performed using the VITEK 2 system or the Kirby-Bauer Disk Diffusion method (Oxoid, UK) according to the recommendations proposed by the Clinical and Laboratory Standards Institute (CLSI).

Statistical analysis

Categorical variables were expressed as frequency counts and percentages with 95% confidence interval (95% CI). Continuous variables were expressed as median and interquartile ranges (IQRs). Comparison of categorical variables was performed using Pearson's chi-squared test or Fisher's exact test, and comparison of continuous variables was performed using the Mann-Whitney U test. In order to identify the risk factors associated with mortality, a multivariate logistic regression model with backward method was generated to control the effects of confounding variables. Variables statistically related ($p < 0.10$) to mortality in the univariate logistic analyses were chosen to build the multivariate model. Results with a 2-tailed p-value < 0.05 were considered to be significant. All statistical analyses were run using SPSS 20.0 software (IBM Corp., Armonk, NY, USA).

Results

Incidence and species distribution

In total, 233 episodes of nosocomial BSIs caused by *Enterococcus* spp. occurred among 224 patients during the 4-year study period. Of the 224 patients who developed enterococcal BSIs, 6 had infections with 2 different species >30 days apart and 3 had 2 infections with the same species >30 days apart. Seven patients who had infections with 2 different species of enterococcus isolated within 48 h were excluded because of the interpretative problem.

For the remaining 226 episodes, classification was available in 224 (99%, 95% CI 98–100%). The most common *Enterococcus* species was *E. faecium*, which comprised 167 (74%, 95% CI 68–80%) of all episodes. *E. faecalis* was the second largest species, comprising 46 (20%, 95% CI 15–25%) of episodes. Of the remaining episodes, 6 (3%, 95% CI 1–5%) due to *E. casseliflavus*, 3 (1%, 95% CI 0–3%) due to *E. gallinarum*, and 2 (1%, 95% CI 0–3%) due to *E. avium*. The number of enterococci isolated in 2015 was the highest, and the least was in 2013. The species ratio in each year is shown in Fig. 1.

The overall incidence of nosocomial enterococcal BSIs was 3.9 episodes per 10,000 admissions and the rate fluctuated from 3.3 to 4.4 episodes per 10,000 admissions during the 4 years (3.7 in 2012, 3.3 in 2013, 4.1 in 2014, and 4.4 in 2015). The overall incidence rates of *E. faecium* and *E. faecalis* were 2.9 episodes and 0.8 episodes per 10,000 admissions, respectively. Incidence of *E. faecalis* BSI showed a rising trend, while that of *E. faecium* was on the decline, as shown in Fig. 2.

Demographic and clinical characteristics

Demographics and clinical data were available for all these 226 incident episodes as shown in Table 1. The median age was 65 years (IQR, 54–75), and 142 (63%, 95% CI 56–69%) of the patients were male. The age distribution was right skewed, with the peak incidence in the 50–59 years group (Figure 3). Malignancy was the most common comorbidity (58%, 95% CI 51–64%), followed by cardiovascular disease (50%, 95% CI 43–57%) and pneumonia (33%, 95% CI 27–39%). The median and range of BMI were all within the normal range. The median CCI score was 3 (IQR, 2–6), and 86.7% of the patients had combined chronic diseases (CCI score ≥ 1). The median APACHE II score was 8 (IQR, 5–18). Some 172 (76%, 95% CI 71–82%) of the episodes occurred in the non-ICU ward, and 54 (24%, 95% CI 18–29%) occurred in the ICU. The median days of hospital stay prior to and

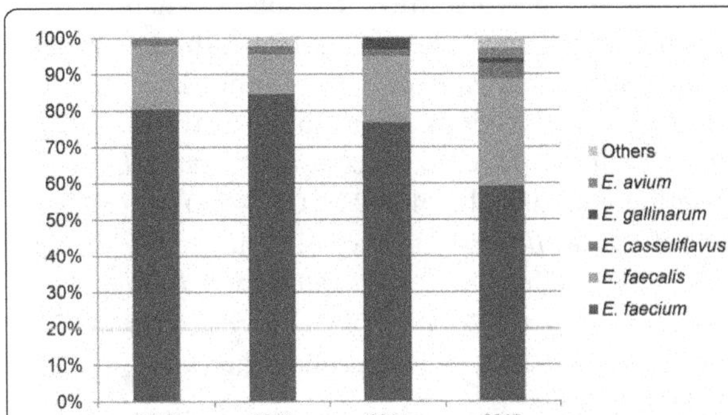

Fig. 1 *Enterococcus* species ratio from 2012 to 2015

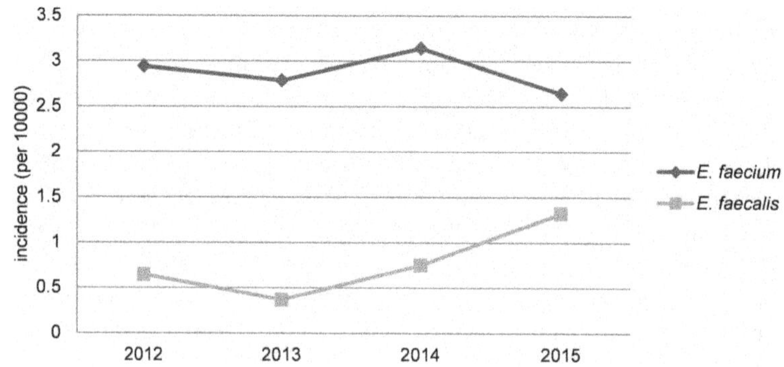

Fig. 2 Incidences of BSIs due to *E. faecium* and *E. faecalis* from 2012 to 2015

after the onset of BSI were 15 and 18, respectively. A total of 210 (93%, 95% CI 90–96%) episodes had prior antibiotic exposure and 182 (81%, 95% CI 75–86%) had invasive medical procedures within the 30 days prior to BSI, such as a central intravenous catheter, Indwelling urinary catheter, and drainage tube.

A comparison of nosocomial BSIs according to *E. faecium* and *E. faecalis* in demographics and clinical characteristics is shown in Table 1. Patients with *E. faecalis* BSIs presented a higher BMI, but the median was in the normal range. Patients with *E. faecium* BSIs showed a higher CCI score than those with *E. faecalis* BSIs (median, 3 vs 2, $p = 0.014$). The median APACHE II score of patients with *E. faecium* BSIs was higher than in those with *E. faecalis* BSIs, but these were not statistically significant.

Microbiology and antimicrobial therapy

The source of nosocomial enterococcal BSIs was mainly related to intra-abdominal and central venous catheter, with the number of 92 (41%, 95% CI 34–47%) and 82 (36%, 95% CI 30–43%), respectively. Foci could not be confirmed for 65 (29%, 95% CI 23–35%) episodes. A total of 21 (9%, 95% CI 5–13%) episodes had polymicrobial infections.

The microbiological data of BSIs due to *E. faecium* and *E. faecalis* are presented in Table 2. There was no difference in the sources of BSI between these 2 species. Patients with *E. faecium* BSIs were more likely to have polymicrobial infections than those with *E. faecalis* (12% vs 2%, $p = 0.048$). No vancomycin-resistant *E. faecalis* isolate was found, and 7 (4%, 95% CI 1–7%) vancomycin-resistant *E. faecium* isolates were identified. *E. faecium* isolates had higher resistance rates than *E. faecalis* to ampicillin (86% vs 9%, $p < 0.001$), erythromycin (78% vs 56%, $p = 0.009$), and ciprofloxacin (86% vs 39%, $p < 0.001$).

Before obtaining the report of antibiotic susceptibility test reports, 98 (43%, 95% CI 37–50%) patients were treated with effective antibiotics. Patients with *E. faecalis* BSIs were more likely to get effective treatment by the empirical use of antibiotics (57% vs 37%, $p = 0.018$).

Outcomes

The median length of hospital stay was 34 days (IQR, 23–55). There was no statistical difference in the length of stay between patients with *E. faecium* BSIs (median, 35) and those with *E. faecalis* BSIs (median, 34). The total 7-day and 30-day mortality rates were 11% (95% CI 7–15%) and 24% (95% CI 18–29%), respectively. The 7-day and 30-day mortality rates for *E. faecium* BSIs were higher than *E. faecalis* BSIs (13% vs 9%, 25% vs 17%), but both had no statistical significance. Patients with malnutrition showed a higher risk of 7-day and 30-day mortality than patients with normal BMI.

Univariate analyses of predictors for 7-day mortality and 30-day mortality are shown separately in Table 3. The 7-day mortality was associated with pneumonia, impaired renal function, CCI, APACHE II score, ICU residence, prior exposure to immunosuppressive agents and central intravenous catheter, and appropriate empirical antimicrobial treatment. The predictors for 30-day mortality were similar to those for 7-day mortality, except for surgery and renal replacement therapy prior to the onset of BSI within 30 days.

In the multivariate logistic regression model (Table 4), the risk factors for 7-day mortality included increasing APACHE II scores (OR 1.2, 95% CI 1.1–1.3), and the use of immunosuppressive agents prior to the onset of enterococcal BSIs (OR 4.6, 95% CI 1.1–19.2); the risk factors for 30-day mortality included impaired renal function (OR 3.3, 95% CI 1.1–9.8), high CCI (OR 1.3, 95% CI 1.1–1.6) and APACHE II scores (OR 1.3, 95% CI 1.2–1.4), and prior exposure to immunosuppressive agents (OR 7.3, 95% CI 1.8–29.0). Appropriate empirical antimicrobial therapy was a protective factor for both 7-day (OR 0.2, 95% CI 0.1–0.7) and 30-day mortality (OR 0.2, 95% CI 0.1–0.4).

Table 1 Demographic and clinical characteristics of patients with enterococcal BSIs

	Total (*n* = 226)	*E. faecium* (*n* = 167)	*E. faecalis* (*n* = 46)	*p*-value
Demographics				
Age	65 (54–75)	65 (55–75)	66 (52–79)	0.450
Male gender	142 (63, 56–69)	104 (62, 55–70)	31 (67, 53–81)	0.524
BMI, median	23 (20–26)	22 (20–25)	24 (23–26)	***0.006***
Comorbidities				
Malignancy	130 (58, 51–64)	95 (57, 49–64)	26 (57, 42–71)	0.965
Cardiovascular disease	113 (50, 43–57)	78 (47, 39–54)	28 (61, 46–76)	0.089
Pneumonia	74 (33, 27–39)	60 (36, 29–43)	14 (30, 17–44)	0.488
Diabetes mellitus	68 (30, 24–36)	45 (27, 20–34)	18 (39, 24–54)	0.109
Impaired liver function	52 (23, 17–29)	41 (25, 18–31)	7 (15, 4–26)	0.180
Cerebrovascular disease	41 (18, 13–23)	34 (20, 14–27)	5 (11, 2–20)	0.141
Impaired renal function	30 (13, 9–18)	22 (13, 8–18)	7 (15, 4–26)	0.720
Hemiplegia	27 (12, 8–16)	24 (14, 9–20)	2 (4, 0–10)	0.066
Neutropenia	14 (6, 3–9)	12 (7, 3–11)	2 (4, 0–10)	0.492
CCI, median	3 (2–6)	3 (2–6)	2 (1–4)	***0.014***
APACHE II score, median	8 (5–11)	8 (5–11)	7 (5–12)	0.501
Hospitalization ward				
Medical	88 (39, 33–45)	68 (41, 33–48)	14 (30, 17–44)	0.204
Surgical	84 (37, 31–44)	56 (34, 26–41)	22 (48, 33–63)	0.075
ICU	54 (24, 18–29)	43 (26, 19–32)	10 (22, 9–34)	0.578
Length of hospital stay, median days				
Prior hospital stay	15 (9–27)	16 (10–28)	14 (7–25)	0.065
Hospital stay after onset of BSIs	18 (8–29)	18 (8–29)	18 (8–33)	0.906
Previous treatment				
Antibiotic exposure	210 (93, 90–96)	160 (96, 93–99)	41 (89, 80–98)	0.082
Total parenteral nutrition	84 (37, 31–44)	60 (36, 29–43)	22 (48, 33–63)	0.142
Mechanical ventilation	87 (38, 32–45)	63 (38, 30–45)	20 (43, 29–58)	0.479
Surgery	74 (33, 27–39)	49 (29, 22–36)	20 (43, 29–58)	0.070
Chemotherapeutic agent	29 (13, 8–17)	24 (14, 9–20)	3 (7, 0–14)	0.153
Immunosuppressive agent	18 (8, 4–12)	16 (10, 5–14)	2 (4, 2–10)	0.259
Renal replacement therapy	15 (7, 3–10)	12 (7, 3–11)	3 (7, 0–14)	0.876
Invasive devices				
Central intravenous catheter	102 (45, 39–52)	82 (49, 41–57)	16 (35, 20–49)	0.084
Indwelling urinary catheter	104 (46, 39–53)	75 (45, 37–53)	25 (54, 39–69)	0.256
Endotracheal intubation	86 (38, 32–44)	60 (36, 29–43)	22 (48, 33–63)	0.142
Peripheral intravenous catheter	69 (31, 24–37)	50 (30, 23–37)	14 (30, 17–44)	0.948
Tracheostomy tube	20 (9, 5–13)	15 (9, 5–13)	4 (9, 0–17)	0.952

Data are presented as n (%,95% CI) or median (IQR)
Significant variables are appeared in bold and italics text

Discussion

This study focused on the incidence and characteristics of nosocomial enterococcal BSI in one of the biggest comprehensive hospitals in China. Two multicentre studies in China reporting on the species distribution and antibiotic resistance of clinical isolates from blood cultures showed that *Enterococcus* spp. were the fourth most common pathogens [3, 4]. But, these 2 studies did not involve the species distribution, clinical information, and prognosis. A single-centre study published recently,

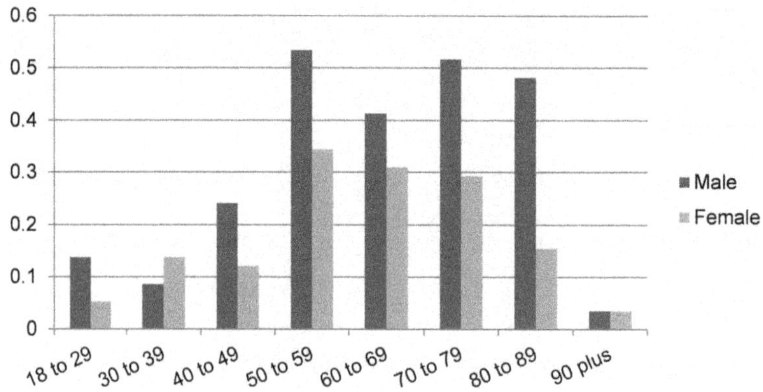

Fig. 3 Age and gender distribution of patients with enterococcal BSIs

also devoted to explore the features of *Enterococcus* spp. BSI in a teaching hospital of China [26]. But the sample size (64 episodes) was smaller than our study, and all nosocomial, health care associated, and community acquired enterococcal BSIs were included.

In our 4-year study, the incidence rate of nosocomial enterococcal BSIs fluctuated from 3.3 to 4.4 episodes per 10,000 admissions. This is similar to an earlier study conducted from 1995 to 2002 at 42 US hospitals [2], but is higher than 2 recent reports from Denmark (1.96/10,000) and Canada (0.69/10,000) [11, 15]. But these were both population-based studies. To our knowledge, there are no such reference data about the incidence of nosocomial enterococcal BSIs in China.

In accordance with other studies, patients with enterococcal BSIs were commonly associated with complications, such as malignant, cardiovascular diseases, diabetes mellitus, or chronic kidney disease [11, 15, 22, 27]. We

Table 2 Comparison of the microbiological characteristics and treatment of patients with *E. faecium* and *E. faecalis* BSIs

	E. faecium (*n* = 167)	*E. faecalis* (*n* = 46)	*p*-value
Source of BSIs			
Intra-abdominal	65 (39, 31–46)	19 (41, 27–56)	0.770
Unknown	53 (32, 25–39)	10 (22, 9–34)	0.188
Central venous catheter	30 (18, 12–24)	10 (22, 9–34)	0.562
Genitourinary	11 (7, 3–10)	3 (7, 0–14)	0.987
Pneumonia	4 (2, 0–5)	3 (7, 0–14)	0.165
Others	4 (2, 0–5)	1 (2, 0–7)	0.930
Type of BSIs			
Polymicrobial	20 (12, 7–17)	1 (2, 0–7)	***0.048***
Antibiotic resistance[a]			
Ampicillin (137 vs 46)[b]	118 (86, 80–92)	4 (9, 0–7)	***<0.001***
Gentamicin (93 vs 21) [b]	49 (53, 42–63)	7 (33, 11–55)	0.109
Tetracycline (105 vs 36) [b]	50 (48, 38–57)	22 (61, 44–78)	0.162
Erythromycin (105 vs 36) [b]	82 (78, 70–86)	20 (56, 39–73)	***0.009***
Ciprofloxacin (137 vs 46) [b]	118 (86, 80–92)	18 (39, 24–54)	***<0.001***
Vancomycin (167 vs 46) [b]	7 (4, 1–7)	0 (0, 0)	0.158
Treatment after the onset of BSIs			
Appropriate antimicrobial treatment	157 (94, 90–98)	43 (93, 86–100)	0.893
Appropriate empirical treatment	62 (37, 30–45)	26 (57, 42–71)	***0.018***

Data are presented as n (%,95% CI) or median (IQR)
Significant variables are appeared in bold and italics text
[a]Not all agents listed tested in all isolates
[b]The numbers in parentheses represent the total numbers of *E. faecium* and *E. faecalis* isolates performed susceptibility test

Table 3 Univariate logistic regression analysis of risk factors for mortality

Variable	7-day mortality				30-day mortality			
	Survivors (n = 201)	Non-survivors (n = 25)	OR (95% CI)	*p*-value	Survivors (n = 172)	Non-survivors (n = 54)	OR (95% CI)	*p*-value
Age, ≥ 70 years	77 (38, 32–45)	13 (52, 31–71)	1.7 (0.8–4.0)	0.191	65 (38, 30–45)	25 (46, 33–60)	1.4 (0.8–2.6)	0.266
Male gender	130 (65, 58–71)	12 (48, 27–69)	0.5 (0.2–1.2)	0.108	113 (66, 59–73)	29 (54, 40–67)	0.6 (0.3–1.1)	0.113
BMI				0.181				0.118
Normal	121 (60, 53–67)	11 (44, 23–65)	1.0		104 (60, 53–68)	28 (52, 38–66)	1.0	
Malnutrition	19 (9, 5–14)	6 (24, 6–42)	3.5 (1.2–10.5)	0.027	14 (8, 4–12)	11 (20, 9–31)	2.9 (1.2–7.1)	0.019
Overweight	53 (26, 20–33)	7 (28, 9–47)	1.5 (0.5–4.0)	0.465	47 (27, 21–34)	13 (24, 12–36)	1.0 (0.5–2.2)	0.943
Obese	8 (4, 1–7)	1 (4, 0–12)	1.4 (0.2–12.0)	0.773	7 (4, 1–7)	2 (4, 0–9)	1.1 (0.2–5.4)	0.943
Comorbidities								
Malignancy	118 (59, 52–66)	12 (48, 27–69)	0.7 (0.3–1.5)	0.310	99 (58, 50–65)	31 (57, 44–71)	1.0 (0.5–1.8)	0.984
Cardiovascular disease	99 (49, 42–56)	14 (56, 35–77)	1.3 (0.6–3.0)	0.526	85 (49, 42–57)	28 (52, 38–66)	1.1 (0.6–2.0)	0.755
Pneumonia	58 (29, 23–35)	16 (64, 44–84)	4.4 (1.8–10.5)	***0.001***[a]	47 (27, 21–34)	27 (50, 36–64)	2.7 (1.4–5.0)	***0.002***[b]
Diabetes mellitus	58 (29, 23–35)	10 (40, 19–61)	1.6 (0.7–3.9)	0.255	46 (27, 20–33)	22 (41, 27–54)	1.9 (1.0–3.6)	0.052[b]
Impaired liver function	43 (21, 16–27)	9 (36, 16–56)	2.1 (0.9–5.0)	0.107	36 (21, 15–27)	16 (30, 17–42)	1.6 (0.8–3.2)	0.187
Cerebrovascular disease	37 (18, 13–24)	4 (16, 1–31)	0.8 (0.3–2.6)	0.768	31 (18, 12–24)	10 (19, 8–29)	1.0 (0.5–2.3)	0.934
Impaired renal function	22 (11, 7–15)	8 (32, 12–52)	3.8 (1.5–9.9)	***0.006***[a]	14 (8, 4–12)	16 (30, 17–42)	4.8 (2.1–10.6)	***0.000***[b]
Hemiplegia	25 (12, 8–17)	2 (8, 0–19)	0.6 (0.1–2.8)	0.523	22 (13, 8–18)	5 (9, 1–17)	0.7 (0.3–1.9)	0.487
Neutropenia	12 (6, 3–9)	2 (8, 0–19)	1.4 (0.3–6.5)	0.692	8 (5, 1–8)	6 (11, 2–20)	2.6 (0.9–7.8)	0.095[b]
CCI	3 (2–5)	4 (3–6)	1.2 (1.0–1.4)	***0.028***[a]	3 (2–5)	4 (3–6.25)	1.3 (1.1–1.4)	***<0.001***[b]
APACHE II score	7 (5–10)	14 (12–17)	1.2 (1.1–1.3)	***<0.001***[a]	6 (5–8.75)	13 (10–17)	1.3 (1.2–1.4)	***<0.001***[b]
ICU residence	53 (26, 20–33)	13 (52, 31–73)	3.0 (1.3–7.0)	***0.010***[a]	42 (24, 18–31)	24 (44, 31–58)	2.5 (1.3–4.7)	***0.005***[b]
Previous treatment								
Antibiotic exposure	185 (92, 88–96)	25 (100)		0.998	156 (91, 86–95)	54 (100)		0.998
Total parenteral nutrition	74 (37, 30–44)	10 (40, 19–61)	1.1 (0.5–2.7)	0.756	58 (34, 27–41)	26 (48, 34–62)	1.8 (1.0–3.4)	0.057[b]
Mechanical ventilation	77 (38, 32–45)	10 (40, 19–61)	1.1 (0.5–2.5)	0.870	66 (38, 31–46)	21 (39, 25–52)	1.0 (0.6–1.9)	0.946
Surgery	69 (34, 28–41)	5 (20, 3–37)	0.5 (0.2–1.3)	0.157	63 (37, 29–44)	11 (20, 9–31)	0.4 (0.2–0.9)	***0.029***[b]
Chemotherapeutic agent	27 (13, 9–18)	2 (8, 0–19)	0.6 (0.1–2.5)	0.449	24 (14, 9–19)	5 (9, 1–17)	0.6 (0.2–1.7)	0.372
Immunosuppressive agent	13 (6, 3–10)	5 (20, 3–37)	3.6 (1.2–11.2)	***0.026***[a]	9 (5, 2–9)	9 (17, 6–27)	3.6 (1.4–9.7)	***0.010***[b]
Renal replacement therapy	11 (5, 2–9)	4 (16, 1–31)	3.3 (1.0–11.3)	0.058[a]	8 (5, 1–8)	7 (13, 4–22)	3.1 (1.1–8.9)	***0.040***[b]
Invasive devices								
Central intravenous catheter	86 (43, 36–50)	16 (64, 44–84)	2.4 (1.0–5.6)	***0.049***[a]	71 (41, 34–49)	31 (57, 44–71)	1.9 (1.0–3.6)	***0.039***[b]
Dwell time of central intravenous catheter	15 (7, 26)	14 (7, 24)	1.0 (1.0–1.0)	0.919	15 (7.5, 26.75)	14 (6.5, 23.25)	1.0 (1.0–1.0)	0.465

Table 3 Univariate logistic regression analysis of risk factors for mortality *(Continued)*

Indwelling urinary catheter	90 (45, 38–52)	14 (56, 35–77)	1.6 (0.7–3.6)	0.291	76 (44, 37–52)	28 (52, 38–66)	1.4 (0.7–2.5)	0.325
Endotracheal intubation	76 (38, 31–45)	10 (40, 19–61)	1.1 (0.5–2.6)	0.832	65 (38, 30–45)	21 (39, 25–52)	1.1 (0.6–2.0)	0.885
Peripheral intravenous catheter	62 (31, 24–37)	7 (28, 9–47)	0.9 (0.4–2.2)	0.771	53 (31, 24–38)	16 (30, 17–42)	1.0 (0.5–1.8)	0.869
Tracheostomy tube	19 (9, 5–14)	1 (4, 0–12)	0.4 (0.1–3.1)	0.381	16 (9, 5–14)	4 (7, 0–15)	0.8 (0.3–2.4)	0.670
Enterococcal species				0.772				0.175
E. faecium	146 (73, 66–79)	21 (84, 69–99)	1.0		122 (71, 64–78)	45 (83, 73–94)	1.0	
E. faecalis	42 (20, 15–26)	4 (16, 1–31)	0.7 (0.2–2.0)	0.472	38 (22, 16–28)	8 (15, 5–25)	0.6 (0.3–1.3)	0.188
Others	13 (6, 3–10)	0 (0)	0.0	0.999	12 (7, 3–11)	1 (2, 0–6)	0.2 (0.0–1.8)	0.159
Source of BSIs								
Abdominal	83 (41, 34–48)	9 (36, 16–56)	0.8 (0.3–1.9)	0.612	72 (42, 34–49)	20 (37, 24–50)	0.8 (0.4–1.5)	0.529
Unknown	56 (28, 22–34)	9 (36, 16–56)	1.5 (0.6–3.5)	0.399	47 (27, 20–33)	18 (33, 20–46)	1.3 (0.7–2.6)	0.396
Central venous catheter	37 (18, 13–24)	4 (16, 1–31)	0.8 (0.3–2.6)	0.768	33 (19, 13–25)	8 (15, 5–25)	0.7 (0.3–1.7)	0.468
Genitourinary	12 (6, 3–9)	2 (8, 0–19)	1.4 (0.3–6.5)	0.692	9 (5, 2–9)	5 (9, 1–17)	1.9 (0.6–5.8)	0.281
Pneumonia	7 (3, 1–6)	1 (4, 0–12)	1.2 (0.1–9.8)	0.895	7 (4, 1–7)	1 (2, 2–6)	0.5 (0.1–3.7)	0.453
Polymicrobial infection	18 (9, 5–13)	3 (12, 0–26)	1.4 (0.4–5.1)	0.622	14 (8, 4–12)	7 (13, 4–22)	1.7 (0.6–4.4)	0.291
Vancomycin-resistant	7 (3, 1–6)	0 (0)	0.0	0.999	5 (3, 0–5)	2 (4, 0–9)	1.3 (0.2–6.8)	0.769
Appropriate emperical antimicrobial treatment	200 (100, 99–100)	13 (52, 31–73)	0.0 (0.0–0.1)	***<0.001***[a]	172 (100)	41 (76, 64–88)	0.2 (0.1–0.5)	***<0.001***[b]

Data are presented as n (%,95% CI) or median (IQR)
Significant variables are appeared in bold and italics text
[a]Variables entered into multivariable logistic regression model of risks factors for 7-day mortality
[b]Variables entered into multivariable logistic regression model of risks factors for 30-day mortality

Table 4 Multivariate logistic regression models of risk factors for mortality

Variable	7-day mortality		30-day mortality	
	OR (95% CI)	*p*-value	OR (95% CI)	*p*-value
Diabetes mellitus	-	-	2.1 (0.9–5.4)	0.103
Impaired renal function	2.1 (0.6–6.9)	0.220	3.3 (1.1–9.8)	***0.030***[b]
CCI	1.2 (0.9–1.5)	0.080	1.3 (1.1–1.6)	***0.003***[b]
APACHE II score	1.2 (1.1–1.3)	***<0.001***[a]	1.3 (1.2–1.4)	***<0.001***[b]
Prior use of immunosuppressive agents	4.6 (1.1–19.2)	***0.036***[a]	7.3 (1.8–29.0)	***0.005***[b]
Appropriate empirical antimicrobial therapy	0.2 (0.0–0.7)	***0.010***[a]	0.2 (0.1–0.4)	***<0.001***[b]

Significant variables are appeared in bold and italics text
[a]Variables entered the final multivariable logistic regression model of risks factors for 7-day mortality
[b]Variables entered the final multivariable logistic regression model of risks factors for 30-day mortality

found that pneumonia was also a major comorbidity of nosocomial enterococcal BSIs at our hospital.

E. faecalis was reported to be the most common pathogen for nosocomial enterococcal BSIs in most investigations, and the ratio of *E. faecium* was no more than 50% [1, 11, 20, 28]. However, a constant increase in *E. faecium* BSI rates was observed [11, 29], and the incidence of *E. faecium* BSIs exceeded *E. faecalis* BSI in 2009 in a 14-year study conducted at a Swiss tertiary hospital [29]. At our hospital, the incidence of nosocomial *E. faecium* BSIs was significantly higher than that of *E. faecalis* BSIs (2.9/10,000 vs 0.8/10,000). The total vancomycin resistance rate of all isolates was 3%, and 4% for *E. faecium* in our study. All of the vancomycin-resistant isolates were *E. faecium*. This vancomycin resistance rate is higher than those in the Danish study (1.9%) [11], but lower than many studies in other countries. The SCOPE project carried out between 1995 and 1996 at 49 US hospitals reported the VRE rate was between 9.5% to 20.6% in nosocomial enterococcal BSIs from different hospitals [30]. The 1997 SENTRY program reported that 14.1% of enterococcal BSIs were VRE in the United States [1]. A prospective nationwide surveillance study at Brazilian hospitals, which published in 2011, showed that the VRE rate was as high as 25% [9]. Therefore, the species distribution and antimicrobial resistance varies geographically.

Abdominal infections, central venous catheters, and unknown sources were the most common foci of enterococcal BSIs in the present study, is similar to the prior studies [28]. However, no infective endocarditis was observed in our study. There may be 2 reasons to explain this difference. First, the study population was different, as we were focused on nosocomial infection. Another reason was that echocardiography was not a routine examination for patients with BSIs in our hospital, so this could lead to missed diagnosis.

Our data showed that patients with nosocomial *E. faecalis* BSIs were more likely to get appropriate empirical treatment than those with *E. faecium* BSIs. This may be explained by the low resistance rate of *E. faecalis* to many antimicrobial agents, such as ampicillin (9%), gentamicin (33%), and ciprofloxacin (39%).

In the present study, the 30-day mortality of nosocomial enterococcal BSIs was 24%, and the early mortality (7-day) accounted for half. This is lower than many prior reports [5, 8, 9, 12, 31], but similar to a study focusing on vancomycin-susceptible enterococcal BSIs [22]. This may be due to selection bias of the study population, or may be a reflection of medical progress. Mortality was higher in patients with higher CCI and APACHE II scores, prior use of immunosuppressive agents, and complicated with impaired renal function. In other reports, the risk factors for mortality of patients with enterococcal BSIs may also include advanced age, pulmonary infection, malignancy, species, polymicrobial infection, ampicillin resistance, high-level gentamicin resistance, and vancomycin resistance [11, 15, 22]. Although controversial, we confirm that the severity of underlying diseases is the most important factor, especially for early morbidity.

The present study has several limitations that should be taken into consideration. First, our study was a retrospective study, the collection of clinical data depended on medical records rather than interviews and clinical examinations at the onset of infection by unified training doctors of our research group. Second, as a single-centre study, it could lead to an inevitable selection bias, and the multivariate logistic analysis might be affected by the small sample size. Third, not all isolates did all the same antimicrobial agent sensitivity test, so we could not incorporate all the antimicrobial agents resistance in predicting mortality risk factors in order to avoid selection bias.

Conclusions

Enterococci were major pathogens for nosocomial BSIs and were associated with high mortality,especially for patients combined with chronic diseases. Increased CCI and APACHE II scores, prior use of immunosuppressive agent and complicated with impaired renal function were risk factors for morality. *E. faecium* were more common than *E. faecalis* at our hospital. For patients with *E. faecium* BSIs who conditions were complicated with serious underlying diseases, vancomycin is the best choice; for patients with *E. faecalis* BSIs, penicillins, aminoglycosides, and fluoroquinolones could also be considered besides vancomycin.

Abbreviations

APACHE II: Acute Physiology and Chronic Health Evaluation II; BMI: Body mass index; BSIs: Bloodstream infections; CCI: Charlson comorbidity index; CI: Confidence interval; IQRs: Interquartile ranges; OR: Odds ratio; PLAGH: Chinese People's Liberation Army General Hospital; RT-NISS: Real-time nosocomial infection surveillance system; VRE: Vancomycin-resistant enterococci

Acknowledgments

We thank all the colleagues in the Infection Management and Disease Control Department for making this study possible.

Funding

This study was funded by grants from the Key Projects in the Military Program during the Twelfth Five-year Plan Period (BWS11J057). The grant agency didn't involve in the design of the study, collection, analysis and interpretation of data, and writing or revising the manuscript.

Authors' contributions

YZ and MD conceived this study, collected clinical data, interpreted the results, wrote and revised the manuscript. YC participated in collecting data and data statistics. LC and QZ participated in the study design and revised the manuscript. All authors read and approved the final manuscript.

Consent for publication

Not applicable.

Competing interests

None of authors declare conflicts of interest relevant to this article.

Author details

[1]Department of Respiratory Medicine, Chinese PLA General Hospital, Fuxing Road No. 28, Beijing 100853, China. [2]Department of Respiratory Medicine, Affiliated Hospital of Chengde Medical University, Nanyingzi Street No. 36, Chengde, Hebei Province 067000, China. [3]Department of Infection Management and Disease Control, Chinese PLA General Hospital, Beijing 100853, China. [4]Department of Respiratory Medicine, The General Hospital of the PLA Rocket Force, Xinjiekou Street No. 16, Beijing 100088, China.

References

1. Pfaller MA, Jones RN, Doern GV, Sader HS, Kugler KC, Beach ML. Survey of blood stream infections attributable to gram-positive cocci: frequency of occurrence and antimicrobial susceptibility of isolates collected in 1997 in the United States, Canada, and Latin America from the SENTRY antimicrobial surveillance program. SENTRY participants group. Diagn Microbiol Infect Dis. 1999;33(4):283–97.
2. Wisplinghoff H, Bischoff T, Tallent SM, Seifert H, Wenzel RP, Edmond MB. Nosocomial bloodstream infections in US hospitals: analysis of 24,179 cases from a prospective nationwide surveillance study. Clin Infect Dis. 2004;39(3): 309–17.
3. Huang YC, Xie Y, Chen ZX, Liu B, Fei Y, Du Y, Shan B, Kang M. Bloodstream infections in southwestern China: 2012 Whire union report on bacterial susceptibility to antibiotics. Sichuan da xue xue bao Yi xue ban. 2015;46(1): 75–81.
4. Guanghui ZD LI, Fu WANG, Zhidong HU, Quan LI, Ziyong SUN. The distribution and antibiotic resistance of clinical isolates from blood culture in 2012 CHINET surveillance program in China. Chin J Chemother. 2014; 14(6):474–81.
5. Nagao M. A multicentre analysis of epidemiology of the nosocomial bloodstream infections in Japanese university hospitals. Clin Microbiol Infect. 2013;19(9):852–8.
6. Deen J, von Seidlein L, Andersen F, Elle N, White NJ, Lubell Y. Community-acquired bacterial bloodstream infections in developing countries in south and southeast Asia: a systematic review. Lancet Infect Dis. 2012;12(6):480–7.
7. DiazGranados CA, Zimmer SM, Klein M, Jernigan JA. Comparison of mortality associated with vancomycin-resistant and vancomycin-susceptible enterococcal bloodstream infections: a meta-analysis. Clin Infect Dis. 2005; 41(3):327–33.
8. Caballero-Granado FJ, Becerril B, Cuberos L, Bernabeu M, Cisneros JM, Pachon J. Attributable mortality rate and duration of hospital stay associated with enterococcal bacteremia. Clin Infect Dis. 2001;32(4):587–94.
9. Marra AR, Camargo LF, Pignatari AC, Sukiennik T, Behar PR, Medeiros EA, Ribeiro J, Girao E, Correa L, Guerra C, Brites C, Pereira CA, Carneiro I, Reis M, de Souza MA, Tranchesi R, Barata CU, Edmond MB. Nosocomial bloodstream infections in Brazilian hospitals: analysis of 2,563 cases from a prospective nationwide surveillance study. J Clin Microbiol. 2011;49(5):1866–71.
10. Linden PK, Pasculle AW, Manez R, Kramer DJ, Fung JJ, Pinna AD, Kusne S. Differences in outcomes for patients with bacteremia due to vancomycin-resistant Enterococcus faecium or vancomycin-susceptible E. Faecium. Clin Infect Dis. 1996;22(4):663–70.
11. Pinholt M, Ostergaard C, Arpi M, Bruun NE, Schonheyder HC, Gradel KO, Sogaard M, Knudsen JD. Incidence, clinical characteristics and 30-day mortality of enterococcal bacteraemia in Denmark 2006-2009: a population-based cohort study. Clin Microbiol Infect. 2014;20(2):145–51.
12. Noskin GA, Peterson LR, Warren JR (1995) Enterococcus faecium and Enterococcus faecalis bacteremia: acquisition and outcome. Clin Infect Dis 1995;20(2):296-301.
13. Peel T, Cheng AC, Spelman T, Huysmans M, Spelman D. Differing risk factors for vancomycin-resistant and vancomycin-sensitive enterococcal bacteraemia. Clin Microbiol Infect. 2012;18(4):388–94.
14. Tavadze M, Rybicki L, Mossad S, Avery R, Yurch M, Pohlman B, Duong H, Dean R, Hill B, Andresen S, Hanna R, Majhail N, Copelan E, Bolwell B, Kalaycio M, Sobecks R. Risk factors for vancomycin-resistant enterococcus bacteremia and its influence on survival after allogeneic hematopoietic cell transplantation. Bone Marrow Transplant. 2014;49(10):1310–6.
15. Billington EO, Phang SH, Gregson DB, Pitout JD, Ross T, Church DL, Laupland KB, Parkins MD. Incidence, risk factors, and outcomes for Enterococcus spp. blood stream infections: a population-based study. Int J Infect Dis. 2014;26:76–82.
16. Berenger BM, Doucette K, Smith SW. Epidemiology and risk factors for nosocomial bloodstream infections in solid organ transplants over a 10-year period. Transpl Infect Dis. 2016;18(2):183–90.
17. Bush LM, Calmon J, Cherney CL, Wendeler M, Pitsakis P, Poupard J, Levison ME, Johnson CC. High-level penicillin resistance among isolates of enterococci. Implications for treatment of enterococcal infections. Ann Intern Med. 1989;110(7):515–20.
18. Patterson JE, Zervos MJ. High-level gentamicin resistance in Enterococcus: microbiology, genetic basis, and epidemiology. Rev Infect Dis. 1990;12(4): 644–52.
19. Barber KE, King ST, Stover KR, Pogue JM. Therapeutic options for vancomycin-resistant enterococcal bacteremia. Expert Rev Anti-Infect Ther. 2015;13(3):363–77.
20. Bhavnani SM, Drake JA, Forrest A, Deinhart JA, Jones RN, Biedenbach DJ, Ballow CH. A nationwide, multicenter, case-control study comparing risk factors, treatment, and outcome for vancomycin-resistant and -susceptible enterococcal bacteremia. Diagn Microbiol Infect Dis. 2000;36(3):145–58.

21. Conde-Estevez D, Grau S, Albanell J, Terradas R, Salvado M, Knobel H. Clinical characteristics and outcomes of patients with vancomycin-susceptible Enterococcus faecalis and Enterococcus faecium bacteraemia in cancer patients. Eur J Clin Microbiol Infect Dis. 2011;30(1):103–8.
22. McBride SJ, Upton A, Roberts SA. Clinical characteristics and outcomes of patients with vancomycin-susceptible Enterococcus faecalis and Enterococcus faecium bacteraemia–a five-year retrospective review. Eur J Clin Microbiol Infect Dis. 2010;29(1):107–14.
23. Du M, Xing Y, Suo J, Liu B, Jia N, Huo R, Chen C, Liu Y. Real-time automatic hospital-wide surveillance of nosocomial infections and outbreaks in a large Chinese tertiary hospital. BMC Med Inform Decis Mak. 2014;14:9.
24. Garner JS, Jarvis WR, Emori TG, Horan TC, Hughes JM. CDC definitions for nosocomial infections. Am J Infect Control. 1988;16:128–40.
25. Satlin MJ, Soave R, Racanelli AC, Shore TB, van Besien K, Jenkins SG, Walsh TJ. The emergence of vancomycin-resistant enterococcal bacteremia in hematopoietic stem cell transplant recipients. Leuk Lymphoma. 2014;55(12): 2858–65.
26. Zheng JX, Li H, Pu ZY, Wang HY, Deng XB, Liu XJ, Deng QW, Yu ZJ. Bloodstream infections caused by Enterococcus spp: A10-year retrospective analysis at a tertiary hospital in China. J Huazhong Univ Sci Technolog Med Sci. 2017;37(2):257–63.
27. Vigani AG, Oliveira AM, Bratfich OJ, Stucchi RS, Moretti ML. Clinical, epidemiological, and microbiological characteristics of bacteremia caused by high-level gentamicin-resistant Enterococcus faecalis. Braz J Med Biol Res. 2008;41(10):890–5.
28. Hamada Y, Magarifuchi H, Oho M, Kusaba K, Nagasawa Z, Fukuoka M, Yamakuchi H, Urakami T, Aoki Y. Clinical features of enterococcal bacteremia due to ampicillin-susceptible and ampicillin-resistant enterococci: an eight-year retrospective comparison study. J Infect Chemother. 2015;21(7):527–30.
29. Weisser M, Capaul S, Dangel M, Elzi L, Kuenzli E, Frei R, Widmer A. Additive effect of Enterococcus faecium on Enterococcal bloodstream infections: a 14-year study in a Swiss tertiary hospital. Infect Control Hosp Epidemiol. 2013;34(10):1109–12.
30. Jones RN, Marshall SA, Pfaller MA, Wilke WW, Hollis RJ, Erwin ME, Edmond MB, Wenzel RP. Nosocomial enterococcal blood stream infections in the SCOPE program: antimicrobial resistance, species occurrence, molecular testing results, and laboratory testing accuracy. SCOPE hospital study group. Diagn Microbiol Infect Dis. 1997;29(2):95–102.
31. Landry SL, Kaiser DL, Wenzel RP. Hospital stay and mortality attributed to nosocomial enterococcal bacteremia: a controlled study. Am J Infect Control. 1989;17(6):323–9.

5

Outbreak of *Fusarium oxysporum* infections in children with cancer: an experience with 7 episodes of catheter-related fungemia

Fabianne Carlesse[1,2], Anna-Paula C. Amaral[2], Sarah S. Gonçalves[3], Hemilio Xafranski[3], Maria-Lucia M. Lee[1], Victor Zecchin[1], Antonio S. Petrilli[1], Abdullah M. Al-Hatmi[4,5], Ferry Hagen[6], Jacques F. Meis[5,6] and Arnaldo L. Colombo[3*]

Abstract

Background: *Fusarium* species are widely spread in nature as plant pathogens but are also able to cause opportunistic fungal infections in humans. We report a cluster of *Fusarium oxysporum* bloodstream infections in a single pediatric cancer center.

Methods: All clinical and epidemiological data related to an outbreak involving seven cases of fungemia by *Fusarium oxysporum* during October 2013 and February 2014 were analysed. All cultured isolates (n = 14) were identified to species level by sequencing of the *TEF1* and *RPB2* genes. Genotyping of the outbreak isolates was performed by amplified fragment length polymorphism fingerprinting.

Results: In a 5-month period 7 febrile pediatric cancer patients were diagnosed with catheter-related *Fusarium oxysporum* bloodstream infections. In a time span of 11 years, only 6 other infections due to *Fusarium* were documented and all were caused by a different species, *Fusarium solani.* None of the pediatric cancer patients had neutropenia at the time of diagnosis and all became febrile within two days after catheter manipulation in a specially designed room. Extensive environmental sampling in this room and the hospital did not gave a clue to the source. The outbreak was terminated after implementation of a multidisciplinary central line insertion care bundle. All *Fusarium* strains from blood and catheter tips were genetically related by amplified fragment length polymorphism fingerprinting. All patients survived the infection after prompt catheter removal and antifungal therapy.

Conclusion: A cluster with, genotypical identical, *Fusarium oxysporum* strains infecting 7 children with cancer, was most probably catheter-related. The environmental source was not discovered but strict infection control measures and catheter care terminated the outbreak.

Keywords: Fusariosis, *Fusarium* sp., *Fusarium oxysporum*, Catheter-related *Fusarium* fungemia, Pediatric invasive fungal infections

* Correspondence: arnaldolcolombo@gmail.com
[3]Division of Infectious Diseases, Escola Paulista de Medicina, Federal University of Sao Paulo (UNIFESP), Rua Pedro de Toledo, 669 e 5° -andar, Sao Paulo CEP 04039-032, Brazil
Full list of author information is available at the end of the article

Background

Due to prolonged survival of patients with cancer, invasive fungal diseases (IFD) emerged as important cause of morbidity and mortality. In pediatric cancer patients, *Candida* species remain as the most important cause of IFD followed by invasive infections by *Aspergillus* spp. and other moulds [1–3].

Epidemiology of fungal infections varies markedly according to the geographic region. In Brazil, *Fusarium* spp. infections have emerged as major pathogens of systemic infections among cancer patients [4]. *Fusarium* species are widely spread in nature as plant pathogens and are also able to cause superficial, locally invasive and disseminated infections in humans [5]. Infection occurs mainly through airborne transmission, skin breakdown due to trauma, burns or insertion of vascular catheters [6, 7]. The clinical presentation relies mostly on the hosts' immune status, with disseminated infections been reported especially in severe immunocompromised individuals leading to high mortality rates [6, 8].

The lack of data concerning the epidemiology and clinical aspects of invasive infections by *Fusarium* spp. in pediatric patients is notable. Here we report a cluster of *Fusarium oxysporum* bloodstream infections from seven pediatric cancer patients documented in a single Brazilian pediatric cancer center.

Methods

We retrospectively studied all clinical and epidemiological data related to an outbreak enrolling seven cases of fungemia by *Fusarium oxysporum* occurring between October 2013 and February 2014 in the Pediatric Oncology Institute (IOP), located in Sao Paulo, Brazil. IOP is a tertiary care hospital specialized in pediatric oncology which admits 300 new cases per year. The outbreak was documented in patients who had been treated with chemotherapy at the same room used for cancer ambulatory chemotherapy. All long-term intravascular catheters are implanted in the surgery room and cared for by a group of trained nurses.

Clinical and epidemiological data were collected by a single investigator who reviewed all electronic medical records in order to complete a clinical form including information related to gender, age, underlying diseases, presence of neutropenia, exposition to invasive medical procedures and immunosuppressive drugs, imaging, culture results, treatment and clinical outcome.

During the outbreak, all catheters were removed and cultured in accordance with procedures standardized in our division based on cultures of catheter tips and material inside the reservoir. A cut-off of $\geq 10^3$ CFU/plate was used to differentiate significant from insignificant colonization as suggested by Brun–Buisson et al. [9, 10]. All patients were screened for putative deep-seated infection by sinus and chest CT as well as echocardiography and eye fundoscopy. After the diagnosis of fusariosis, at least two serum samples were collected from each patient to check for galactomannan levels and patients were followed for another 90 days for clinical signs and symptoms.

Laboratory procedures

Isolates

All *Fusarium* spp. cultured from blood and catheter samples (swab, flush and tip) were initially identified by morphological characteristics [11] and further identified to species level by sequencing *TEF1* and *RPB2* genes [12].

Besides clinical strains, we cultured environmental samples including air-filters, tap water samples, swab of room surfaces, and different intravenously administered drugs [13, 14]. We finally also evaluated all health care workers for the presence of onychomycosis or other superficial fungal infections.

Molecular identification of *Fusarium* isolates

Genomic DNA of all *Fusarium* isolates was extracted with the PrepMan Ultra Sample Preparation Reagent kit (Applied Biosystems, Palo Alto, CA, USA) according to the manufacturer's instructions. PCRs were performed for the amplification of the largest subunit of RNA polymerase (*RPB2*) and the translation elongation factor-1α (*TEF1α*) following the methods published by Salah et al. [15]. The primer pairs for *TEF1α* were EF1 & EF2 [16] and for *RPB2* were RPB2-7cR & RPB2 -5F [17]. PCR products were sequenced with the same primers used for amplification. The ABI Prism® Big DyeTM Terminator v. 3.0 Ready Reaction Cycle Sequencing Kit (Applied Biosystems) was used for sequencing PCR according to the manufacturer's instructions. The samples were run on an ABI 3730XL automatic sequencer (Applied Biosystems). A BLAST search of *TEF1* and *RPB2* sequences against the database FUSARIUM-ID (http://isolate.fusariumdb.orgl/), the *Fusarium* database (http://www.cbs.knaw.nl/*fusarium*) and GenBank databases (www.ncbi.nlm.nih.gov) were used as an initial step to identify isolates to species and/or species complex. The *TEF1* and *RPB2* nucleotide sequences of all isolates were deposited in GenBank.

Amplified fragment length polymorphism

Amplified fragment length polymorphism (AFLP) fingerprinting was performed as described recently [18]. Briefly, ~50 ng of genomic DNA was digested by using the HpyCH4IV and MseI restriction enzymes (New England Biolabs, Ipswich, MA, U.S.A.) and in the same reaction specific adaptors were ligated to each of the two sticky ends of the DNA fragments. The samples were after a 1 h incubation at room temperature diluted with 10 mM Tris-HCl, 1.0 µl of this diluted product was used as input for the PCR that contains the selective primers HpyCH4IV-C (5′-Flu-

GTAGACTGCGTACCCGTAC-3′) and MseI-TGAG (5′-GATGAGTCCTGACTAATGAG). After the PCR was performed, the amplicons were 20× diluted using ddH_2O and 1.0 μl of it was mixed with 8.9 μl ddH_2O and 0.1 μl LIZ600 internal size marker (Promega, Leiden, The Netherlands) followed by a heating step for 1 min at 100 °C. Fragment analysis was performed on an ABI3500xL Genetic Analyzer (Applied Biosystems, Foster City, CA, U.S.A.) according to the manufacturer's instructions. Subsequently, the raw data was imported into Bionumerics v7.5 (Applied Maths, Sint Martems-Latum, Belgium), after processing the data a dendrogram was generated by using the UPGMA algorithm.

Results

From October 2013 to February 2014 we were caught by surprise with the occurrence of seven episodes of microbiologic documented catheter-related *F. oxysporum* bloodstream infections (CR-BSI) in our division. This finding led us to believe that we were facing an outbreak because only six cases of invasive fusariosis had been diagnosed in our hospital in the 11 years previously, all caused by *Fusarium solani* species complex strains.

Demographic and clinical data of all seven patients are depictured in Table 1. Ages ranged from 0 to 8 years (3 males), 6 out 7 were treated with chemotherapy for solid tumors, and one for acute lymphoid leukemia (ALL). Two patients (solid tumors) had underwent an autologous stem cell transplantation more than 14 days before and none of the patients received corticosteroids or other immunosuppressive agents. Only one patient had a neutrophil count below 500 cells/mm^3 at the moment of the infection. Fever was the only trigger to collect blood cultures and vascular catheters were removed promptly at the time fungemia was identified. The six intravascular devices removed included 5 totally surgically implanted (Porth-a-Cath) catheters and one peripherally inserted catheter (PICC). All fungemic episodes were documented following 2 days after the last catheter puncture by the nurse. No single patient had any additional skin breakdown or onychomycosis that could explain the portal of entrance for *Fusarium* spp. All catheter tips, reservoir and blood cultures collected through the CVC of the 7 patients yielded *Fusarium oxysporum*. Although they had no signs or symptoms of any organ involvement, further laboratorial investigation was conducted to exclude fungal invasion of target organs. All children had a chest computer tomography (CT), sinus magnetic resonance image, eye fundoscopy and echocardiography done without any evidence of a deep-seated fungal infection. All serum samples were galactomannan negative. Catheters were promptly removed after blood cultures became positive and all patients had good clinical response to antifungal therapy. Oral voriconazole was the therapy of choice for six patients (7 mg/kg/dose) and adequate serum levels (≥1 mg/L) were measured in all patients. One child was treated with liposomal amphotericin B (5 mg/kg/day) due to age restrictions (9 months) for using voriconazole.

It is important to note that during the whole period this cluster occurred, the hospital building was being enlarged, counting with an extensive construction area.

All environmental samples and different intravenous preparations in search for sources of *Fusarium* spp. were negative. Healthcare workers who had previous contact with the patients were checked for the presence of any cutaneous or nail lesions suggestive of fungal infections but nothing was found.

Molecular identification of *Fusarium* isolates

A total of 16 *Fusarium* spp. clinical isolates were identified to genus level by colony and microscopic characteristics of the isolates. Upon molecular identification, based on *TEF1* and *RPB2* partial genes analysis, all *Fusarium* isolates were found to be members of the *F. oxysporum* species complex. All environmental samples were culture negative.

A phylogenetic tree (Additional file 1: Figure S1) was constructed with a total of 20 sequences for two genes, with three strains from the *Fusarium solani* species complex (FSSC) i.e. *F. falciforme* (NRRL32542), *F. keratoplasticum* (FRC-S2477) and *F. petroliphilum* (NRRL32856) as outgroup. The generated tree was separated into two clades. Clade 1 included all members of the *F. oxysporum* species complex (FOSC) and clade 2 represented the *F. solani* species complex (FSSC), the final result of the identification process was that 16 isolates were confirmed as members of FOSC.

Typing results by amplified fragment length polymorphism

All *Fusarium* strains obtained from blood and catheter tips were considered genetically related by AFLP fingerprinting, suggesting that all isolates had a common source. Cluster analysis revealed the presence of two clusters, one with a 95% similarity that includes isolates BRAZIL 1127 (Patient 2 catheter tip culture), 1129 (Patient 2 reservoir culture), 1131 (Patient 2 blood culture) and 1134 (Patient 3 catheter tip culture), and a second one with all other Brazilian isolates that exhibited similarity of 97% (Fig. 1). The reference *F. oxysporum* isolates CBS192.31 and CBS180.29, had a similarity of 90% and 80%, respectively, to the Brazilian isolates.

Discussion

In Brazil, invasive fusariosis is the most common cause of systemic mould infections in hematologic cancer patients [4] and has been associated with a poor prognosis [19]. There is a gap in knowledge with regard to the epidemiology of fusariosis in pediatric patients. Most papers

Table 1 Demographics and clinical characteristics of 7 patients with catheter-related fungemia due to *Fusarium oxysporum*

Case	Underlying diseases	HSCT	Age (years)	Gender	Neutropenia	CVC	GMI	Time interval between CVC placement and infection	Chest CT	ECHO	Fundoscopic exam	Therapy	Duration (days)	Outcome
1	Solid tumor	Auto	3	Male	Yes	Port-a-cath	Negative	665 days	Normal	Normal	Normal	Voriconazole	21	Alive
2	Solid tumor	No	2	Female	No	Port a cath	Negative	89 days	Normal	Normal	Normal	Voriconazole	21	Alive
3	Solid tumor	No	1	Male	No	Port a cath	Negative	114 days	Normal	Normal	Normal	Voriconazole	21	Alive
4	Solid tumor	No	9 months	Female	No	Port a cath	Negative	125 days	Normal	Normal	Normal	L-Ampho B	16	Alive
5	Solid tumor	Auto	1	Female	No	Port a cath	Negative	112 days	Normal	Normal	Normal	Voriconazole	21	Alive
6	Solid tumor	No	2	Female	No	Port a cath	Negative	282 days	Normal	Normal	Normal	Voriconazole	21	Alive
7	ALL in remission	No	8	Male	No	PICC	Negative	158 days	Normal	Normal	Normal	Voriconazole	14	Alive

ALL acute lymphoblastic leukemia, *Auto* Autologous, *CVC* central venous catheter, *PICC* peripherally inserted central catheter, *GMI* galactomannan index, *ECHO* echocardiography, *Chest CT* chest computed tomography, *L-Ampho B* liposomal amphotericin B

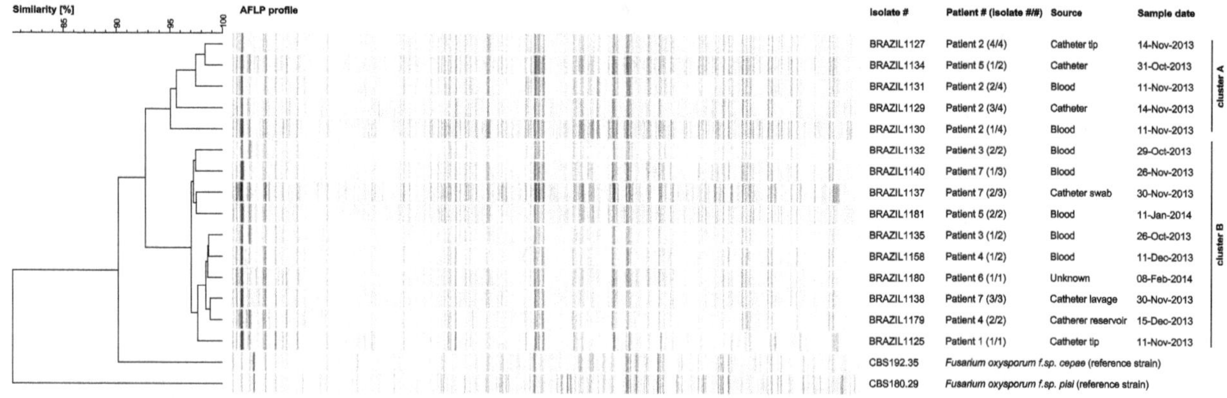

Fig. 1 AFLP fingerprint analysis was performed on 16 clinical *Fusarium oxysporum* species complex isolates. The dendrogram was generated by using the Pearson correlation similarity coefficient followed by single linkage cluster analysis

represent single case reports, with the exception of two outbreaks that were also documented in Brazilian medical centers and a review paper [20–22]. Information provided by the largest pediatric series of fusariosis published in the medical literature shows that the most common underlying condition was leukemia. Lung, blood and skin were the most commonly reported sites of infection and mortality rates are usually higher than 50% [22].

There is a consensus in the literature that the respiratory tract is the main portal of entry for this fungal infection, followed by skin breakdown due trauma and/or burns [23–31]. Despite some reports suggesting that fusariosis may also be acquired by contamination of a central venous catheter, the real prevalence and the natural history of intravascular catheter related fusariosis remains unclear [32–36].

Velasco and colleagues reported four immunocompromised children between 4 and 12 years, having neuroblastoma (n = 1) or hematologic malignancies (n = 3) who developed catheter-related *Fusarium* spp. infections without neutropenia. Fungemia was followed by skin lesions in only one patient and there was no clinical or radiological evidence of respiratory tract involvement. All patients survived after cathether removal and treatment with conventional amphotericin B [21].

Recently, Colombo et al. [35] described a case of a 13-year-old boy in Italy diagnosed with ALL readmitted 1 month after the start of chemotherapy due to intermittent fever of unknown origin, without any clinical or radiological evidence of invasive infection. Patient had his Broviac central venous catheter removed and blood cultures taken from the CVC were positive only for *F. solani* species complex. In addition, scanning electron microscopy of the catheter tip demonstrated the formation of a large mycelium in the catheter lumen that yielded a positive culture of *F. solani* complex. This finding represents a strong support for the hypothesis that fungemia was related to fungal colonization of the catheter. Fungemia resolved without any evidence of deep-seated infection after prompt CVC removal and therapy with voriconazole.

We report an outbreak of *F. oxysporum* infection enrolling 6 children with solid cancers and one with ALL in complete remission without persistent neutropenia. Fever was the only clinical manifestation of infection and the trigger to collect blood cultures in all episodes. Patients were carefully examined, and no single event of fungal deep tissue infection was documented. Finally, in the absence of respiratory infection as well as any type of skin breakdown that could be the port of entry, we are convinced that the intravascular catheter was the source of all episodes of *F. oxysporum*. Indeed, by typing all isolates with AFLP we confirmed our hypothesis that the 7 cases of *F oxysporum* were related, and all cultures of catheter tips and reservoirs had similar or identical genotypes to isolates obtained from blood cultures. Because all environmental investigations were negative for the presence of *Fusarium* spp., we were not able to identify the presumed common source of all infections. On the other hand, we may not exclude the possibility that medical devices were colonized by *Fusarium* during inappropriate management of intravascular catheters by health care workers or by the contamination of intravascular fluids.

Disseminated fusariosis is a difficult to treat fungal infection with an overall mortality ranging between 50% and 80% mostly due to uncontrolled hematologic malignant disease, prolonged neutropenia and the exposition to corticosteroids [19, 37]. Indeed, during a recent outbreak among children with cancer, fungemia and deep-seated infections due to *Fusarium* the mortality rate was 50% [20].

In contrast, in the present series, and as documented by previous reports of catheter related fusariosis [21, 33], we observed a complete clinical recovery of all patients after removal of the intravascular catheter and initiation of appropriate antifungal therapy. The good outcome documented with our patients may be explained also because there was no neutropenia or exposition to corticosteroids at the time they developed fusariosis.

F. oxysporum was the etiologic agent responsible for all fungemias documented in the present outbreak. This finding is in accordance with previous reports where seven out ten cases of *Fusarium* spp. fungemias and intravascular catheter related infections were due non-*solani Fusarium* species [21, 23, 33–36, 38].

Measures taken to control the outbreak were lowering the level of humidity in the CVC storage room and the implementation of a multidisciplinary quality-improvement intervention, including a central line insertion care bundle, consisting of hand hygiene, maximal sterile barrier use upon insertion and use of chlorhexidine skin disinfection. After the introduction of these actions, no further cases were noted.

In conclusion, *Fusarium* fungemia may be acquired by intravascular catheter colonization without any further deep-seated infections. In case of *Fusarium* outbreaks, especially involving non-*F. solani* species, clinicians should be aware that contamination of central venous catheter may be the potential source of infection.

Conclusions

We described 7 episodes of *Fusarium oxysporum* fungemia where we presented strong clinical and laboratorial documentation supporting the hypothesis that the portal of entry for all cases of fusariosis was the intravascular central catheter. In case of *Fusarium* outbreaks, especially involving non-*F. solani* species, clinicians should be aware that contamination of central venous catheter may be a potential source. Finally, we added information suggesting that the clinical outcome of catheter related fungemia due to *Fusarium* may be favorable in patients without neutropenia who were submitted to prompt CVC removal and early initiation of antifungal therapy.

Abbreviations

AFLP: Amplified fragment length polymorphism; ALL: Acute lymphoid leukemia; CFU: Colony forming unit; CR-BSI: Catheter-related blood stream infections; CT: Computer tomography; CVC: Central venous catheter; FOSC: Fusarium solani species complex; FSSC: Fusarium solani species complex; IFD: Invasive fungal diseases; PICC: Peripherally inserted central catheter

Acknowledgements

The authors wish to thank the staff of the Laboratório Especial de Micologia-UNIFESP as well as the clinical teams of the Oncology Pediatric Institute (IOP-GRAACC) involved for all their commitment in managing the outbreak.

Funding

No funding.

Authors' contributions

FC and ALC performed epidemiological data analysis and initial draft preparation. FC, APCA, MLML, VZ, and ASP took care of patients and were involved in outbreak control. SSG, HX, FH and AMA, performed molecular studies. JFM and ALC provided expert advice and methodology. FC, JFM, and ALC finalized the draft. All authors read and approved the final manuscript.

Consent for publication

Not applicable.

Competing interests

FC received educational grants from Pfizer, United Medical and Astellas. ALC received educational grants from Pfizer, Gilead, United Medical and Astellas, and funding for research from Pfizer and Astellas. JFM received grants from Astellas, Basilea and Merck. He has been a consultant to Astellas, Basilea and Merck and received speaker's fees from Merck, United Medical and Gilead. All other authors no conflict of interest.

Author details

[1]Oncology Pediatric Institute (IOP-GRAACC), Escola Paulista de Medicina, Federal University of Sao Paulo (UNIFESP), Sao Paulo, Brazil. [2]Department of Pediatrics, Escola Paulista de Medicina, Federal University of Sao Paulo (UNIFESP), Sao Paulo, Brazil. [3]Division of Infectious Diseases, Escola Paulista de Medicina, Federal University of Sao Paulo (UNIFESP), Rua Pedro de Toledo, 669 e 5° -andar, Sao Paulo CEP 04039-032, Brazil. [4]Westerdijk Fungal Biodiversity Centre, Utrecht, The Netherlands. [5]Center of Expertise in Mycology Radboudumc/CWZ, Nijmegen, The Netherlands. [6]Department of Medical Microbiology and Infectious Diseases, Canisius Wilhelmina Hospital (CWZ), Nijmegen, The Netherlands.

References

1. Castagnola E, Caviglia I, Pistorio A, Fioredda F, Micalizzi C, Viscoli C, et al. Bloodstream infections and invasive mycoses in children undergoing acute leukaemia treatment: a 13-year experience at a single Italian institution. Eur J Cancer. 2005;41(10):1439–45.
2. Castagnola E, Cesaro S, Giacchino M, Livadiotti S, Tucci F, Zanazzo G, et al. Fungal infections in children with cancer: a prospective, multicenter surveillance study. Pediatr Infect Dis J. 2006;25(7):634–9.
3. Hale KA, Shaw PJ, Dalla-Pozza L, MacIntyre CR, Isaacs D, Sorrell TC. Epidemiology of paediatric invasive fungal infections and a case-control study of risk factors in acute leukaemia or post stem cell transplant. Br J Haematol. 2010;149(2):263–72.
4. Nucci M, Garnica M, Gloria AB, Lehugeur DS, Dias VC, Palma LC, et al. Invasive fungal diseases in haematopoietic cell transplant recipients and in patients with acute myeloid leukaemia or myelodysplasia in Brazil. Clin Microbiol Infect. 2013;19(8):745–51.
5. Al-Hatmi AM, Meis JF, de Hoog GS. *Fusarium*: Molecular diversity and intrinsic drug resistance. PLoS Pathog. 2016;12(4):e1005464.
6. Nucci M, Anaissie EJ, Queiroz-Telles F, Martins CA, Trabasso P, Solza C, et al. Outcome predictors of 84 patients with hematologic malignancies and *Fusarium* infection. Cancer. 2003;98(2):315–9.
7. Raad I, Tarrand J, Hanna H, Albitar M, Janssen E, Boktour M, et al. Epidemiology, molecular mycology, and environmental sources of *Fusarium* infection in patients with cancer. Infect Control Hosp Epidemiol. 2002;23(9):532–7.
8. Dignani MC, Anaissie E. Human fusariosis. Clin Microbiol Infect. 2004; 10(Suppl 1):67–75.
9. Douard MC, Arlet G, Longuet P, Troje C, Rouveau M, Ponscarme D, et al. Diagnosis of venous access port-related infections. Clin Infect Dis. 1999;29(5):1197–202.
10. Brun-Buisson C, Abrouk F, Legrand P, Huet Y, Larabi S, Rapin M. Diagnosis of central venous catheter-related sepsis. Critical level of quantitative tip cultures. Arch Intern Med. 1987;147(5):873–7.

11. Azor M, Gene J, Cano J, Manikandan P, Venkatapathy N, Guarro J. Less-frequent *Fusarium* species of clinical interest: correlation between morphological and molecular identification and antifungal susceptibility. J Clin Microbiol. 2009;47(5):1463–8.
12. Al-Hatmi AM, Hagen F, Menken SB, Meis JF, de Hoog GS. Global molecular epidemiology and genetic diversity of *Fusarium*, a significant emerging group of human opportunists from 1958 to 2015. Emerg Microbes Infect. 2016;5(12):e124.
13. Mesquita-Rocha S, Godoy-Martinez PC, Goncalves SS, Urrutia MD, Carlesse F, Seber A, et al. The water supply system as a potential source of fungal infection in paediatric haematopoietic stem cell units. BMC Infect Dis. 2013;13:289.
14. Edel-Hermann V, Sautour M, Gautheron N, Laurent J, Aho S, Bonnin A, et al. A clonal lineage of *Fusarium oxysporum* circulates in the tap water of different French hospitals. Appl Environ Microbiol. 2016;82(21):6483–9.
15. Salah H, Al-Hatmi AM, Theelen B, Abukamar M, Hashim S, van Diepeningen AD, et al. Phylogenetic diversity of human pathogenic *Fusarium* and emergence of uncommon virulent species. J Inf Secur. 2015;71(6):658–66.
16. O'Donnell K, Kistler HC, Cigelnik E, Ploetz RC. Multiple evolutionary origins of the fungus causing Panama disease of banana: concordant evidence from nuclear and mitochondrial gene genealogies. Proc Natl Acad Sci U S A. 1998;95(5):2044–9.
17. Reeb V, Lutzoni F, Roux C. Contribution of RPB2 to multilocus phylogenetic studies of the euascomycetes (Pezizomycotina, Fungi) with special emphasis on the lichen-forming Acarosporaceae and evolution of polyspory. Mol Phylogenet Evol. 2004;32(3):1036–60.
18. Al-Hatmi AM, Mirabolfathy M, Hagen F, Normand AC, Stielow JB, Karami-Osbo R, et al. DNA barcoding, MALDI-TOF, and AFLP data support *Fusarium ficicrescens* as a distinct species within the *Fusarium fujikuroi* species complex. Fungal Biol. 2016;120(2):265–78.
19. Nucci M, Anaissie E. *Fusarium* infections in immunocompromised patients. Clin Microbiol Rev. 2007;20(4):695–704.
20. Litvinov N, da Silva MT, van der Heijden IM, Graca MG, Marques de OL, Fu L, et al. An outbreak of invasive fusariosis in a children's cancer hospital. Clin Microbiol Infect. 2015;21(3):268–7.
21. Velasco E, Martins CA, Nucci M. Successful treatment of catheter-related fusarial infection in immunocompromised children. Eur J Clin Microbiol Infect Dis. 1995;14(8):697–9.
22. Schwartz KL, Sheffield H, Richardson SE, Sung L, Morris SK. Invasive fusariosis: A single pediatric center 15-year experience. J Pediatric Infect Dis Soc. 2015;4(2):163–70.
23. Chaulk CP, Smith RW, Feagler JR, Verdirame J, Commers JR. Fungemia due to *Fusarium solani* in an immunocompromised child. Pediatr Infect Dis. 1986;5(3):363–6.
24. Schneller FR, Gulati SC, Cunningham IB, O'Reilly RJ, Schmitt HJ, Clarkson BD. *Fusarium* infections in patients with hematologic malignancies. Leuk Res. 1990;14(11–12):961–6.
25. Okuda C, Ito M, Sato Y, Oka K, Hotchi M. Disseminated cutaneous *Fusarium* infection with vascular invasion in a leukemic patient. J Med Vet Mycol. 1987;25(3):177–86.
26. Lozano M, Ribera JM, Puig J, Rives A, Sierra J, Granena A, et al. *Fusarium solani* bronchopneumonia in a patient with acute myeloblastic leukemia. Enferm Infecc Microbiol Clin. 1990;8(2):124–5.
27. Alvarez-Franco M, Reyes-Mugica M, Paller AS. Cutaneous *Fusarium* infection in an adolescent with acute leukemia. Pediatr Dermatol. 1992;9(1):62–5.
28. Nucci M, Anaissie E. Cutaneous infection by *Fusarium* species in healthy and immunocompromised hosts: implications for diagnosis and management. Clin Infect Dis. 2002;35(8):909–20.
29. Nucci M, Varon AG, Garnica M, Akiti T, Barreiros G, Trope BM, et al. Increased incidence of invasive fusariosis with cutaneous portal of entry, Brazil. Emerg Infect Dis. 2013;19(10):1567–72.
30. Varon AG, Nouer SA, Barreiros G, Trope BM, Magalhaes F, Akiti T, et al. Superficial skin lesions positive for *Fusarium* are associated with subsequent development of invasive fusariosis. J Inf Secur. 2014;68(1):85–9.
31. Boutati EI, Anaissie EJ. *Fusarium*, a significant emerging pathogen in patients with hematologic malignancy: ten years' experience at a cancer center and implications for management. Blood. 1997;90(3):999–1008.
32. Nucci M, Marr KA, Vehreschild MJ, de Souza CA, Velasco E, Cappellano P, et al. Improvement in the outcome of invasive fusariosis in the last decade. Clin Microbiol Infect. 2014;20(6):580–5.
33. Raad I, Hachem R. Treatment of central venous catheter-related fungemia due to Fusarium oxysporum. Clin Infect Dis. 1995;20(3):709–11.
34. Kiehn TE, Nelson PE, Bernard EM, Edwards FF, Koziner B, Armstrong D. Catheter-associated fungemia caused by *Fusarium chlamydosporum* in a patient with lymphocytic lymphoma. J Clin Microbiol. 1985;21(4):501–4.
35. Colombo A, Maccari G, Congiu T, Basso P, Baj A, Toniolo A. Colonization of a central venous catheter by the hyaline fungus *Fusarium solani* species complex: A case report and SEM imaging. Case Rep Med. 2013;2013:618358.
36. Eljaschewitsch J, Sandfort J, Tintelnot K, Horbach I, Ruf B. Port-a-cath-related *Fusarium oxysporum* infection in an HIV-infected patient: treatment with liposomal amphotericin B. Mycoses. 1996;39(3–4):115–9.
37. Tortorano AM, Richardson M, Roilides E, Diepeningen AV, Caira M, Munoz P, et al. ESCMID and ECMM joint guidelines on diagnosis and management of hyalohyphomycosis: *Fusarium* spp., *Scedosporium* spp. and others. Clin Microbiol Infect. 2014;20(Suppl 3):27–46.
38. Ammari LK, Puck JM, McGowan KL. Catheter-related *Fusarium solani* fungemia and pulmonary infection in a patient with leukemia in remission. Clin Infect Dis. 1993;16(1):148–50.

6

Hospital clones of methicillin-resistant *Staphylococcus aureus* are carried by medical students even before healthcare exposure

Ido Orlin[1], Assaf Rokney[2], Avi Onn[1,3], Daniel Glikman[1,4†] and Avi Peretz[1,5*†]

Abstract

Background: Methicillin-resistant *Staphylococcus aureus* (MRSA) strains are prevalent in healthcare and the community. Few studies have examined MRSA carriage among medical students.
The aim of this study is to examine *Staphylococcus aureus* (SA) carriage, and particular MRSA, over time in cohort medical students

Methods: Prospective collection of nasal swabs from medical students in Israel and assessment of SA carriage. Three samples were taken per student in preclinical and clinical parts of studies. Antibiotic susceptibilities were recorded and MRSA typing was performed by staphylococcal cassette chromosome *mec* (SCC*mec*) types, Panton Valentine Leukocidin (PVL) encoding genes, and *spa* types. Clonality was assessed by pulsed-field gel electrophoresis.

Results: Among 58 students, SA carriage rates increased from 33% to 38% to 41% at baseline (preclinical studies), 13 and 19 months (clinical studies), respectively ($p = 0.07$). Methicillin-susceptible SA (MSSA) carriage increased in the clinical studies period (22 to 41%, $p = 0.01$). Overall, seven students (12%) carried 13 MRSA isolates. MRSA isolates were PVL negative and were characterized as SCC*mec*II-t002, SCC*mec*IV-t032, or t12435 with untypable SCC*mec*. MRSA carriage during the pre-clinical studies was evident in 4/7 students. Two students carried different MRSA clones at various times and persistent MRSA carriage was noted in one student. Simultaneous carriage of MRSA and MSSA was not detected.

Conclusions: MSSA carriage increased during the clinical part of studies in Israeli medical students. Compared with previous reports, higher rates of MRSA carriage were evident. MRSA strains were genotypically similar to Israeli healthcare-associated clones; however, carriage occurred largely before healthcare exposure, implying community-acquisition of hospital strains.

Keywords: Methicillin-resistance, Review, *Staphylococcus aureus*, Carriage, Medical students, Community-associated, Healthcare-associated

* Correspondence: Aperetz@poria.health.gov.il
†Equal contributors
[1]The Faculty of Medicine in the Galilee, Bar-Ilan University, Galilee, Israel
[5]Clinical Microbiology Laboratory, Padeh Poriya Medical Center, Poriya, Hanna Senesh 818/2, Tiberias, Israel
Full list of author information is available at the end of the article

Background

Staphylococcus aureus (SA) is a versatile pathogen capable of colonizing humans and mammals, and causing skin and invasive diseases such as endocarditis, osteomyelitis, and severe sepsis. Methicillin-resistant SA (MRSA) was reported in 1961, soon after the introduction of the semisynthetic penicillin, methicillin [1]. Until the 1990s, MRSA strains were associated mostly with hospitals and infected patients who had contact with the healthcare system, hence the name healthcare-associated MRSA (HA-MRSA). These strains were typically resistant to multiple antimicrobials (multi-drug resistant – MDR) and carried large staphylococcal cassette chromosome *mec* (SCC*mec*) elements, mostly types I-III [2]. Beginning in the late 1990s, community-associated strains of MRSA (CA-MRSA) were described with increasing incidence, colonizing and infecting patients who had no recent contact with the healthcare system. These strains were usually non-MDR, carried small SCC*mec* elements, mostly types IV and V, and also carried the genes encoding the Panton-Valentine leukocidin (PVL), a pore-forming toxin rarely found among SA isolates [1]. Nowadays, in many geographic regions there are no longer lineages, genetic markers, or susceptibility phenotypes that are indicative for specific epidemiological origins such as HA-MRSA or CA-MRSA [1].

The primary reservoir of SA is the anterior nares, but the organism can be isolated from multiple sites. The prevalence and incidence of SA nasal carriage vary according to the population studied. According to multiple cross-sectional surveys, the mean carriage rate across the general population is 37% [3]. Regarding MRSA carriage in the era of CA-MRSA, the overall MRSA carriage rate in the United States has increased from 0.8% in 2001–2002 to 1.5% in 2003–2004, and it is particularly important in the hospital environment because colonized and infected patients represent the most important reservoir of MRSA in healthcare facilities [4, 5].

The carriage of MRSA among healthcare workers (HCW) due to the relation of their exposure to patients harboring these strains is a well-known phenomenon [6]. Medical students seem to be no exception, as their clinical study environment involves various medical settings such as hospitals and community clinics, which may contribute to their carriage status. In a non-systematic review of the English literature we found several studies, conducted worldwide, investigating SA carriage among medical students (Table 1) [7–32]. These studies reported MRSA carriage rates of 0–5.4% and SA carriage rates of 14–45% (excluding a small study from India reporting a higher carriage rate and a study from Canada of dental students [12, 15]). Only in a minority of these studies assessed the difference of SA carriage between pre-clinical and clinical medical students and most investigations assessed carriage at a single time-point only [7, 9, 21–23, 26, 27, 31]. Of these, three studies demonstrated higher SA carriage rates in the clinical studies stage [9, 23, 26]. Furthermore, only a single study from Thailand had prospectively examined the change in SA carriage in the same group of medical students over multiple sampling times [26]. Therefore, we aimed to prospectively examine the change in SA carriage among medical students transitioning from pre-clinical to clinical education with a focus on MRSA. Moreover, we aimed to characterize MRSA isolates from medical students using SCC*mec* and *spa* typing as well as PFGE.

Methods

Study population

The study population included medical students at the Faculty of Medicine in the Galilee of Bar-Ilan University, in Safed, Israel. The Faculty has two academic classes: 4-year and 3-year tracks. The 3-year track students finished 3 years of pre-clinical medical education in medical faculties across Europe (such as Hungary, Italy, and Lithuania). Almost all of these students reported no patient encounters during their studies, as most of their education was lecture-based. The 4-year track students have graduated from various pre-med Israeli academic institutions. As no dormitories are available, most students live separately. The study was approved by the local Ethics Committees of Baruch Padeh Medical Center, Poriya, and Bar-Ilan University.

Sampling

Samples were collected three times for each participant during 2012–2014. Sampling was made by a sterile swab (COPAN, Italy) from the nostrils, independently by the participant. First sampling was performed towards the end of pre-clinical studies, with second and third samplings collected at 13 and 19 months post-initial sampling while students were rotating in clinical clerkships. All samples were kept at room temperature for a maximum of 24 h before being transferred to the microbiology laboratory.

Staphylococcus aureus identification

Microbiological examinations were performed at the Baruch Padeh Medical Center Microbiology Laboratory in Poriya, Israel. Primary culture was performed by striking technique in order to perform culture and colony isolation on a selective chromogenic growth medium (Chromagar MRSA/MSSA, hylabs, Israel). Confirmatory tests for SA included gram staining, catalase test, and rapid agglutination test for simultaneous detection of the fibrinogen affinity antigen (clumping factor), protein

Table 1 Staphylococcus aureus carriage among medical students in published papers

Year	Reference	Country	Population	SA Carriage, n (%)			MRSA Carriage, n (%)			Notes
				Total	Pre-clinical group	Clinical group	Total	Pre-clinical group	Clinical group	
1994	Stubbs et al. [7]	Australia	$N = 808$	261/808 (30%)	68/193 (35%)	252/615 (40%)	0	0	0	
2004	Berthelot et al. [8]	France	$N = 124$	34/124 (27%)	N/A	N/A	1/124) (1%)	N\A	N/A	
2007	Güçlü et al. [9]	Turkey	$N = 179$	50/179 (28%)	12/179 (15%)	38/179 (76%)[a]	N/A	N/A	N/A	
2007	Higuchi et al. [10]	Japan	$N = 98$	36/98 (36%)	N/A	N/A	0	0	0	
2007	Adesida et al. [11]	Nigeria	$N = 182$	26/182 (14%)	N/A	N/A	0	0	0	
2008	Baliga et al. [12]	India	$N = 50$	44/50 (88%)	N/A	N/A	12/50 (24%)	N/A	N/A	
2009	Slifka et al. [13]	USA	$N = 182$	62/182 (34%)	N/A	N/A	5/182 (3%)	2/95(2%)	3/87 (3%)	
2011	Ma et al. [14]	China	$N = 2103$[b]	212/2103 (10%)	N/A	N/A	22/2103 (1%)	N/A	N/A	SCC*mec* I, ST88 PVL- ($n = 1$); SCC*mec* II, ST5 PVL+ ($n = 1$) PVL- ($n = 1$); SCC*mec* III, ST 239 PVL- ($n = 1$); SCC*mec* IVa, ST88 PVL+ ($n = 5$), PVL-($n = 3$), ST30 ($n = 1$), ST1, PVL+ ($n = 1$); SCC*mec* IVn, ST59 ($n = 2$); SCC*mec* IVc, ST30, PVL+ ($n = 2$) SCC*mec* V, ST59 PVL+ ($n = 2$), ST90 PVL- ($n = 1$); non typable ($n = 1$)
2011	Roberts et al. [15]	Canada	$N = 61$[c]	N/A	N/A	N/A	13/61 (21%)	N/A	N/A	SCC*mec* IV, ST1159 ($n = 1$); 12 NT*[,HA] [ST8,ST30 ($n = 3$), ST39, ST45, ST101, ST109, ST256 ($n = 2$), ST 1474, ST1474]
2011	Chamberlain et al. [16]	USA	$N = 132$	62/132 (47%)	N/A	N/A	7/132 (5%)	N/A	N/A	
2011	Kitti et al. [17]	Thailand	$N = 200$	30/200 (15%)	N/A	N/A	2/200 (1%)	N/A	N/A	SCC*mec* II ($n = 2$)
2012	Gualdoni et al. [18]	Austria	$N = 79$	20/79 (25%)	N/A	N/A	0	N/A	N/A	
2012	Bettin et al. [19]	Colombia	$N = 387$	96/387 (25%)	N/A	N/A	6/387 (2%)	N/A	N/A	SCC*mec* I, PVL- ($n = 1$); SCC*mec* IV, PVL+ ($n = 5$) [CA]
2012	Mahmutović Vranić et al. [20]	Bosnia	$N = 387$	39/387 (11%)	N/A	N/A	0	N/A	N/A	
2012	Chen et al. [21]	Taiwan	$N = 322$	55/322 (17%)	24/167 (14%)	31/155 (20%)	7/322 (2%)	4/167 (2%)	3/155 (2%)	SCC*mec* IV, ST59 ($n = 2$), N/A MLST ($n = 4$), PVL − ($n = 6$)[CA] SCC*mec* V_T, ST59, PVL+ ($n = 1$)[CA]
2012	Syafinaz et al. [22]	Malaysia	$N = 209$	21/209 (10%)	14/111 (13%)	7/97 (7%)	0	0	0	
2013	Bellows et al. [23]	USA	$N = 94$	15/94 (16%)	3/42 (7%)	12/52 (23%)[a]	3/94 (3%)	0	3/52 (6%)	

Table 1 Staphylococcus aureus carriage among medical students in published papers *(Continued)*

2013	Cirković et al. [24]	Serbia	$N = 533$	N/A	N/A	N/A	2/533 (0.4%)	N/A	N/A	SCC*mec* IV, ST80[CA] SCC*mec* V,ST152[CA]
2013	Trépanier et al. [25]	Canada	$N = 497^d$	N/A	N/A	N/A	1/497 (0.2%)	1/247 (0.4%)	0	
2014	Treesirichod et al. [26]	Thailand	$N = 128$	42/127 (33%)	38/128 (30%)	2nd sample 39/128 (31%) 3rd sample 50/127 (39%)[a]	0	0	0	3 prospective samples
2015	Zakai et al. [27]	Saudi Arabia	$N = 182$	60/182 (32%)	32/32 (100%)	28/150 (19%)	10/182 (5%)	0/32	10/150 (7%)	
2015	Collazos Marín et al. [28]	Colombia	$N = 216$	54 (25%)	N/A	N/A	9/216 (4%)	N/A	N/A	4/9 (44%)[CA]
2015	Ho et al. [29]	China	$N = 1149$	526/1149 (45%)	N/A	N/A	6/1149 (1%)	N/A	N/A	SCC*mec* IV,t437 (n = 3)[CA] : PVL+ ($n = 1$) t11642 ($n = 1$)[CA], t1081 ($n = 1$)[HA], t267 ($n = 1$)[HA]
2016	Baek et al. [30]	South Korea	$N = 159^c$	N/A	N/A	N/A	5/159 (3%)	N/A		SCC*mec* IV ($n = 4$) SCC*mec* I (n = 1)
2016	Okamo et al. [31]	Tanzania	$N = 314$	66/314 (21%)	33/166 (20%)	33/148 (22%)	1/314 (0.3%)	N/A	N/A	
2016	Ansari et al. [32]	Nepal	$N = 200$	30/200 (15%)	N/A	N/A	8/200 (4%)	N/A	N/A	

N/A not available, *CA-MRSA* community-associated methicillin-resistant *Staphylococcus aureus*, *HA-MRSA* hospital-associated methicillin-resistant *Staphylococcus aureus*, *SA Staphylococcus aureus*, SCC*mec* Staphylococcal Cassette Chromosome *mec*

[a] $p < 0.05$

[b] Medical interns

[c] Dental students

[d] Divided to 250 medical residents and 247 undergrad students including interns

[HA] suggested by article as HA-MRSA

[CA] Suggested by article as CA-MRSA

[*] Not SCC*mec* type I-V

A, and the capsular polysaccharides (Pastorex™ Staph Plus, BIO RAD, France).

Susceptibility tests

Antimicrobial susceptibility tests were performed by disc diffusion method on Muller-Hinton agar (BD Diagnostics, Sparks, MD) in accordance with the Clinical and Laboratory Standards Institute (CLSI) guidelines for rifampicin, vancomycin, erythromycin, gentamicin, cefotaxime, clindamycin, penicillin, oxacillin, mupirocin, fusidic acid, tetracycline, trimethoprim-sulfamethoxsazole (TMP-SMX), and cefoxitin [33]. MDR for MRSA was defined as resistance to at least three antimicrobial agents in addition to β-lactams.

Molecular characteristics

Typing of MRSA strains was performed at the National *Staphylococcus aureus* Reference Center, Central Laboratories, Israel Ministry of Health, Jerusalem, Israel.

PCR detection of *mec*A and PVL genes

PCR reactions in a total volume of 23 mL included 10.5 mL DDW, 12.5 mL PCR mix (ReddyMix, Tamar Laboratory Supplies, Mevaseret Zion), MecA1 and MecA2 primers or Luk-PV-1 and Luk-PV-2 primers (1 mM each). Thermocycling conditions were set at 94 °C for 2 min followed by 30 cycles of 94 °C for 30 s, 55 °C for 30 s, 72 °C for 60 s, followed by a final step of 72 °C for 2 min [34, 35].

Detection of SCC*mec* types

SCC*mec* types were detected using the method of Zhang et al. [35]. PCR reactions were performed in a total volume of 20 mL, including 9.5 mL DDW, 9.5 mL PCR mix (ReddyMix, Tamar Laboratory Supplies, Mevaseret Zion), and 1 mL primer mix with a final concentration as recommended [35]. Thermocycling conditions were set at 95 °C for 5 min, followed by 11 cycles of 94 °C for 45 s, 65 °C for 45 s, 72 °C for 1.5 min, followed by 26 - cycles of 94 °C for 45 s, 55 °C for 45 s, 72 °C for 1.5 min, and a final step of 72 °C for 10 min [35].

spa typing

spa typing was performed in a 20 mL reaction including 9.5 mL DDW, 9.5 mL PCR mix (ReddyMix, Tamar Laboratory Supplies, Mevaseret Zion), and primers 1514R, 1113 F (4pmol each). Thermocycling conditions were set at 94 °C for 5 min, followed by 35 cycles of 94 °C for 45 s, 60 °C for 45 s, 72 °C for 90 s, followed by a final extension step of 72 °C for 10 min. Cycle sequencing was carried out using the BigDye Terminator v1.1 chemistry (Applied Biosystems, Foster City, CA, USA) according to manufacturer's protocol. Cycle sequencing products were purified by gel using Performa DTR according to the manufacturer's recommendation. Electrophoresis was carried out on a 3730 × l Genetic Analyzer (Applied Biosystems) and the analysis was done using sequencing Analysis v.5.3.1 software (Applied Biosystems). *spa* typing analysis was performed using BioNumerics 7.5 software [36].

PFGE

Agarose-embedded (Lonza, USA) SA DNA was digested with SmaI (Fermentas, Lithuania) followed by gel electrophoresis in the CHEF MAPPER (Bio-Rad) system. Electrophoresis conditions were 14 °C, 0.5 × Tris-borate-EDTA buffer (Sigma, Switzerland), initial pulse 5 s, final pulse 50 s, 6 V, 18 h. *Salmonella Braenderup* H9812 restricted with XbaI (Fermentas, Lithuania) was used as a marker. PFGE restriction patterns were analyzed by the BioNumerics software (Applied Maths). The pulsotypes were compared using the band-based DICE similarity coefficient with 1% optimization and tolerance. The un-weighted pair group method with arithmetic mean (UPGMA) algorithm was used for cluster analysis [37].

Statistical analysis

Statistical analysis was performed using SPSS for windows version 21 (IBM Analytics). Proportion tests, Chi-square tests, and Wilcoxon signed ranks test were used for the univariate analysis using $\alpha = 0.05$ and 95% confidence interval (CI). Statistical significance was based on $p \leq 0.05$.

Results

A total of 58/109 students of the 2012 class (53%) participated in our study: 31 students of the 4-year track and 27 students of the 3-year track. There were 30 females and 28 males; the age range was 23–35 years. All 58 students participated during the entire study; three samples were taken from each of these students. Overall, 65 SA isolates were cultured from 32 students in the entire study period: 13 MRSA strains from seven students and 52 MSSA strains from 28 students.

First sample (pre-clinical sampling)

Overall, 19 (33%) SA isolates were cultured from 7 (12%) students of the three-year track and 12 (20%) students of the 4-year track (Figs. 1 and 2). Four (7%) MRSA isolates were identified: three from students of the 4-year track (10%) and one from a student of the 3-year track (4%). No significant differences in the rates of MSSA and MRSA isolation between the medical tracks were noted ($p = 0.5$; Fig. 2).

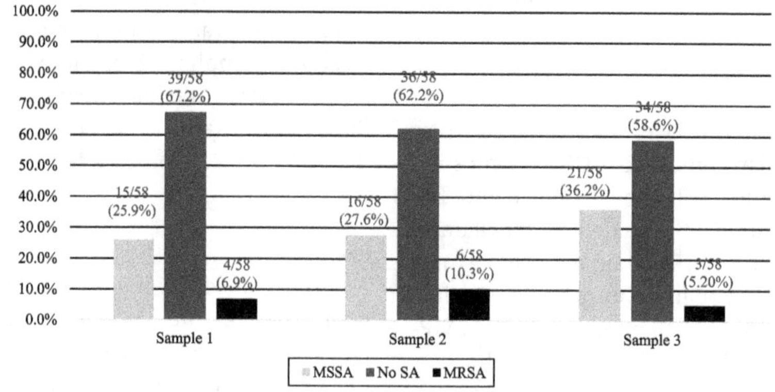

Fig. 1 Staphylococcus aureus carriage rates among medical students by sample

Second sample (first clinical sampling)

Thirteen months after the first pre-clinical samples, 22 SA (38%) isolates were cultured from 30% (eight of 27) of the 3-year track students and 45% (14 of 31) of the 4-year track students (Figs. 1 and 2). Further analysis revealed 16 MSSA (28%) and 6 MRSA isolates (10%) (Fig. 1). No significant differences were noted in the rates of MSSA and MRSA isolation between the medical tracks ($p = 0.47$) or between the first and second samples ($p = 0.76$; Fig. 2).

Third sample (second clinical sampling)

The last sample took place 6 months following the second sample and included 24 (41%) SA isolates cultured from 44% (12 of 27) of the 3-year track students and 39% (12 of 31) of the 4-year track students (Figs. 1 and 2). Overall, 21 MSSA (36%) and three MRSA isolates (5%) were identified. No significant differences in the rates of MSSA and MRSA isolation between the medical tracks were noted ($p = 0.74$). Compared with the second sample, an increase in the carriage rate of MSSA was noted in students of the 3-year track ($p = 0.01$; Fig. 2). Non-significant increases in the overall SA carriage between the pre-clinical sample and the third sample ($p = 0.21$) and between the second sample and the third sample ($p = 0.07$) were noted.

Phenotypic and genotypic characterization of MRSA isolates

The *mec*A gene was detected in all MRSA isolates. According to PFGE analysis, three closely-related clones of MRSA strains were identified (Fig. 3, Table 2) [37]. The first clone was isolated exclusively from the 4-year track students; this clone carried SCC*mec* IV, was PVL negative, and typed as *spa* type t032. The second clone was isolated from a single student of the 3-year track and was PVL negative, *spa* type t12435, with an untypable SCC*mec*. The third clone was cultured from students in both medical tracks and carried SCC*mec* II, was PVL negative, and typed as *spa* type t002.

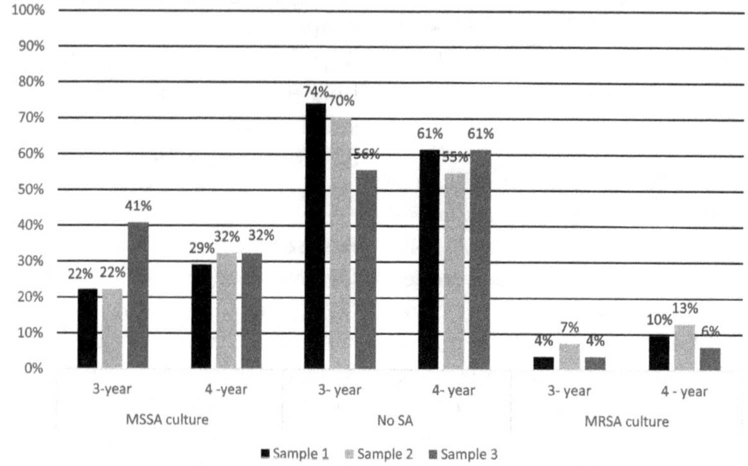

Fig. 2 Carriage rates of Staphylococcus aureus isolates according to medical track and sampling time

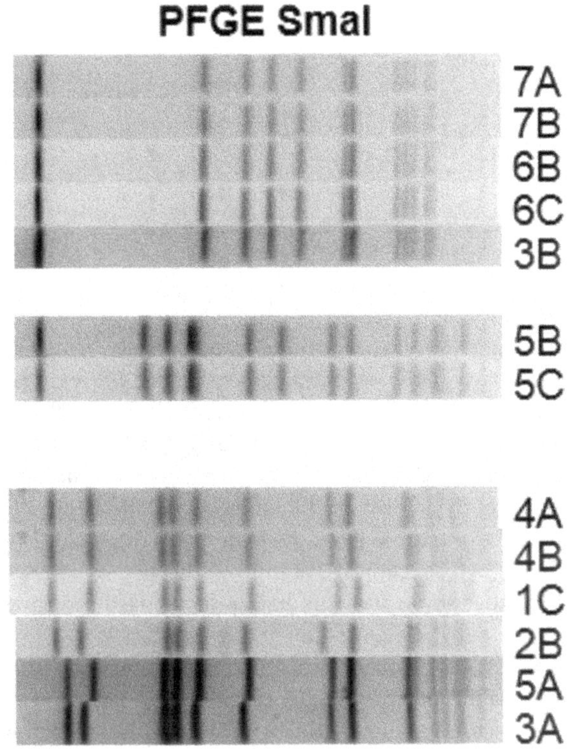

Fig. 3 Pulsed-field gel electrophoresis analysis of methicillin-resistant Staphylococcus aureus strains found in the study. * The numbers represent the students with MRSA carriage as mentioned in Fig. 4; the *capital letters* represent the sample time. For example: 1C is a clone cultured from student 1 on the third sample of the study

Overall, 38% of MRSA isolates (5 out of 13) were resistant to clindamycin whereas only 6% of MSSA isolates were clindamycin resistant ($p = 0.01$; Table 3). Clindamycin resistance rates differed among the various MRSA clones: half of SCC*mec* II, t002 isolates were resistant while none were resistant in the SCC*mec* IV, t032 clone. All MRSA isolates were susceptible to TMP-SMX, tetracycline, rifampicin, fusidic acid, mupirocin, and vancomycin, and were non-MDR.

Carriage of MRSA over multiple sampling times

Five of the seven (71%) students who were colonized with MRSA carried the bacterium in more than one sample (Fig. 4); two students carried different MRSA clones at various sampling times. Four students (57%) had MRSA carriage during the pre-clinical studies. None of the students carried MRSA and MSSA simultaneously.

Table 2 Summary of molecular characteristics of carried methicillin-resistant *Staphylococcus aureus* strains

	3-year track ($n = 4$)	4-year track ($n = 9$)	Total ($n = 13$)
SCC*mec* II, t002	2	5	7
SCC*mec* IV, t032	0	4	4
t12435[a]	2	0	2

[a]Untypable SCC*mec*
All MRSA Isolates were PVL-negative
Staphylococcal Cassette Chromosome *mec* (SCC*mec*)

Discussion

The carriage of SA increased in medical students along the sampling time (33, 38, and 41%, respectively). A non-significant increase ($p = 0.07$) was noted in the overall rise of SA carriage. However, a statistically significant increase in the MSSA carriage among the 3-year track students was evident when the second sample was compared with the third; both were taken during the clinical stages of studies. Thus, it is possible that a larger sample would also lead to a significant overall rise in SA carriage between the preclinical and clinical parts of the studies. This was indeed observed in three of eight studies comparing preclinical and clinical medical students [9, 23, 26].

In the multiple samplings we performed, up to 10% of the students carried MRSA. This rate is higher than observed in other studies looking at medical students, where carriage rates of 0–5.4% were noted (Table 1). In fact, according to a systematic review of MRSA carriage among healthcare workers in Europe and the United States, it is close to the reported carriage rates of nursing staff [6]. Possible explanations for this difference in rates of MRSA carriage among medical students may be from various sampling times in the studies, MRSA prevalence rates in hospitals and communities in different countries, and the relatively small sample size of studies.

The MRSA strains we isolated are compatible with HA-MRSA strains. We base this observation on the molecular characteristics of the strains and epidemiologic studies from Israel. Both SCC*mec* II, t002 and SCC*mec* IV, t032 are common hospital MRSA strains in Israel [38, 39]. Indeed, SCC*mec* II, t002 is reported to be the second most common clone in Israeli hospitals [38]. Although mostly described in CA-MRSA strains, up to 30% of HA-MRSA isolates in Israel carry SCC*mec* types IV and V [38, 39]. A recent report of community-onset MRSA in Israel demonstrated SCC*mec* IV, t032 to represent nearly 30% of SCC*mec* IV isolates; thus this strain is commonly isolated both in Israeli hospitals and in patients from the community [40]. In contrast, typical CA-MRSA strains in Israel have different genotypes: USA300 (SCC*mec* IV, t008, PVL+) and SCC*mec* IV, t991, PVL- [40]. The third strain in our study, t12435, is relatively rare, being isolated only a few times from hospitalized patients in northern Israel according to data from the Israeli National *Staphylococcus aureus* Reference Center. Although non-MDR phenotype of MRSA is commonly described among CA-MRSA strains, this phenotype was also common among SCC*mec* IV, t032

Table 3 Antibiotic resistance rates of Staphylococcus aureus isolates

	3-year program		4-year program		Total	
	MSSA ($n = 23$)	MRSA ($n = 4$)	MSSA ($n = 29$)	MRSA ($n = 9$)	MSSA ($n = 52$)	MRSA ($n = 13$)
Ciprofloxacin	0%	0%	3%	22%	2%	15%
Clindamycin	4%	100%	7%	11%	6%	38%
Erythromycin	60%	25%	21%	22%	38%	23%
Gentamicin	17%	75%	3%	44%	10%	54%

All isolates were susceptible to trimethoprim-sulfamethoxazole (TMP-SMX), fusidic acid, mupirocin, tetracycline, rifampin, and vancomycin
MSSA Methicillin-susceptible *Staphylococcus aureus*, *MRSA* Methicillin-resistant *Staphylococcus aureus*

isolates from Israeli hospitals with relatively low clindamycin resistance rates [1, 2, 40]. Our findings differ from other reports of MRSA in medical students: predominantly CA-MRSA clones (as suggested by the authors) were isolated from medical students in China, Serbia, Canada, Colombia and Taiwan, suggesting these countries have a different MRSA epidemiology [15, 19, 21, 24, 28, 29].

Two additional observations are worth mentioning: we did not find new, non-local MRSA clones among the students, although the 3-year track students arrived from various countries in Europe. This probably implies acquisition of MRSA clones in Israel but can also represent acquisition of global MRSA strains from Europe [41]. The second observation is that although students carried MRSA isolates compatible with HA-MRSA clones, the acquisition of the majority of MRSA isolates, including two of three clones, took place before the clinical part of the studies, namely before the exposure to the healthcare system occurred. Indeed, 80% of community-onset MRSA isolates among patients insured by a large health maintenance organization in Israel were recently shown to be of nosocomial origin [40]. This can explain the acquisition of HA-MRSA clones by students before clinical rotations. Another explanation may be that some students had unrecognized healthcare exposure early in their studies.

In assessing carriage over time, we observed that in two students multiple MRSA clones were carried on different occasions. Compared with MSSA, less is known about the natural history of MRSA carriage and therefore comparison to MSSA data may seem tempting. However, this comparison is problematic as the variety of genotypes and prevalence in the community is larger

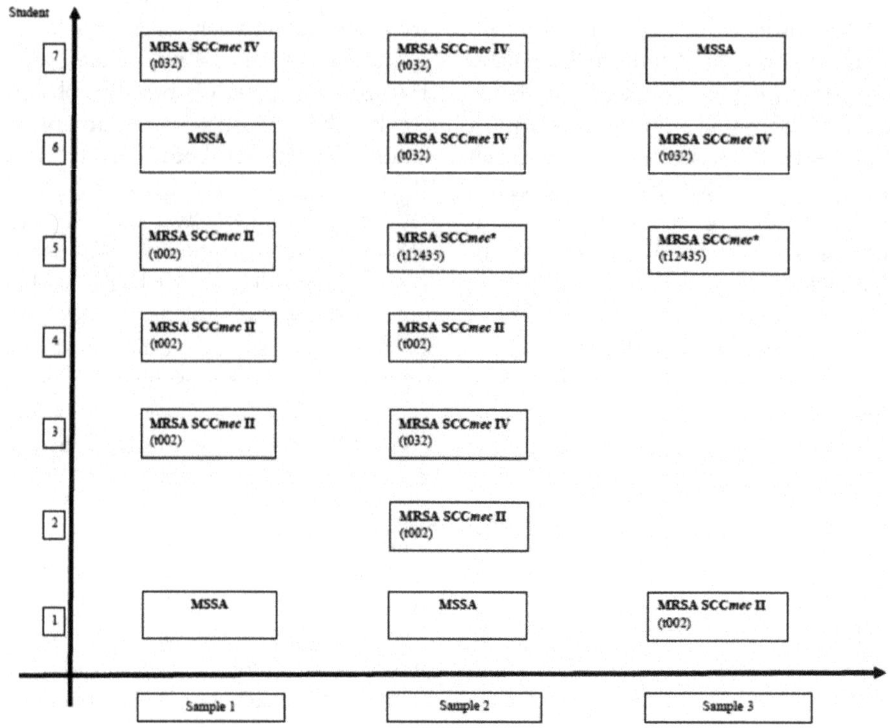

Fig. 4 Time-line of methicillin-resistant S. aureus carriage

for MSSA in most geographic locales [1, 3]. Carrying multiple genotypes of MRSA over time may imply acquisition of a new strain from a fellow student or during healthcare exposure. Furthermore, we noticed that only one of seven students colonized with MRSA can be defined as a persistent carrier and even so with multiple genotypes. Lastly, we observed that there was no simultaneous carriage of MRSA and MSSA isolates. Simultaneous carriage of MRSA and MSSA was previously reported either as a rare occurrence, assuming competition for colonization space and nutrients, or in contrast, as a relatively common occurrence [42, 43].

Our study had some limitations. The number of students participating was relatively small and the sampling was not done simultaneously in all students. The nose was the only site tested. Additionally, only one medical school participated. This may limit the power of the study and the generalization for all areas of Israel. The strengths of the study are in the prospective collection of data over multiple times in preclinical and clinical parts of the students' education, the participation of all students during the whole study, and the genotyping of MRSA strains.

Conclusion

MSSA carriage rates increased during the clinical part of the studies in medical students in Israel. Higher rates of MRSA carriage were evident in this study compared with previous reports of medical students. MRSA strains carried were genotypically similar to healthcare-associated clones in Israel; however, MRSA carriage occurred in the majority of students before healthcare exposure, probably representing community-acquisition of hospital strains. Until official recommendations regarding screening and interventions for MRSA in medical students will be published, a call for good personal hygiene is in place.

Abbreviations

CA-MRSA: Community-associated methicillin-resistant *Staphylococcus aureus*; HA-MRSA: Healthcare-associated methicillin-resistant *Staphylococcus aureus*; MRSA: Methicillin-resistant *Staphylococcus aureus*; PVL: Panton-Valentine Leukocidin; SA: *Staphylococcus aureus*

Acknowledgement

Not applicable

Funding

No funding was obtained for this study.

Authors' contributions

All authors have read and approved the final version of the manuscript. IO participated in the design of the study, collected data, helped in drafting the manuscript, and reviewed the final draft. AR participated in the design of the study, performed the molecular studies, helped in drafting the manuscript, and reviewed the final draft. AO participated in the design of the study, helped in drafting the manuscript, and reviewed the final draft. DG and AP conceived the study, collected and analyzed data, helped in drafting the manuscript, and wrote the final draft.

Authors' information

Ido Orlin

The article was written as part of the requirements of the School of Medicine in the Galilee, Bar-Ilan University, for an MD degree

Competing interests

The authors declare that they have no competing interests.

Consent for publication

Not applicable.

Author details

[1]The Faculty of Medicine in the Galilee, Bar-Ilan University, Galilee, Israel. [2]National Staphylococcus aureus Reference Center, Central Laboratories, Israel Ministry of Health, Jerusalem, Israel. [3]Pediatric Gastrointestinal Unit, Padeh Poriya Medical Center, Poriya, Tiberias, Israel. [4]Pediatric Infectious Diseases Service, Galilee Medical Center, Nahariya, Israel. [5]Clinical Microbiology Laboratory, Padeh Poriya Medical Center, Poriya, Hanna Senesh 818/2, Tiberias, Israel.

References

1. David M, Daum R. Community-associated methicillin-resistant Staphylococcus aureus: epidemiology and clinical consequences of an emerging epidemic. Clin Microbiol Rev. 2010;23(3):616–87.
2. David M, Glikman D, Crawford S, et al. What is community-associated methicillin-resistant Staphylococcus aureus? J Infect Dis. 2008;197(9): 1235–43.
3. Kluytmans J, van Belkum A, Verbrugh H. Nasal carriage of Staphylococcus aureus: epidemiology, underlying mechanisms, and associated risks. Clin Microbiol Rev. 1997;10(3):505–20.
4. Glick S, Samson D, Huang E, et al. Screening for methicillin-resistant Staphylococcus aureus: A comparative effectiveness review. Am J Infect Control. 2014;42:148–55.
5. Gorwitz RJ, Kruszon-Moran D, McAllister SK, et al. Changes in the prevalence of nasal colonization with Staphylococcus aureus in the United States, 2001-2004. J Infect Dis. 2008;197(9):1226–34.
6. Dulon M, Peters C, Schablon A, et al. MRSA carriage among healthcare workers in non-outbreak settings in Europe and the United States: a systematic review. BMC Infect Dis. 2014;14:363.
7. Stubbs E, Pegler M, Vickery A, Harbour C. Nasal carriage of Staphylococcus aureus in Australian (pre-clinical and clinical) medical students. J Hosp Infect. 1994;27(2):127–34.
8. Berthelot P, Grattard F, Fascia P, et al. Is nasal carriage of methicillin-resistant Staphylococcus aureus more prevalent among student healthcare workers? Infect Control Hosp Epidemiol. 2004;25:364–5.
9. Güçlü E, Yavuz T, Tokmak A, et al. Nasal carriage of pathogenic bacteria in medical students: effects of clinic exposure on prevalence and antibiotic susceptibility. Eur Arch Otorhinolaryngol. 2007;264:85–8.
10. Higuchi W, Isobe H, Iwao Y, et al. Extensive multidrug resistance of coagulase-negative staphylococci in medical students. J Infect Chemother. 2007;13:63–6.
11. Adesida S, Abioye O, Bamiro B, et al. Associated risk factors and pulsed field gel electrophoresis of nasal isolates of Staphylococcus aureus from medical students in a tertiary hospital in Lagos, Nigeria. Braz J Infect Dis. 2007;11:63–9.
12. Baliga S, Bansil R, Suchitra U, et al. Nasal carriage of methicillin-resistant Staphylococcus aureus in medical students. J Hosp Infect. 2008;68:91–2.
13. Slifka J, Nettleman M, Dybas L, et al. Is acquisition of methicillin-resistant Staphylococcus aureus an occupational hazard for medical students? Clin Infect Dis. 2009;49:482–3.

14. Ma X, Sun D, Wang S, et al. Nasal carriage of methicillin-resistant Staphylococcus aureus among preclinical medical students: epidemiologic and molecular characteristics of methicillin-resistant S. aureus clones. Diagn Microbiol Infect Dis. 2011;70:22–30.
15. Roberts C, Soge O, Horst A, et al. Methicillin-resistant Staphylococcus aureus from dental school clinic surfaces and students. Am J Infect Control. 2011; 39:628–32.
16. Chamberlain R, Singh K. Prevalence of methicillin resistant Staphylococcus aureus in nasal samples from preclinical second-year medical students. Mo Med. 2011;108(5):373–6.
17. Kitti T, Boonyonying K, Sitthisak S. Prevalence of methicillin-resistant Staphylococcus aureus among university students in Thailand. Southeast Asian J Trop Med Public Health. 2011;42:1498–504.
18. Gualdoni A, Lingscheid T, Tobudic S, et al. H. Low nasal carriage of drug-resistant bacteria among medical students in Vienna. GMS Krankenhhyg Interdiszip. 2012;7:Doc04.
19. Bettin A, Causil C, Reyes N. Molecular identification and antimicrobial susceptibility of Staphylococcus aureus nasal isolates from medical students in Cartagena, Colombia. Braz J Infect Dis. 2012;16:329–34.
20. Mahmutović Vranić S, Puškar M. Staphylococcus aureus carriage among medical students. Med Glas (Zenica). 2012;9:325–9.
21. Chen C, Chen Y, Huang C. Nasal carriage rate and molecular epidemiology of methicillin-resistant Staphylococcus aureus among medical students at a Taiwanese university. Int J Infect Dis. 2012;16:e799–803.
22. Syafinaz M, Nur Ain Z, Nadzirahi N, et al. Staphylococcus aureus nasal carriers among medical students in a medical school. Med J Malaysia. 2012; 67:636–8.
23. Bellows C, Smith A, Wheeler J, Morici L. Nasal carriage of methicillin-resistant Staphylococcus aureus among students at a Louisiana medical university. Braz J Infect Dis. 2013;17:118–9.
24. Cirković I, Djukić S, Vuković D, et al. Nasal carriage of methicillin-resistant Staphylococcus aureus among medical students of Belgrade University. Srp Arh Celok Lek. 2013;141:349–53.
25. Trépanier P, Tremblay C, Ruest A. Methicillin-resistant Staphylococcus aureus colonization among medical residents. Can J Infect Dis Med Microbiol. 2013; 24:e39–41.
26. Treesirichod A, Hantagool S, Prommalikit O. Nasal carriage and antimicrobial susceptibility of Staphylococcus aureus among medical students at the HRH Princess Maha Chakri Sirindhorn Medical Center, Thailand: a follow-up study. J Infect Public Health. 2014;7:205–9.
27. Zakai A. Prevalence of methicillin-resistant Staphylococcus aureus nasal colonization among medical students in Jeddah, Saudi Arabia. Saudi Med J. 2015;36:807–12.
28. Collazos Marín F, Estupiñan Arciniegas G, Chavez Vivas M. Characterization of Staphylococcus aureus isolates that colonize medical students in a hospital of the city of Cali, Colombia. Int J Microbiol. 2015;2015:358489.
29. Ho P-L, Lai EL, Chow K-H. Carriage of methicillin-susceptible and -resistant Staphylococcus aureus by medical students in Hong Kong. J Hosp Infect. 2015;91(2):184–5.
30. Baek S, Baek H, Yoo J. Higher nasal carriage rate of methicillin-resistant Staphylococcus aureus among dental students who have clinical experience. J Am Dent Assoc. 2015;147:348–53.
31. Okamo B, Moremi N, Seni J, et al. Prevalence and antimicrobial susceptibility profiles of Staphylococcus aureus nasal carriage among pre-clinical and clinical medical students in a Tanzanian University. BMC Res Notes. 2016;9:47.
32. Ansari S, Gautam R, Shrestha S, et al. Risk factors assessment for nasal colonization of Staphylococcus aureus and its methicillin resistant strains among pre-clinical medical students of Nepal. BMC Res Notes. 2016;9:214.
33. Clinical and Laboratory Standards Institute/NCCLS. Performance Standards for Antimicrobial Susceptibility Testing; Twenty-Fourth Informational Supplement. Wayne: Clinical and Laboratory Standards Institute; 2014. CLSI/NCCLS Document M100-S24.
34. McClure A, Conly M, Lau V, et al. Novel multiplex PCR assay for detection of the staphylococcal virulence marker Panton-Valentine leukocidin genes and simultaneous discrimination of methicillin-susceptible from -resistant staphylococci. J Clin Microbiol. 2006;44(3):1141–4.
35. Zhang K, McClure A, Elsayed S, et al. Novel multiplex PCR assay for characterization and concomitant subtyping of staphylococcal cassette chromosome mec types I to V in methicillin-resistant Staphylococcus aureus. J Clin Microbiol. 2005;43(10):5026–33.
36. Harmsen D, Claus H, Witte W, et al. Typing of methicillin-resistant Staphylococcus aureus in a university hospital setting by using novel software for spa repeat determination and database management. J Clin Microbiol. 2003;41(12):5442–8.
37. Tenover C, Arbeit D, Goering V, et al. Interpreting chromosomal DNA restriction patterns produced by pulsed-field gel electrophoresis: criteria for bacterial strain typing. J Clin Microbiol. 1995;33(9):2233–9.
38. Adler A, Chmelnitsky I, Shitrit P, et al. Molecular epidemiology of methicillin-resistant Staphylococcus aureus in Israel: dissemination of global clones and unique features. J Clin Microbiol. 2012;50(1):134–7.
39. Shitrit P, Openhaim M, Reisfeld S, et al. Characteristics of SCCmec IV and V Methicillin-Resistant Staphylococcus aureus (MRSA) in Israel. Isr Med Assoc J. 2015;17(8):470–5.
40. Biber A, Parizade M, Taran D, et al. Molecular epidemiology of community-onset methicillin-resistant Staphylococcus aureus infections in Israel. Eur J Clin Microbiol Infect Dis. 2015;34(8):1603–13.
41. Grundmann H, Aanensen DM, van den Wijngaard CC, et al. Geographic distribution of *Staphylococcus aureus* causing invasive infections in Europe: A molecular-epidemiological analysis. PLoS Med. 2010;7:e1000215.
42. Dall'Antonia M, Coen PG, Wilks M, et al. Competition between methicillin-sensitive and -resistant Staphylococcus aureus in the anterior nares. J Hosp Infect. 2005;61:62–7.
43. Mongkolrattanothai K, Gray BM, Mankin P, et al. Simultaneous carriage of multiple genotypes of Staphylococcus aureus. J Med Microbiol. 2011;60: 317–22.

7

Clinical and molecular characteristics, risk factors and outcomes of Carbapenem-resistant *Klebsiella pneumoniae* bloodstream infections in the intensive care unit

Xia Zheng[1], Jian-feng Wang[2], Wang-lan Xu[3], Jun Xu[1] and Juan Hu[1*]

Abstract

Background: To analyze the clinical characteristics and outcomes of carbapenem-resistant *Klebsiella pneumoniae* (CRKp) and carbapenem-susceptible *K. pneumoniae* (CSKp) bloodstream infections (BSIs), and to study the risk factors for development of CRKp BSI and *K. pneumoniae* BSI-related mortality.

Methods: A retrospective case control study of patients with *K. pneumoniae* BSI was conducted in the intensive care unit of the First Affiliated Hospital, Medical of College, Zhejiang University from January 2013 to December 2014. Carbapenem resistance was defined in accordance with the Clinical and Laboratory Standards Institute 2016 guidelines. Risk factors for the development of CRKp BSI and risk factors for mortality due to *K. pneumoniae* BSI were assessed. Virulence genes were detected by polymerase chain reaction assay.

Results: In total, 48 patients were enrolled in the study, including 31 (65%) patients with CRKp BSI and 17 (35%) patients with CSKp BSI. CSKp infection was associated with more severe clinical symptoms, particularly a higher serum creatinine level (165.06 ± 127.01 in the CSKp group vs. 93.77 ± 84.35 μmol/L in the CRKp group, $p = 0.039$), but there was no significant difference in prognosis between the CSKp and CRKp groups. On multivariate analysis, indwelling central venous catheter ($p = 0.045$) was the only factor independently associated with CRKp bacteremia. However, the mortality of *K. pneumoniae* BSI patients was not correlated with carbapenem resistance. In addition, the isolates had diverse clonality and different origins. The frequency of detection of the *allS* and *magA* virulence genes was higher in the CSKp group than in the CRKp group (*alls* $p = 0.04$; *magA* $p = 0.047$).

Conclusions: Patients in the CSKp group experienced more severe clinical symptoms, although mortality did not differ significantly between the CRKp and CSKp groups. An indwelling central venous catheter was the only factor independently associated with CRKp BSI. The mortality of patients with *K. pneumoniae* BSI was not associated with carbapenem resistance. The frequency of virulence genes was higher in the CSKp group than in the CRKp group.

Background

Klebsiella pneumoniae, a member of the family Enterobacteriaceae, is a causative organism of various infections, including serious community-onset infections, such as necrotizing pneumonia, pyogenic liver abscesses, and endogenous endophthalmitis [1, 2]; and nosocomial infections, particularly urinary tract infections (UTIs), respiratory tract infections, and bloodstream infections (BSIs) [1, 3, 4]. Due to abuse of antimicrobial agents in developing countries, the incidence of carbapenem-resistant Enterobacteriaceae (CRE) is of considerable concern. *K. pneumoniae* is the most prevalent Enterobacteriaceae species, accounting for 71.9% of 242 CRE strains in a retrospective study conducted in a tertiary hospital in Hangzhou, China [5]. Surveillance of antibiotic resistance by the China CHINET showed that 2.9% and 2.8% of *Klebsiella* spp. were resistant to imipenem and meropenem, respectively, in 2005 compared to 10.5% and 13.4%, respectively, in 2014 [6]. The production of carbapenemases (e.g., KPC, NDM, VIM, OXA-

* Correspondence: 21218046@zju.edu.cn
[1]Intensive Care Unit, The First Affiliated Hospital, College of Medicine, Zhejiang University, 79 Qingchun Road, Hangzhou 310003, People's Republic of China
Full list of author information is available at the end of the article

48-like) is the most common mechanism of resistance among *K. pneumoniae* isolates. Other mechanisms include alterations in outer membrane permeability, mediated by loss of porins and the upregulation of efflux systems [7].

The mortality rate of carbapenem-resistant *Klebsiella pneumoniae* (CRKp) infections in North America, South America, Europe, and Asia is reportedly 33.24%, 46.71%, 50.06%, and 44.82%, respectively [8]. Similarly, a study done in Shanghai, China showed that the 28-day mortality and in-hospital mortality rates of CRKp BSI patients were significantly higher than those of patients with carbapenem-susceptible *K. pneumoniae* (CSKp) BSIs (33.3% vs. 16%, $p = 0.04$; 42.4% vs. 24.6%, $p = 0.005$, respectively) [9]. Although CRKp is reportedly associated with prolonged hospitalization and mortality [8, 10–12] because such patients typically receive inappropriate empiric therapy, other studies found no such relationship [13–15].

There are various risk factors for CRKp BSI. A study conducted in a teaching hospital in Shanghai, China suggested that skin and soft tissue infection (odds ratio [OR] 26.63 and ICU-acquired infection (OR 5.82) was a risk factor for CRKp BSI [9]. multisite colonization (hazard ratio [HR] 13.73), ICU stay (HR 3.14) and previous BSI (HR 6.62) was associated with the development of CRKp BSI in colonized patients [16]. Primary liver disease and hepatitis C virus infection or hepatocellular cancer were significantly associated with development of CRKp in intensive care unit (ICU) patients after orthotopic liver transplantation [17]. Even no exposure independently predicted CRKp BSI in carriers of CRKp [18].

Similarly, several factors are reportedly associated with mortality related to *K. pneumoniae* BSI. The lung as the probable source of infection (OR 4.23) and a high Sequential Organ Failure Assessment (SOFA) score (OR 1.40) were strong prognostic factors for crude 28-day *K. pneumoniae* BSI mortality in a teaching hospital in Shanghai, China [9]. Septic shock (HR 3.86), acute respiratory failure (HR 2.32), inadequate initial antimicrobial therapy (HR 1.87) and carbapenem resistance by *K. pneumoniae* isolates (HR 1.85) were independently associated with mortality in onco-hematological patients [19]. In a univariate analysis, Acute Physiology and Chronic Health Evaluation (APACHE II) score, SOFA score, and CRKp BSI were predictive of ICU mortality after orthotopic liver transplantation [17].

It is generally accepted that CRKp BSIs are associated with high mortality, mostly because of the paucity of antimicrobials active against CRKp and the multiple comorbidities of patients [20]. Severe infection causes organ dysfunction and/or failure via complex mechanisms, including pathogenic microorganisms, an excessive inflammatory response, and immune dysfunction. However, antimicrobial resistance does not always lead to organ dysfunction and/or failure [21]. The immune system plays an important role in disease manifestations, with multiple contributing factors, some of which may not be accounted for by routinely collected data. At present, whether the systemic manifestations of infection and frequency of bacterial virulence genes differ between CRKp and CSKp BSI patients is unclear. Therefore, the objective of our study was to compare the prognosis and clinical characteristics of patients with CRKp and CSKp infections in the ICU, identify risk factors for the development of CRKp BSI and mortality of *K. pneumoniae* BSI, and assess the frequency of bacterial virulence genes in patients with CRKp and CSKp BSI.

Methods

Study design and patients

This retrospective case-control study was conducted at the First Affiliated Hospital of the Medical College, Zhejiang University, a 2500-bed tertiary-care teaching hospital, and included all adult patients with BSI caused by *K. pneumoniae* and hospitalized in the 30-bed medical ICU from January 1, 2013 to December 31, 2014.

The patients were identified using the records of the clinical microbiology laboratory. All patients with a positive blood culture for *K. pneumoniae* was included in the study. Infective symptoms and signs were compatible with systemic inflammatory response syndrome (SIRS; i.e., fever or hypothermia, respiratory rate > 20 breaths per minute, tachycardia >90 beats/min, and white blood cell count >11,000 ml or <4000/ml, using the 1999 criteria). If more than one episode occurred in the same patient, only the first episode was included in the study [22].

Cases with incomplete medical records were excluded from the study. From 2013, the identification and antimicrobial susceptibility testing of all blood *K. pneumoniae* isolates were performed using Vitek 2 panels (bioMerieux, France); isolates were stored at −80 °C [23]. Reserved strains were retrospectively tested for the presence of specific virulence genes.

The patients were divided into the CRKp and CSKp groups. Carbapenem resistance was defined as a minimum inhibitory concentration of ≥4 mg/L for meropenem or imipenem or ≥2 mg/L for ertapenem; other strains were defined as carbapenem-susceptible. Data interpretation was performed in accordance with the Clinical and Laboratory Standards Institute (CLSI) 2016 guidelines.

To identify risk factors for the development of CRKp BSI and m related ortality, the following data were recorded: demographics (sex, age), comorbidities, history of surgery, hospital or ICU admission in the last 30 days, use of steroids or immune modulators, antibiotic exposure history, and indwelling prosthetic material. In addition, for assessment of severe infection, APACHE II scores, liver function, kidney function, and inflammatory markers, at admission and at the time of positive blood culture, were recorded [17, 19].

The primary outcomes were crude survival rates at 7, 14, and 28 days. Secondary outcomes were current ICU stay duration, bacterial clearance rate, and duration of mechanical ventilation [24].

Multilocus sequence typing and pulsed-field gel electrophoresis

According to the multilocus sequence typing (MLST) scheme of *K. pneumonia*, seven conserved housekeeping genes (*gapA*, *infB*, *mdh*, *pgi*, *phoE*, *rpoB*, and *tonB*) were amplified and sequenced [25]. Pulsed-field gel electrophoresis (PFGE) was performed using *Xba*I (Dalian Takara Bio Inc., China), as described previously. To identify isolates associated with outbreaks, PFGE band patterns were interpreted according to the criteria proposed by Tenover et al. [26, 27].

Detection of virulence genes by polymerase chain reaction

The K1, K2, K5, K20, K54, and K57 capsular serotypes were detected by polymerase chain reaction (PCR), as described previously. Virulence genes (*magA*, *rmpA*, *rmpA2*, and *allS*) were detected by PCR using primers, as described previously. PCR products were interpreted and sequenced [23].

Statistical analysis

Statistical analyses were performed using SPSS software (ver. 18.0; SPSS Inc., USA). Continuous variables are presented as means ± SD and were evaluated by Student's *t*-test or the Mann-Whitney U test, as appropriate. A chi-squared test or Fisher's exact test was used for categorical variables, and multivariate analyses were performed using logistic regression models to identify independent risk factors for the outcome variables. All biologically plausible variables significant at $p < 0.10$ in univariate analysis were entered into a multivariate forward logistic regression analysis. A p value <0.05 was considered to indicate statistical significance.

Results

Demographics of the study population

Between January 1, 2013 and December 31, 2014, 48 patients had at least one episode of *K. pneumoniae* BSI in the ICU of our hospital. Thirty-three bloodstream isolates were included in this study; the others were excluded due to incomplete clinical information. The mean age in the CRKp and CSKp groups was 57.61 ± 14.78 and 62.71 ± 16.34 years, respectively (p = 0.306). Male patients accounted for 79% of the patients (56% in the CRKp group and 23% in the CSKp group, p = 0.502). To assess the frequency of bacterial virulence genes, 33 isolates (21 resistant and 12 susceptible) were obtained from 33 patients (17 and 4 male patients from the CRKp and CSKp groups, respectively [p = 0.357]). The mean age of these patients was 58.14 ± 15.16 and 65.58 ± 15.57 years, respectively (p = 0.190).

Clinical symptoms and prognostic factors of *K. pneumoniae* BSI

APACHEII score, peripheral blood leukocyte count, and C-reactive protein level were higher in the CSKp group than in the CRKp group at the time of bacteremia, albeit not significantly so. Many indexes showed the deteriorative tendencies in CSKp, including coagulation function, liver and kidney function, however only the static difference occurred in serum creatinine level (165.06 ± 127.01 in the CSKp group vs. 93.77 ± 84.35 μmol/L in the CRKp group, p = 0.039) (Table 1).

The prognostic factors of the CRKp and CSKp BSI patients are presented in Table 2. The duration of mechanical ventilation of the CRKp and CSKp groups was 18.50 ± 31.91 and 28.72 ± 31.06 days, respectively (p = 0.127). The current ICU stay duration was similar between the CRKp and CSKp groups (21.47 ± 33.67 vs. 31.74 ± 30.75 days, respectively [p = 0.073]). The bacterial clearance rate was 32% and 35% in the CRKp and CSKp groups, respectively (p = 0.718). The survival rate of the CRKp group was 74% at 7 days, 68% at 14 days, and 61% at 28 days, compared to 65% at 7 days, 59% at 14 days, and 47% at 28 days in the CSKp group (p = 0.489, 0.537, and 0.342, respectively).

Risk factors for the development of CRKp BSI

In univariate analyses, development of CRKp BSI was significantly associated with central venous catheterization and an indwelling urinary catheter, but not with

Table 1 Clinical symptoms of *K. pneumoniae* BSI

Variable	CSKp (n = 17)	CRKp (n = 31)	P
APACHEII score(mean ± SD)	18.18 ± 7.48	15.03 ± 6.38	0.089
WBC 10E9/L (mean ± SD)	14.24 ± 13.63	13.99 ± 9.66	0.497
leukocytes count (mean ± SD)	81.20 ± 14.60	88.02 ± 7.95	0.180
CRP(mg/l)(mean ± SD)	162.49 ± 118.07	113.74 ± 79.63	0.191
ALT (mean ± SD)	152.88 ± 399.23	49.84 ± 50.05	0.359
AST (mean ± SD)	490.82 ± 1655.64	49.63 ± 48.54	0.088
Total bilirubin (mean ± SD)	73.06 ± 142.17	62.68 ± 128.66	0.754
Direct bilirubin (mean ± SD)	43.29 ± 83.58	39.48 ± 86.63	0.779
PT (s) (mean ± SD)	17.71 ± 10.54	15.05 ± 5.27	0.439
Creatinine (mean ± SD)	165.06 ± 127.01	93.77 ± 84.35	0.039
Urea nitrogen (mean ± SD)	14.42 ± 9.88	14.40 ± 10.05	0.931

Abbreviations: *CSKp* carbapenem-susceptible *Klebsiella pneumoniae*, *CRKp* carbapenem-resistant *Klebsiella pneumoniae*, *WBC* white blood cell, *CRP* C-reactive protein, *ALT* alanine transaminase, *AST* aspartate transaminase, *PT* prothrombin time

Table 2 Clinical outcomes of *K. pneumoniae* BSI

Variable	CSKp (n = 17)	CRKp (*n* = 31)	*P*
Duration of mechanical ventilation (mean ± SD)(d)	18.50 ± 31.91	28.72 ± 31.06	0.127
Current ICU stay	21.47 ± 33.67	31.74 ± 30.75	0.073
Bacterial clearance rate	6(35%)	10(32%)	0.718
7-day survival rate	11(65%)	23(74%)	0.489
14-day survival rate	10(59%)	21(68%)	0.537
28-day survival rate	8(47%)	19(61%)	0.342

Abbreviations: *CSKp* carbapenem-susceptible *Klebsiella pneumoniae, CRKp* carbapenem-resistant *Klebsiella pneumoniae, ICU* intensive care unit

comorbidities (including diabetes mellitus, hypertension, coronary heart disease,chromic liver disease, chronic renal failure, solid organ tumor, history of surgery, prior healthcare-associated exposure, exposure to glucocorticoids and/or immunosuppressive drugs, trachea cannula or tracheotomy, an indwelling nasogastric tube, a drainage tube at multiple sites, and APACHE II score at admission). Hepatic and renal function at admission showed a trend towards being associated with the development of CRKp BSI. Although the majority of CRKp BSI patients had been exposed to antimicrobials before the positive culture, only exposure to tigecycline, imipenem and meropenem were included in the multivariate analysis of CRKp BSI (Table 3).

Variables significant at $p < 0.10$ in the univariate analyses were included in the multivariate analysis, and were as follows: an indwelling central venous catheter, indwelling urinary catheter, exposure to linezolid, imipenem and meropenem, and liver and kidney function at admission. In the multivariate analysis, central venous catheterization was the only independent factor for CRKp BSI. Exposure to imipenem and meropenem were likely related to CRKp BSI, but the association was not significant due to the small sample (Table 4).

Risk factors for mortality of *K. pneumoniae* BSI patients

In univariate analyses, the mortality of *K. pneumoniae* BSI patients was significantly associated with the APACHE II score on the day of bacteremia, but not with CRKp. Liver failure on the day of bacteremia and trachea cannula showed a trend towards being associated with a higher mortality rate. Variables significant at $p < 0.10$ in the univariate analyses were included in the multivariate analysis. However, no factor was identified as being associated with the mortality of *K. pneumoniae* BSI patients in the multivariate analysis, likely due to the small sample size (Table 5).

Molecular characteristics of CRKp and CSKp BSI

The PFGE patterns revealed that the 33 isolates had different origins (Fig. 1). MLST revealed considerable clonal diversity; 18 sequence types (STs) were detected (Fig. 2), of which ST11 comprised the majority.

The CSKp isolates harbored the *rmpA2, allS, K1,* and *magA* virulence genes, while the CRKp isolates possessed *rmpA2, magA,* and *K5,* but not *allS* or *K1. rmpA, K2, K20, K54,* and *K57* were not detected. The frequency of detection of *allS* and *magA* was higher in the CSKp group than in the CRKp group (*allS* $p = 0.04$; *magA* $p = 0.047$) (Table 6).

Discussion

CRKp BSI is a global public health problem that has been increasing in recent times, and is responsible for considerable morbidity [20, 28, 29]. The incidence of *K. pneumoniae* BSIs in ICU patients exceeds that of *Escherichia coli* BSIs [30, 31]. The mortality rate of critical patients with *K. pneumoniae* BSIs in the ICU was reported to rise up to 67.6% [30].

Population-based screening for *K. pneumoniae* bacteremia was conducted in the Calgary Health Region (population, 1.2 million) from 2000 to 2007. Dialysis, solid-organ transplantation, chronic liver disease, and cancer were risk factors for *K. pneumoniae* bacteremia [10]. CRE surveillance in Michigan healthcare facilities showed that cardiovascular disease, renal failure, and diabetes mellitus were the most frequently reported comorbidities, and risk factors for CRE included surgery within the previous 90 days, recent infection or colonization with a multidrug-resistant organism, and recent exposure to antimicrobials, particularly third- or fourth-generation cephalosporins [32]. The more frequent hospital contact associated with serious comorbidities may result in exposure to, and possibly infection by, nosocomial microorganisms. Moreover, severe chronic comorbidities were more frequent among patients with CRKp BSIs, but chronic comorbidities were not risk factors for CRKp BSI [33]. Similarly, in this study, comorbidities were not independent risk factors for CRKp BSI.

Glucocorticoids and immunosuppressors were not independent risk factors for CRKp BSI; however, previous studies reported different results. In one study, only prior carbapenem administration ($p = 0.003$), was significantly associated with CRKp infection, and another study revealed that the type of antibiotic used before infection—such as third-generation cephalosporins, macrolides and quinolones—was an independent risk factor for CRKp ($p < 0.05$) [11, 12]. Indeed, prior use of macrolides and antibiotic exposure for ≥14 days were the only factors independently associated with nosocomial CRKp bacteremia [33]. In another case-case control study, exposure to quinolones was not associated with CRKp infection, and colonization by CRKp and use of carbapenems were risk factors for infection with CRKp [34]. However, in our study, no antibiotic was a risk factor for CRKp BSI. Different in definitions, the duration

Table 3 Univariate analysis of risk factors for CRKp BSI

Variable	CSKp (n = 17)	CRKp (n = 31)	Univariate analysis		
			Adjusted OR	95% CI	*P*-value
Sex (male, n)	11(65%)	27(87%)	0.611	0.144—2.596	0.502
Age (y) (mean ± SD)	62.71 ± 16.34	57.61 ± 14.78			0.306
Co- morbidities					
Diabetes mellitus	5 (29%)	9 (29%)	0.982	0.268—3.602	0.978
Hypertension	9 (53%)	15 (48%)	0.833	0.255—2.724	0.763
Coronary heart disease	1 (6%)	3 (10%)	1.714	0.164—17.886	1
Chronic liver disease	3(18%)	6(19%)	1.120	0.242-5.186	1
Chronic renal failure	2 (12%)	4 (13%)	1.111	0.182—6.796	0.909
Solid organ tumor	4 (24%)	7 (23%)	0.948	0.233—3.850	0.940
HIV	0	0	NA	NA	NA
Surgery in the past medical history[a]	3 (18%)	5 (16%)	0.897	0.186—4.322	0.893
Prior healthcare-associated exposure	7 (41%)	9 (29%)	0.584	0.169—2.017	0.393
Prior medicine exposure					
Glucocorticoid	7 (41%)	13 (42%)	1.032	0.311—3.428	0.959
Immunosuppressor[b]	1 (6%)	2 (6%)	1.103	0.093—13.135	1
Prior use of antimicrobials					
Penicillin	3 (18%)	10 (32%)	2.105	0.480—9.237	0.318
Second cephalosporin	1 (6%)	4 (13%)	2.240	0.228—22.051	0.838
extended-spectrum cephalosporins	7 (41%)	15 (48%)	1.224	0.351—4.269	0.750
Aminoglycosides	1 (6%)	3 (10%)	1.615	0.153—17.016	1
Quinolones	1 (6%)	3 (10%)	1.615	0.153—17.016	1
Tigecycline	0	4 (13%)	0.625	0.492—0.795	0.613
Imipenem	1 (6%)	11(39%)	8.556	0.984—74.408	*0.064*
Meropenem	1 (6%)	12 (39%)	9.882	1.141—85.619	*0.068*
Ertapenem	0	0	NA	NA	NA
Linezolid	1 (6%)	12 (39%)	9.882	1.141—85.619	*0.068*
Glycopeptides Vancomycin	1 (6%)	8 (26%)	5.333	0.599—47.468	0.216
Teicoplanin	1 (6%)	5 (16%)	2.917	0.309—27.560	0.333
Invasive procedure before					
Central venous catheterization	10(59%)	30 (97%)	21.000	2.294—192.225	*0.003*
Trachea cannula	4(24%)	10 (32%)	1.548	0.401—5.971	0.525
Tracheotomy	5(29%)	12 (39%)	1.516	0.426—5.393	0.519
Urinary catheter	7(41%)	23 (74%)	4.107	1.168—14.436	*0.024*
stomach tube	14(82%)	27 (87%)	1.446	0.283—7.384	0.656
Intrathoracic drain	0(0)	4 (13%)	0.614	0.485—0.776	0.282
Abdominal cavity drainage-tube	5(29%)	15 (48%)	2.250	0.639—7.923	0.202
External ventricular drainage tube care	0(0)	1 (3%)	0.612	0.490—0.765	1
Liver function on admission	5(35%)	3 (10%)	0.257	0.053—1.252	*0.079*
Renal function on admission	7(41%)	4(13%)	0.275	0.071—1.070	*0.055*
APACHE II score on admission	12.29 ± 7.32	9.45 ± 4.60			0.334

Abbreviations: CSKp carbapenem-susceptible *Klebsiella pneumoniae, CRKp* carbapenem-resistant *Klebsiella pneumoniae, OR* odds ratio, *CI* confidence interval, *HIV* human immunodeficiency virus, *APACHE* Acute Physiology and Chronic Health Evaluation

[a]History of surgery and non-invasive procedures, such as endoscopy or colonoscopy, are excluded from this category

[b]Immunosuppressors: Immunosuppressive drugs, immunosuppressive agents or antirejection medications are drugs that inhibit or prevent activity of the immune system, including cytostatics, antibodies, drugs acting on immunophilins, etc. (https://en.wikipedia.org/wiki/Immunosuppressive_drug)

Table 4 Multivariate analysis of risk factors for CRKp BSI

Variable	Adjusted OR	95% CI	*P*-value
Indwelling central venous catheters	14.343	1.063—193.444	0.045
Exposure to meropenem	11.968	0.756—69.720	0.086
Exposure to imipenem	7.258	0.945—151.497	0.055

Abbreviations: *OR* odds ratio, *CI* confidence interval

of exposure to antibiotics, or different drug-treatment populations among these studies may account for the divergent findings.

In terms of invasive procedures, only an indwelling central venous catheter and urinary catheter were associated with CRKp BSI in univariate analyses. In the multivariate analysis, an indwelling central venous catheter was the only factor independently associated with CRKp BSI, partly consisted with the past studies [35, 36]. However, previous studies indicated that other variables, such as mechanical ventilation and a nasogastric tube, were related to CRKp BSI [36–38].

Liver and kidney function indices at admission were higher in the CSKp group than in the CRKp group in this study, similar to some previous studies [15, 39]. However, reduced liver and kidney function was not associated with CRKp BSIs.

To improve outcomes, and where there is a need to avoid unnecessary antibiotics so as to reduce CRKp emergence, greater efforts should be made to ensure that initial appropriate antibiotic therapy is delivered to

Table 5 Univariate analysis of the 28-day mortality rate of *K. pneumoniae* BSI patients in the ICU

Variable	Died (n = 21)	Survived (n = 27)	Univariate analysis		
			P	OR	95% CI
Sex (male, n)					
Age (y) (mean ± SD)	57.74 ± 16.63	61.57 ± 13.69	0.448		
APACHE II score at admission	11.50 ± 5.53	10.07 ± 4.95	0.406		
APACHE II score on the day of bacteremia	18.29 ± 7.36	14.48 ± 6.11	0.031		
Liver failure[a] at admission	7	8	0.784	1.188	0.348—4.051
Kidney failure[b] at Admission	4	7	0.574	0.672	0.168—2.694
Liver failure on the day of bacteremia	11	7	0.06	3.143	0.933—10.584
Kidney failure on the day of bacteremia	6	6	0.614	1.400	0.377—5.195
Co-infection	14	20	0.575	0.700	0.2—2.445
CRKp	12(57.1%)	19(70.3%)	0.342	0.561	0.170—1.856
Diabetes mellitus	5(23.8%)	9(23.3%)	0.371	0.556	0.152—2.027
Hypertension	10(47.6%)	14(51.9%)	0.771	0.844	0.270—2.644
Coronary heart disease	2(9.5%)	2(7.4%)	0.792	1.316	0.170—10.208
Chronic renal failure	2(9.5%)	4(14.8%)	0.582	0.605	0.1—3.672
Solid organ tumor	4(19%)	7(25.9%)	0.574	0.672	0.168—2.694
Surgery in the past medical history	2(9.5%)	6(22.2%)	0.242	0.368	0.066—2.050
Prior healthcare-associated exposure	8(38.1%)	8(29.6%)	0.537	1.462	0.437—4.889
Glucocorticoid	8	12	0.658	0.769	0.240—2.460
Immunosuppressor	2(9.5%)	1(3.7%)	0.409	2.737	0.231—32.430
Central venous catheterization	17(81%)	23(85.2%)	0.696	0.739	0.161—3.383
Trachea cannula	9(42.9%)	5(18.5%)	0.066	3.3	0.899—12.108
Tracheotomy	6(27.3%)	11(40.7%)	0.325	0.545	0.162—1.833
Urinary catheter	13(61.9%)	17(16.9%)	0.940	0.956	0.295—3.102
Abdominal cavity drainage- tube	6(28.6%)	14(51.9%)	0.105	0.371	0.111—1.247
Stomach tube	18(85.7%)	23(85.2%)	0.959	1.043	0.305—0.593
Intrathoracic drain	0	4(14.8%)	0.121	0.523	0.394—0.693
External ventricular drainage tube care	1(4.7%)	0	0.438	0.426	0.305—0.593

Abbreviations: *OR* odds ratio, *CI* confidence interval, *CRKp* carbapenem-resistant *Klebsiella pneumoniae*

[a]Liver failure was defined as a serum bilirubin level of >3 mg/dl and/or prothrombin time (PT) of <50% on day 5 after surgery or thereafter; in patients with jaundice, it was defined as an increase in the serum bilirubin level or a PT < 50% on day 5 or thereafter [49]

[b]Kidney failure was defined as a creatinine level of ≥2 mg/dl or requirement for dialysis [33]

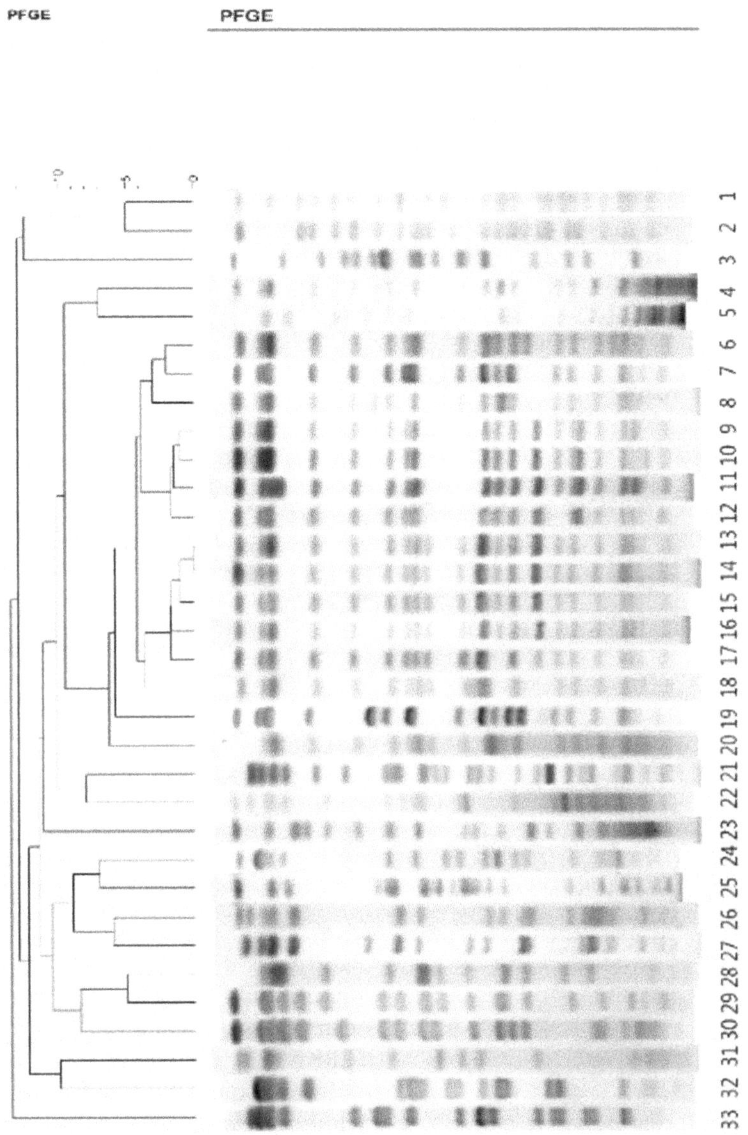

Fig. 1 Pulsed-field gel electrophoresis (PFGE) results. Pulsotypes of 33 *K. pneumoniae* blood isolates. The PFGE patterns revealed that the 33 isolates had different origins

critically ill infected patients, and antibiotic de-escalation should be practiced to avoid unnecessary antibiotic exposure [40]. Moreover, control of the infection source is important for reducing the incidence of BSI. Central line (CL)-associated BSIs in ICUs result in increased morbidity and mortality, and are largely preventable; thus, preventive measures for catheter-related infection are important. Such measures can be applied at central line insertion and maintenance. For example, use of maximal sterile barrier precautions and/or avoiding the femoral vein were applied to reduce the risk of central venous catheter-related bloodstream infection. Moreover, use of central lines should be reduced wherever possible, such as by daily assessment of the need for a CL and timely removal of an unnecessary CL [41].

Infection-related mortality involves a number of factors, including host defense, virulence of the pathogen, source location and control, and the efficacy of available antimicrobials. A recent meta-analysis showed that patients with CRKp had a significantly higher mortality rate than those with CSKp (42.14 vs. 21.12, $p < 0.001$) [8]; this suggests that antimicrobial resistance is related to mortality. However, severe infections are not necessarily caused by drug-resistant bacteria, i.e., antimicrobial resistance is not linked with infection-induced organ dysfunction or failure, or with mortality,

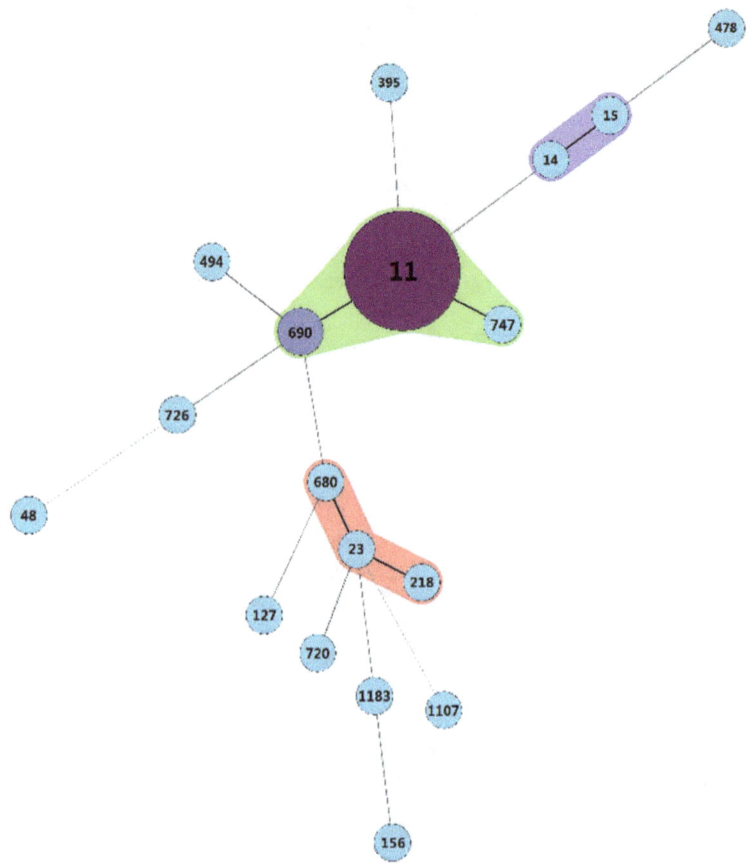

Fig. 2 Multilocus sequence typing (MLST) results. Eighteen sequence types (STs) of 33 *K. pneumoniae* blood isolates. MLST indicated considerable clonal diversity; 18 STs were detected, of which ST11 comprised the majority

Table 6 Frequency rates of bacterial virulence genes in 33 isolates

Variable	CSKp (*n* = 12)	CRKp (n = 21)	P
rmpA2	3	4	0.686
Alls	3	0	0.04
K1	1	0	0.364
K5	0	1	1
magA	4	1	0.047
K1+ magA	1	0	0.364
rmpA2 + magA	1	0	0.364
alls + magA	1	0	0.364
rmpA	0	0	–
K2	0	0	–
K20	0	0	–
K54	0	0	–
K57	0	0	–

Abbreviations: *CSKp* carbapenem-susceptible *Klebsiella pneumoniae*, *CRKp* carbapenem-resistant *Klebsiella pneumoniae*

in critically ill patients. Therefore, the difference in clinical features and risk factors between CSKp and CRKp BSIs is intriguing.

In our study, the CSKp BSI patients had more severe clinical characteristics, such as higher APACHE II scores and lower alanine transaminase (AST) levels. Indeed, the serum creatinine level at the time of the positive culture was significantly higher in the CSKp group than in the CRKp group. However, CSKp BIS patients had only a trend towards a higher mortality rate. Therefore, although CS-Kp infection can lead to worse clinical symptoms, the mortality rate is similar between the two groups, despite there being fewer therapeutic options for CRKp BSI.

The risk factors for mortality due to CSKp and CRKp infection were evaluated in this study. The mortality of *K. pneumoniae* BSI patients was associated with a higher APACHE II score, liver failure, and trachea cannula on the day of bacteremia, but not with carbapenem resistance. In another study, multivariate analyses revealed that carbapenem resistance was not a risk factor for mortality due to *K. pneumoniae* bacteremia [33]. The mortality rate of CRKp patients was significantly higher than that of CSKp patients in that study, which contradicts our findings and those of a study conducted in Israel in 2012 [42]. The risk factors for mortality due to *K. pneumoniae* BSI vary among studies, and include bedridden status, chronic liver disease, Charlson comorbidity index ≥5, mechanical ventilation, hemodialysis [33], and Pitt bacteremia score [42].

PFGE and MLST revealed that the isolates had considerable clonality; the 33 isolates were of different origins. No suspected outbreaks occurred during the study period. We assessed the frequency of 10 virulence genes in the CSKp and CRKp BSI isolates. *magA* is involved in the production of the K1 capsule, which is an important virulence factor [43]. A previous study confirmed local emergence of *K. pneumoniae* invasive syndrome and implicated *magA* and *rmpA* in its pathogenesis [44]. A number of putative virulence factors, including *magA* and *rmpA*, are associated with hypermucoviscous *K. pneumoniae* (hvKP), which can cause serious infections [45, 46]. Alarmingly, multidrug-resistant, including carbapenem-resistant hvKP isolates have emerged [23, 47, 48]; thus, we assessed the frequency rates of various virulence genes in the CRKp and CSKp groups. The frequency rates of *allS* and *magA* were higher in the CSKp group than in the CRKp group, despite the small number of subjects. Therefore, further studies of virulence genes, possibly using whole-genome sequencing (which is becoming less costly and more rapid) and involving larger populations, are warranted.

Our study had several limitations. First, relatively few patients were enrolled, which hampered the multivariate analysis and ability to draw firm conclusions. Second, some *K. pneumoniae* isolates were not stored. Third, the therapeutic regimen for *K. pneumoniae* BSI was not taken into consideration. Fourth, in the ICU setting, a heterogeneous population can limit the statistical analysis. Fifth, the role of the immune system was not analyzed. Despite these limitations, however, we identified several differences between the CRKp and CSKp groups, and explored the impact of carbapenem resistance and bacterial virulence genes on the outcomes of patients with *K. pneumoniae* BSIs.These data can lay the groundwork for future research in this field.

Conclusions

An indwelling central venous catheter is a risk factor for CRKp BIS. Liver and kidney function at admission were lower in the CSKp group than in the CRKp group in this study. The mortality rate and frequency of bacterial virulence genes were similar between the CSKp and CRKp groups. Mortality due to *K. pneumoniae* BSI was not related to carbapenem resistance in univariate analysis. Further study is required to verify the correlation between CRKp-mortality mortality and the virulence genes of *K. pneumoniae* isolates.

Abbreviations

ALT: Alanine transaminase; APACHE II: Acute Physiology and Chronic Health Evaluation; AST: Aspartate transaminase; BSIs: Bloodstream infections; CI: Confidence interval; CL: Central line; CLSI: Clinical and laboratory standards institute; CRE: Carbapenem-resistant Enterobacteriaceae; CRKp: Carbapenem-resistant *K. pneumoniae*; CRP: C-reactive protein; CSKp: Carbapenem-susceptible *K. pneumoniae*; HIV: Human immunodeficiency virus; HR: Hazard ratio; hvKP: Hypermucoviscous *K. pneumoniae*; ICU: Intensive care unit; MLST: Multilocus sequence typing; OR: Odds ratio; PCR: Polymerase chain reaction; PFGE: Pulsed-field gel electrophoresis; PT: Prothrombin time; SIRS: Systemic inflammatory response syndrome; SOFA: Sequential organ failure assessment; ST: Sequence typing; UTIs: Urinary tract infections; UTIs: Urinary tract infections; WBC: White blood cell

Acknowledgments

Not applicable.

Funding

No funding.

Authors' contributions

XZ contributed to the writing of the manuscript; JFW analyzed bacterial virulence genes; WX analyzed and interpreted the clinical data; JX analyzed the antimicrobial susceptibility results; JH performed the statistical analysis; all authors read and approved the final manuscript.

Consent for publication

Not applicable.

Competing interests

The authors declare that they have no competing interests.

Author details

[1]Intensive Care Unit, The First Affiliated Hospital, College of Medicine, Zhejiang University, 79 Qingchun Road, Hangzhou 310003, People's Republic of China. [2]Department of Respiratory Diseases, The Affiliated Hospital of Hangzhou Normal University, Hangzhou, Zhejiang, No. 126 Wenzhou Road, Hangzhou 310009, People's Republic of China. [3]Intensive Care Unit, Hospital of Zhejiang General Corps of Armed Police Forces, No. 16 Nanhu Road, Jiaxing, 314000 Zhejiang, People's Republic of China.

References

1. Broberg CA, Palacios M, Miller VL. Klebsiella: a long way to go towards understanding this enigmatic jet-setter. F1000prime reports. 2014;6:64.
2. Siu LK, Yeh KM, Lin JC, Fung CP, Chang FY. *Klebsiella pneumoniae* liver abscess: a new invasive syndrome. The Lancet Infectious diseases.2012;12:881–7.
3. Hansen DS, Gottschau A, Kolmos HJ. Epidemiology of Klebsiella bacteraemia: a case control study using Escherichia Coli bacteraemia as control. J Hosp Infect. 1998;38:119–32.
4. Daikos GL, Markogiannakis A, Souli M, Tzouvelekis LS. Bloodstream infections caused by carbapenemase-producing Klebsiella Pneumoniae: a clinical perspective. Expert Rev Anti-Infect Ther. 2012;10:1393–404.
5. Yang Y, Chen J, Lin D, Xu X, Cheng J, Sun C. Prevalence and drug resistance characteristics of carbapenem-resistant Enterobacteriaceae in Hangzhou, China. Front Med. 2017; 10.1007/s11684-017-0529-4.

6. Xu A, Zhuo C, Su DH, Hu FP, Zhu DM, Wang F, Jiang XF, Xu YC, Zhang XJ, Sun ZY, Chen ZJ, Ni YX, Sun JY, Hu ZD, Li J, Zhang ZX, Ji P, Wang CQ, Wang AM, Yang Q, Xu YH, Shen JL, Shan B, Du Y, Zhang H, Kong J, Wei LH, Wu L, Xie Y, Kang M, Hu YJ, Ai XM, Yu YS, Lin J, Huang WX, Jia B, Chu YZ, Tian SF, Han YQ, Guo SF. Changing susceptibility of Klebsiella strains in hospitals across China:data from the CHINET antimicrobial resistance surveillance program, 2005-2014. Chin J Infect Chemother. 2016;16:267–74.
7. Pitout JD, Nordmann P, Poirel L. Carbapenemase-producing Klebsiella Pneumoniae, a key pathogen set for global Nosocomial dominance. Antimicrob Agents Chemother. 2015;59:5873–84.
8. Xu L, Sun X, Ma X. Systematic review and meta-analysis of mortality of patients infected with carbapenem-resistant Klebsiella Pneumoniae. Ann Clin Microbiol Antimicrob. 2017;16:18.
9. Tian L, Tan R, Chen Y, Sun J, Liu J, Qu H, Wang X. Epidemiology of Klebsiella Pneumoniae bloodstream infections in a teaching hospital: factors related to the carbapenem resistance and patient mortality. Antimicrob Resist Infect Control. 2016;5:48.
10. Meatherall BL, Gregson D, Ross T, Pitout JD, Laupland KB. Incidence, risk factors, and outcomes of Klebsiella Pneumoniae bacteremia. Am J Med. 2009;122:866–73.
11. Schwaber MJ, Klarfeld-Lidji S, Navon-Venezia S, Schwartz D, Leavitt A, Carmeli Y. Predictors of carbapenem-resistant Klebsiella Pneumoniae acquisition among hospitalized adults and effect of acquisition on mortality. Antimicrob Agents Chemother. 2008;52:1028–33.
12. Gallagher JC, Kuriakose S, Haynes K, Axelrod P. Case-case-control study of patients with carbapenem-resistant and third-generation-cephalosporin-resistant Klebsiella Pneumoniae bloodstream infections. Antimicrob Agents Chemother. 2014;58:5732–5.
13. Falagas ME, Rafailidis PI, Kofteridis D, Virtzili S, Chelvatzoglou FC, Papaioannou V, Maraki S, Samonis G, Michalopoulos A. Risk factors of carbapenem-resistant Klebsiella pneumoniae infections: a matched case control study. J Antimicrob Chemother. 2007;6.
14. Liu SW, Chang HJ, Chia JH, Kuo AJ, Wu TL, Lee MH. Outcomes and characteristics of ertapenem-nonsusceptible Klebsiella Pneumoniae bacteremia at a university hospital in northern Taiwan: a matched case-control study. J Microbiol Immunol Infect. 2012;45:113–9.
15. Ny P, Nieberg P, Wong-Beringer A. Impact of carbapenem resistance on epidemiology and outcomes of nonbacteremic Klebsiella Pneumoniae infections. Am J Infect Control. 2015;43:1076–80.
16. Giacobbe DR, Del Bono V, Bruzzi P, Corcione S, Giannella M, Marchese A, Magnasco L, Maraolo AE, Pagani N, Saffioti C, Ambretti S, Cardellino CS, Coppo E, De Rosa FG, Viale P, Viscoli C, ISGRI-SITA (Italian Study Group on Resistant Infections of the Società Italiana Terapia Antinfettiva). Previous bloodstream infections due to other pathogens as predictors of carbapenem-resistant Klebsiella Pneumoniae bacteraemia in colonized patients: results from a retrospective multicentre study. Eur J Clin Microbiol Infect Dis. 2017;36:663–9.
17. Mouloudi E, Massa E, Papadopoulos S, Iosifidis E, Roilides I, Theodoridou T, Piperidou M, Orphanou A, Passakiotou M, Imvrios G, Fouzas I, Papanikolaou V, Gritsi-Gerogianni N. Bloodstream infections caused by carbapenemase-producing Klebsiella Pneumoniae among intensive care unit patients after orthotopic liver transplantation: risk factors for infection and impact of resistance on outcomes. Transplant Proc. 2014;46:3216–8.
18. Amit S, Mishali H, Kotlovsky T, Schwaber MJ, Carmeli Y. Bloodstream infections among carriers of carbapenem-resistant Klebsiella Pneumoniae: etiology, incidence and predictors. Clin Microbiol Infec. 2015;21:30–4.
19. Trecarichi EM, Pagano L, Martino B, Candoni A, Di Blasi R, Nadali G, Fianchi L, Delia M, Sica S, Perriello V, Busca A, Aversa F, Fanci R, Melillo L, Lessi F, Del Principe MI, Cattaneo C, Tumbarello M. HaematologicMalignancies associated bloodstream infections surveillance (HEMABIS) registry - Sorveglianza Epidemiologica Infezioni Funginein Emopatie Maligne(SEIFEM) group, Italy. Bloodstream infections caused by Klebsiella Pneumoniae in onco-hematological patients: clinical impact of carbapenem resistance in a multicentre prospective survey. Am J Hematol. 2016;91:1076–81.
20. Cristina ML, Alicino C, Sartini M, Faccio V, Spagnolo AM, Del Bono V, Cassola G, De Mite AM, Crisalli MP, Ottria G, Schinca E, Lo Pinto G, Bottaro LC, Viscoli C, Orsi A, Giacobbe DR, Icardi G, Genoan Klebsiella pneumoniae research group. Epidemiology, management, and outcome of carbapenem-resistant Klebsiella Pneumoniae bloodstream infections in hospitals within the same endemic metropolitan area. J Infect Public Health. 2017; 10.1016/j.jiph.2017.06.003.
21. Naimi TS, LeDell KH, Como-Sabetti K, Borchardt SM, Boxrud DJ, Etienne J, Johnson SK, Vandenesch F, Fridkin S, O'Boyle C, Danila RN, Lynfield R. Comparison of community- and health care-associated methicillin-resistant Staphylococcus Aureus infection. JAMA. 2003;290:2976–84.
22. Vardakas KZ, Matthaiou DK, Falagas ME, Antypa E, Koteli A, Antoniadou E. Characteristics, risk factors and outcomes of carbapenem-resistant Klebsiella Pneumoniae infections in the intensive care unit. J Infect. 2015;70:592–9.
23. Yao B, Xiao X, Wang F, Zhou L, Zhang X, Zhang J. Clinical and molecular characteristics of multi-clone carbapenem-resistant hypervirulent (hypermucoviscous) Klebsiella Pneumoniae isolates in a tertiary hospital in Beijing, China. Int J Infect Dis. 2015;37:107–12.
24. Vasilev K, Reshedko G, Orasan R, Sanchez M, Teras J, Babinchak T, Dukart G, Cooper A, Dartois N, Gandjini H, Orrico R, Ellis-Grosse E; 309 Study Group. A phase 3, open-label, non-comparative study of tigecycline in the treatment of patients with selected serious infections due to resistant gram-negative organisms including Enterobacter species, Acinetobacter Baumannii and Klebsiella Pneumoniae. J Antimicrob Chemother. 2008;62 Suppl 1:i29–40.
25. Li W, Sun G, Yu Y, Li N, Chen M, Jin R, Jiao Y, Wu H. Increasing occurrence of antimicrobial-resistant hypervirulent (hypermucoviscous) Klebsiella Pneumoniae isolates in China. Clin Infect Dis. 2014;58:225–32.
26. Duck WM, Steward CD, Banerjee SN, McGowan JE Jr, Tenover FC. Optimization of computer software settings improves accuracy of pulsed-field gel electrophoresis macrorestriction fragment pattern analysis. J Clin Microbiol. 2003;41:3035–42.
27. Endimiani A, Depasquale JM, Forero S, Perez F, Hujer AM, Roberts-Pollack D, Fiorella PD, Pickens N, Kitchel B, Casiano-Colón AE, Tenover FC, Bonomo RA. Emergence of blaKPC-containing Klebsiella Pneumoniae in a long-term acute care hospital: a new challenge to our healthcare system. J Antimicrob Chemother. 2009;64:1102–10.
28. Cristina ML, Sartini M, Ottria G, Schinca E, Cenderello N, Crisalli MP, Fabbri P, Lo Pinto G, Usiglio D, Spagnolo AM. Epidemiology and biomolecular characterization of carbapenem-resistant klebsiella pneumoniae in an Italian hospital. J Prev Med Hyg. 2016;57:E149–E56.
29. Raz-Pasteur A, Hussein K, Finkelstein R, Ullmann Y, Egozi D. Blood stream infections (BSI) in severe burn patients–early and late BSI: a 9-year study. Burns. 2013;39:636–42.
30. Delle Rose D, Sordillo P, Gini S, Cerva C, Boros S, Rezza G, Meledandri M, Gallo MT, Prignano G, Caccese R, D'Ambrosio M, Citterio G, Rocco M, Leonardis F, Natoli S, Fontana C, Favaro M, Celeste MG, Franci T, Testore GP, Andreoni M, Sarmati L. Microbiologic characteristics and predictors of mortality in bloodstream infections in intensive care unit patients: A 1-year, large, prospective surveillance study in 5 Italian hospitals. Am J Infect Control. 2015;43:1178–83.
31. Tabah A, Koulenti D, Laupland K, Misset B, Valles J, Bruzzi de Carvalho F, Paiva JA, Cakar N, Ma X, Eggimann P, Antonelli M, Bonten MJ, Csomos A, Krueger WA, Mikstacki A, Lipman J, Depuydt P, Vesin A, Garrouste-Orgeas M, Zahar JR, Blot S, Carlet J, Brun-Buisson C, Martin C, Rello J, Dimopoulos G, Timsit JF. Characteristics and determinants of outcome of hospital-acquired bloodstream infections in intensive care units: the EUROBACT International Cohort Study. Intensive Care Med. 2012;38:1930–45.
32. Brennan BM, Coyle JR, Marchaim D, Pogue JM, Boehme M, Finks J, Malani AN, VerLee KE, Buckley BO, Mollon N, Sundin DR, Washer LL, Kaye KS. Statewide surveillance of carbapenem-resistant enterobacteriaceae in Michigan. Infect Control Hosp Epidemiol. 2014;35:342–9.
33. Hussein K, Raz-Pasteur A, Finkelstein R, Neuberger A, Shachor-Meyouhas Y, Oren I, Kassis I. Impact of carbapenem resistance on the outcome of patients' hospital-acquired bacteraemia caused by Klebsiella pneumoniae. J Hosp Infect. 2013;83:307–13.
34. Gomez Rueda V, Zuleta Tobon JJ. Risk factors for infection with carbapenem-resistant Klebsiella pneumoniae: a case-case-control study. Colombia medica (Cali, Colombia). 2014;45:54–60.
35. Diaz A, Ortiz DC, Trujillo M, Garces C, Jaimes F, Restrepo AV. Clinical characteristics of carbapenem-resistant Klebsiella pneumoniae infections in Ill and colonized children in Colombia. Pediatr Infect Dis J. 2016;35:237–41.
36. Akgul F, Bozkurt I, Sunbul M, Esen S, Leblebicioglu H. Risk factors and mortality in the carbapenem-resistant Klebsiella pneumoniae infection: case control study. Pathog Global Health. 2016;110:321–5.
37. Candevir Ulu A, Kurtaran B, Inal AS, Komur S, Kibar F, Yapici Cicekdemir H, Bozkurt S, Gürel D, Kılıç F, Yaman A, Aksu HS, Taşova Y. Risk factors of carbapenem-resistant Klebsiella pneumoniae infection: a serious threat in ICUs. Med Sci Monit. 2015;21:219–24.
38. Mills JP, Talati NJ, Alby K, Han JH. The epidemiology of carbapenem-resistant Klebsiella pneumoniae colonization and infection among long-term acute care hospital residents. Infect Control Hosp Epidemiol. 2016;37:55–60.

39. Vardakas KZ, Matthaiou DK, Falagas ME, Antypa E, Koteli A, Antoniadou E. Characteristics, risk factors and outcomes of carbapenem-resistant Klebsiella pneumoniae infections in the intensive care unit. J Infec. 2015;70:592–9.
40. Markley JD, Bernard S, Bearman G, Stevens MP. De-escalating antibiotic use in the inpatient setting: strategies, controversies, and challenges. Curr Infect Dis Rep. 2017;19.
41. Valencia C, Hammami N, Agodi A, Lepape A, Herrejon EP, Blot S, et al. Poor adherence to guidelines for preventing central line-associated bloodstream infections (CLABSI): results of a worldwide survey. Antimicrob Resist Infect. 2016;5:49.
42. Ben-David D, Kordevani R, Keller N, Tal I, Marzel A, Gal-Mor O, Maor Y, Rahav G. Outcome of carbapenem resistant Klebsiella pneumoniae bloodstream infections. Clin Microbiol Infec. 2012;18:54–60.
43. Yeh KM, Chang FY, Fung CP, Lin JC, Siu LK. magA is not a specific virulence gene for Klebsiella pneumoniae strains causing liver abscess but is part of the capsular polysaccharide gene cluster of K. pneumoniae serotype K1. J Med Microbiol. 2006;55:803–4.
44. Chang L, Bastian I, Warner M. Survey of Klebsiella pneumoniae bacteraemia in two South Australian hospitals and detection of hypermucoviscous phenotype and magA/rmpA genotypes in K. pneumoniae isolates. Infection. 2013;41:559–63.
45. Fang CT, Chuang YP, Shun CT, Chang SC, Wang JT. A novel virulence gene in Klebsiella pneumoniae strains causing primary liver abscess and septic metastatic complications. J Exp Med. 2004;199:697–705.
46. Yu WL, Ko WC, Cheng KC, Lee HC, Ke DS, Lee CC, Fung CP, Chuang YC. Association between rmpA and magA genes and clinical syndromes caused by Klebsiella pneumoniae in Taiwan. Clin Infect Dis. 2006;42:1351–8.
47. Yang Z, Liu W, Cui Q, Niu W, Li H, Zhao X, Wei X, Wang X, Huang S, Dong D, Lu S, Bai C, Li Y, Huang L, Yuan J. Prevalence and detection of Stenotrophomonas maltophilia carrying metallo-beta-lactamase blaL1 in Beijing, China. Front Microbiol. 2014;5:692.
48. Zhang Y, Zeng J, Liu W, Zhao F, Hu Z, Zhao C, Wang Q, Wang X, Chen H, Li H, Zhang F, Li S, Cao B, Wang H. Emergence of a hypervirulent carbapenem-resistant Klebsiella pneumoniae isolate from clinical infections in China. J Infect. 2015;71:553–60.
49. Capussotti L, Vigano L, Giuliante F, Ferrero A, Giovannini I, Nuzzo G. Liver dysfunction and sepsis determine operative mortality after liver resection. Br J Surg. 2009;96:88–94.

Evaluation of automated systems for aminoglycosides and fluoroquinolones susceptibility testing for Carbapenem-resistant *Enterobacteriaceae*

Zhichang Zhao[1†], Fangjun Lan[2†], Maobai Liu[1], Weiyuan Chen[3], Liya Huang[3], Qili Lin[3] and Bin Li[2*]

Abstract

Background: Automated systems (MicroScan WalkAway 96 Plus, Phoenix 100, and Vitek 2 Compact) are widely used in clinical laboratories nowadays. The aim of this study is to evaluate the performance of these three systems for susceptibility testing of aminoglycosides and fluoroquinolones against Carbapenem-resistant *Enterobacteriaceae* (CRE).

Methods: A total of 75 CRE isolates were used in this study. Quinolone resistance determinants (QRDs) (*qnrA*, *qnrB*, *qnrC*, *qnrD*, *qnrS*, *aac(6')-Ib-cr*, *oqxAB* and *qepA*) and aminoglycoside resistance determinants (ARDs) (*aac(6')-Ib*, *armA*, *npmA*, *rmtA*, *rmtB*, *rmtC*, *rmtD* and *rmtE*) of these CRE were screened by PCR. The MICs of aminoglycosides (gentamicin and amikacin) and fluoroquinolones (ciprofloxacin and levofloxacin) to CRE obtained with the automated systems were compared with the reference method (agar dilution method).

Results: Totally, 97.3% (73/75) of CRE harbored QRDs. The *qnr* gene was the most common QRD determinant identified in 68 (96.7%), followed by *aac (6')-Ib-cr* in 56 (74.7%), *oqxAB* in 23 (30.7%), and *qepA* in 2 (2.7%), respectively. 22.7% (17/75) of CRE harbored ARD determinants. *rmtA*, *rmtB* and *npmA* were identified among these isolates in 6 (8.0%), 6 (8.0%) and 5 (6.7%), respectively. A total of 900 results were obtained in this study. Overall, the total error rate was 9.89%. Twenty-eight very major errors (3.11%), 22 major errors (2.44%) and 39 minor errors (4.33%) were identified against agar dilution method. The very major errors were almost evenly distributed between results for fluoroquinolones (2.89%) and aminoglycosides (3.33%), while the major errors and minor errors were more commonly found in the results of fluoroquinolones (3.11% and 6.44%, respectively) than aminoglycosides (1.78% and 2.22%, respectively).

Conclusions: Our study shows that testing difficulties in susceptibility testing do exist in automated systems. We suggest clinical laboratories using automated systems should consider using a second, independent antimicrobial susceptibility testing method to validate aminoglycosides and fluoroquinolones susceptibility.

Keywords: Automated identification systems, Carbapenem-resistant *Enterobacteriaceae*, Aminoglycosides, Fluoroquinolones

* Correspondence: leonlee307@hotmail.com
†Equal contributors
[2]Department of Clinical Laboratory, Fujian Medical University Union Hospital, 29 Xinquan Rd, Fuzhou, Fujian 350001, People's Republic of China
Full list of author information is available at the end of the article

Background

Carbapenem-resistant *Enterobacteriaceae* (CRE) has spread throughout the world nowadays [1–3]. CRE usually show high levels of resistance to many types of antibiotics. Infections caused by CRE will pose a serious threat to patients for the limited therapeutic options. Therefore, CRE infections are always associated with poor outcomes and high mortality rate at the present time [4–6]. The most optimal treatment options for CRE infections have not been well defined. Current treatment options include the use of some older agents either in monotherapy or in combination therapy, such as aminoglycosides and fluoroquinolones [7, 8]. Aminoglycosides and fluoroquinolones are two different important types of antimicrobial agents for the treatment of life-threatening bacterial infections. Aminoglycosides have demonstrated in vitro activity against CRE, and are often used as part of combination regimens [9, 10]. While fluoroquinolones are sometimes used to combat urinary tract infection caused by CRE [11].

The task of clinical laboratories and microbiologists to perform proper antimicrobial susceptibility test and interpretation constitutes an important initial step in implementing appropriate treatments and antibiotic use policies [12]. In this regard, the accuracy of different antimicrobial susceptibility testing methods may allow physicians to prescribe safe and effective antibiotics to treat infections. Automated systems have been used widely in many clinical laboratories for species identification of the pathogens and susceptibility testing. These systems could decrease the labor and save time compared to those for standardized methods. But probable errors reported by automated systems maybe have serious implications for the clinical outcome for patients with multiple drug resistant bacteria infections, such as CRE infections. Unfortunately, there is no information on the accuracy of these systems in detecting the susceptibility to aminoglycosides and fluoroquinolones with CRE currently.

In China, according to the CHINET report, the incidence of CRE has increased remarkably in the last 10 years [13]. In most Chinese hospitals, the susceptilbility of CRE to aminoglycosides and fluoroquinolones are detected using automated systems. Phoenix 100, Vitek-2 Compact and MicroScan WalkAway 96 Plus are the most common automated identification systems currently used in our country. The aim of the present study was to assess the performance of three automated instruments for the susceptibility testing of aminoglycosides and fluoroquinolones against CRE isolates.

Methods

Clinical isolates

A total of 75 carbapenem-resistant *Enterobacteriaceae* were included in this study. They were collected at Fujian Medical University Union Hospital in Fuzhou, China, and some were reported previously [14].

Antimicrobial susceptibility tests

Aminoglycosides (gentamicin and amikacin) and fluoroquinolones (ciprofloxacin and levofloxacin) susceptibility tests were conducted simultaneously following the manufacturers' instructions using the three different automated systems: MicroScan WalkAway 96 Plus (SIEMENS AG FWB, Germany) with NC 50 cards, Phoenix 100 (Becton, Dickinson and Company, USA) with NMIC/ID-4 panels and Vitek-2 Compact (Bio Mérieux, France) with AST-GN16 cards. All the assays were accomplished in the research laboratory of Fujian Medical University Union Hospital, China. The susceptibility breakpoints of the three commercial systems were interpreted as recommended by the Clinical and Laboratory Standards Institute(CLSI) [15]. Reference MIC values for the tested isolates were determined by agar dilution method with Mueller-Hinton agar according to CLSI guidelines [15]. *E. coli* ATCC25922 was used as quality control strain.

Detection of quinolone resistance determinants (QRDs) and aminoglycoside resistance determinants (ARDs)

In this study, QRDs refer to plasmid mediated quinolone resistance genes. All the 75 CRE were screened for the presence of QRDs (*qnrA*, *qnrB*, *qnrC*, *qnrD*, *qnrS*, *aac(6')-Ib-cr*, *oqxAB* and *qepA*) and ARDs (*aac(6')-Ib*, *armA*, *npmA*, *rmtA*, *rmtB*, *rmtC*, *rmtD* and *rmtE*) with PCR using primers as previously described [16, 17]. PCR products were purified and sequenced on an ABI PRISM 3730 automated sequencer (Applied Biosystems, Foster City, USA).

Evaluation of concordance among methods

The results were analyzed by using the standard agar dilution method as the reference method. Categorical agreement was defined as a result from any of the three automated system methods that belonged to the same interpretive category (i.e., susceptible, intermediate, or resistant) as that determined with the standard agar microdilution method. Essential agreement was defined as when the same MIC values (within ±1 dilution) were obtained by the automated systems and the reference method. In this study, when both MIC values obtained with automated systems and reference method were under or over the limit concentrations in the automated system, these results were considered to "agreement". A "very major error" was defined as a result in the susceptible category when an organism was considered resistant by the reference method, but susceptible by the test method. A "major error" was defined when an organism considered susceptible by the reference method was resistant by the test method. A "minor error" was defined when an organism was considered susceptible or resistant either by the reference or the test method, while intermediate by the other method. All tests showing very major errors or major errors were repeated in duplicate by both reference and test methods.

Results

Prevalence of the QRDs and ARDs among CRE

In total, 97.3% (73/75) of CRE harbored QRDs. The *qnr* gene was the most common QRD determinant identified in 68 (96.7%), followed by *aac (6')-Ib-cr* in 56 (74.7%), *oqxAB* in 23 (30.7%), and *qepA* in 2 (2.7%), respectively. Among the 68 *qnr* positive CRE, *qnrA*, *qnrB*, *qnrS* was detected in 64 (94.1%), 17 (25.0%), and 9 (13.2%), respectively. *qnrC* and *qnrD* were not found in this study (Table 1).

22.7% (17/75) of CRE harbored ARD determinants. *rmtA*, *rmtB* and *npmA* were identified among these isolates in 6 (8.0%), 6 (8.0%) and 5 (6.7%), respectively. A*ac(6')-Ib*, *armA*, *npmA*, *rmtC*, *rmtD* and *rmtE* were not detected in the present study.

Resistance rates with reference agar dilution method

Generally, based on the agar dilution method, the rates of resistance of CRE to CIP, LEV, GEN and AMK were 53.3% (40/75), 37.3% (28/75), 81.3% (61/75) and 14.7% (11/75), respectively (Table 2). The MIC ranges were 0.125–512 μg/ml for CIP, 0.125–128 μg/ml for LEV, 1–512 μg/ml for GEN and 1–512 μg/ml for AMK. The MIC_{50} was 8 μg/ml for CIP, 2 μg/ml for LEV, 128 μg/ml for GEN and 8 μg/ml for AMK.

Performance on susceptibility of three automatic systems

A total of 900 results were obtained in this study, corresponding to 300 for Phoenix, 300 for WalkAway and 300 for Vitek. Overall, the total error rate was 9.89% (89/900).

Twenty-eight very major errors (3.11%), 22 major errors (2.44%) and 39 minor errors (4.33%) were identified in this study against agar dilution method (Table 3). The very major errors were almost evenly distributed between results for fluoroquinolones (2.89%) and aminoglycosides (3.33%), while the major errors and minor errors were more commonly found in the results of quinolones (3.11% and 6.44%, respectively) than aminoglycosides (1.78% and 2.22%, respectively). Very major errors were 3.67% of the total number of results for Vitek-2, 2.33% for BD Phonix and 3.33% for WalkAway. Major errors were 2.67% for Vitek-2, 2.00% for BD Phonix and 2.67% for WalkAway. Finally, minor errors were 6.00% for Vitek-2, 4.00% for BD Phonix and 3.00% for WalkAway. As to fluoroquinolones, most of the minor errors were susceptible findings interpreted as in intermediate, and resistance results interpreted as intermediate. The agreement in clinical categories was only

Table 1 Seventy five carbapenem-resistant *Enterobacteriaceae* isolates containing QDRs and ADRs that were detected in this study

Species (no. of isolates)	QDRs and ADRs expressed	No. of isolates
Escherichia coli (18)	*qnrA*	2
	qnrA + oqxB	1
	aac(6')-Ib-cr + qnrA	6
	aac(6')-Ib-cr + qnrB	1
	aac(6')-Ib-cr + NPMA	2
	aac(6')-Ib-cr + qnrA + RmtB	2
	aac(6')-Ib-cr + qnrA + NPMA	3
	oqxB + qnrA	1
Enterobacter cloacae (20)	*aac(6')-Ib-cr + qnrA + qnrB*	9
	aac(6')-Ib-cr + qnrA + qnrB + qnrS	1
	aac(6')-Ib-cr + qnrB + qnrS	1
	aac(6')-Ib-cr + qnrA + oqxB + oqxA+ RmtA	1
	aac(6')-Ib-cr + qnrA	2
	aac(6')-Ib-cr + qnrA + qepA	1
	aac(6')-Ib-cr	2
	qnrA	2
	aac(6')-Ib-cr + qnrA + qnrS	1
Klebsiella pneumoniae (31)	*qnrA*	3
	qnrA + RmtB	1
	qnrA + RmtA	2
	qnrA + qnrB + oqxA + oqxB	1
	qnrA + oqxA+ RmtA	1
	qnrA + qnrS + oqxB	1
	qnrA + qnrS + oqxA + oqxB + RmtA	1
	aac(6')-Ib-cr + qnrA	1
	aac(6')-Ib-cr + qnrA + oqxA	1
	aac(6')-Ib-cr + qnrA + oqxB	3
	aac(6')-Ib-cr + qnrA + qepA	1
	aac(6')-Ib-cr + qnrA + qnrS + oqxB	1
	aac(6')-Ib-cr + qnrA + oqxA + oqxB	8
	aac(6')-Ib-cr + qnrA + qnrS+ oqxA + oqxB	1
	aac(6')-Ib-cr + qnrA + qnrB + oqxB+ RmtA	1
	aac(6')-Ib-cr + qnrA + qnrB + qnrS + oqxB + oqxA + RmtA	1
	aac(6')-Ib-cr + qnrA + oqxB + oqxA + NPMA	1
	aac(6')-Ib-cr + oqxB+ oqxA	1
	oqxA + oqxB	1
Klebsiella oxytoca (4)	*aac(6')-Ib-cr + qnrA*	3
	aac(6')-Ib-cr + qnrB+ qnrS	1
Enterobacter aerogenes (1)	*aac(6')-Ib-cr + qnrB + qnrS*	1

Table 2 Susceptibility of CRE based on testing methods in this study (N = 75)

Testing method[a]	Testing results (%, [no. of strains])											
	CIP			LEV			GEN			AMK		
	S	I	R	S	I	R	S	I	R	S	I	R
ADM	37.3% (28)	9.3% (7)	53.3% (40)	52.0% (39)	10.7% (8)	37.3% (28)	17.3% (13)	1.3% (1)	81.3% (61)	74.7% (56)	10.7% (8)	14.7%(11)
Vitek-2	40.0% (30)	8.0% (6)	52.0% (39)	52.0% (39)	1.3% (1)	46.7% (35)	20.0% (15)	2.7% (2)	77.3% (58)	86.7% (65)	0	13.3%(10)
Phoenix	33.3% (25)	8.0% (6)	53.3% (40)	42.7% (32)	8.0% (6)	48.0% (36)	18.7% (14)	4.0% (3)	77.3% (58)	84.0% (63)	1.3% (1)	14.7% (11)
Microscan	29.3% (22)	8.0% (6)	62.7% (47)	45.3% (34)	6.7% (5)	48.0% (36)	22.7% (17)	4.0% (3)	73.3% (55)	80.0% (60)	5.3% (4)	14.7% (11)

[a]ADM, agar dilution method

76.0 to 85.4% for CIP and LEV. While as to aminoglycosides, most of the minor errors were resistance results interpreted as intermediate, or susceptible findings interpreted as in intermediate. The agreement in clinical categories was 86.7 to 92.0% for GEN and AMK.

Discussion

CRE have become to one of the most difficult-to-treat pathogens for nosocomial infections due to the lack of treatment options [18, 19]. CRE are usually resistant to many commonly prescribed antimicrobials but may still remain susceptible to one or more antibiotics [20]. Aminoglycosides and fluoroquinolones are sometimes used as a choice to combat CRE infections currently [21, 22]. In China, automated systems are widely used nowadays not only in identification of bacteria, but to perform the antimicrobial susceptibility test as a routine in clinical microbiology laboratory. The present study was conducted to evaluate the performance of automated systems for the susceptibility testing on the two types of antibiotics (aminoglycosides and fluoroquinolones).

In this study, we found that QRD and ARD determinants were widely disseminated among CRE, which were similar to previous studies (Table 1) [23–26]. The resistance rates to fluoroquinolones were about 50% (53.3% to CIP and 37.3% to LEV) based on the reference method, which was lower that in previous larger surveillance data from China [27]. The discrepancy probably due to the detection methods used in the previous study. In this study, the automated systems gave similar resistance rates to CIP, while the resistance rates to LEV were higher obtained with automated systems than that got from reference method. Meanwhile, the resistance rates to aminoglycosides vary with the specific drug (81.7% to GEN and 14.7% to AMK) based on the reference method, which were in line with many previous studies [24, 27]. In this study, the automated systems gave similar resistance rates to both GEN and AMK compared with the reference method.

Previous studies showed that automated systems were thought to be reliable for antibiotic susceptibility test, including aminoglycosides and fluoroquinolones [28, 29]. However, according to the US FDA's recommendation, the performance of susceptibility tests is considered adequate when the total error rate is <10%, with ≤1.5% of errors being very major errors and ≤3.0% being major errors, and when the overall essential MIC agreement is >90% [30]. Taking these values as a reference, the three automated systems cannot be considered reliable for susceptibility testing of aminoglycosides and

Table 3 Summary of the results on CRE obtained with automated methods compared to the results with reference method

Antibiotics	System (concns in mg/l)	% agreement in clinical categories	% essential agreement	No. of errors of different types (%)		
				Very major	Major	Minor
CIP	WalkAway (0.12, 1, 2)	76.0	81.3	2 (0.2)	4 (0.4)	4 (0.4)
	BD Phoenix (0.12, 0.25,0.5, 1,2)	80.0	88.0	2 (0.2)	1 (0.1)	4 (0.4)
	Vitek-2 (0.25, 0.5,1, 2, 4)	85.4	84.0	3 (0.3)	2 (0.2)	7 (0.8)
LEV	Walkaway (4, 8)	78.7	86.7	2 (0.2)	2 (0.2)	3 (0.3)
	BD Phoenix (2, 4, 8)	77.3	84.0	1 (0.1)	2 (0.2)	4 (0.4)
	Vitek-2 (1, 2,4, 8, 16)	81.3	81.3	3 (0.3)	3 (0.3)	7 (0.8)
GEN	Walkaway (4, 8)	86.7	89.3	5 (0.6)	1 (0.1)	2 (0.2)
	BD Phoenix (2, 4, 8)	90.7	90.7	3 (0.3)	2 (0.2)	3 (0.3)
	Vitek-2 (1, 2,4, 8, 16)	89.3	90.7	3 (0.3)	2 (0.2)	3 (0.3)
AMK	Walkaway (8, 16, 32)	92.0	94.7	1 (0.1)	1 (0.1)	0
	BD Phoenix (8, 16, 32)	90.7	89.3	1 (0.1)	1 (0.1)	1 (0.1)
	Vitek-2 (8, 16, 32)	88.0	84.0	2 (0.2)	1 (0.1)	1 (0.1)

fluoroquinolones against CRE in our study for the high very major error rate and overall essential MIC agreement (Table 3).

Our study has several limitations. The study was carried out at a single research laboratory. To reduce biases, the measurements were performed in biological duplicates by blinded researchers on different days. Another limitation was the relatively small sample size. For this reason, we were unable to obtain comprehensive evaluation of the three automated systems for aminoglycoside and fluoroquinolones susceptibility testing for CRE. Lastly, only one reference method was chosen in this study. More accurate methods (such as broth dilution method, E-test) should be used to confirm the AST results.

Conclusions

This is the first study assessing the accuracy of automated systems in detecting the susceptibility of aminoglycosides and fluoroquinolones to CRE. Our limited study suggests that testing difficulties in susceptibility testing do exist in automated systems. These findings warn us that reporting errors could result in serious implications for the clinical outcome for patients. We suggest clinical laboratories using automated systems should consider using a second, independent antimicrobial susceptibility testing method to validate aminoglycosides and fluoroquinolones susceptibility.

Abbreviations

ARDs: Aminoglycoside resistance determinant; CRE: Carbapenem resistant *Enterobacteriaceae*; MIC: Minimum inhibitory concentration; QRDs: Quinolone resistance determinants

Acknowledgements

Not applicable.

Funding

This study was supported by the Fujian Provincial Funds for Distinguished Young Scientists in Colleges and Universities, China (grant no. JA13134), and the Medical Elite Cultivation Program of Fujian, China (grant no. 2015-ZQN-ZD-15).

Authors' contributions

BL designed the experiment and wrote the manuscript. ZZ, WC, LH and QL performed the experiments. FL and ML participated in data analysis and review of the draft manuscript. All authors read and approved the final manuscript.

Consent for publication

Not applicable.

Competing interests

The authors declare that they have no competing interests.

Author details

[1]Department of Pharmacy, Fujian Medical University Union Hospital, Fuzhou, Fujian 350001, China. [2]Department of Clinical Laboratory, Fujian Medical University Union Hospital, 29 Xinquan Rd, Fuzhou, Fujian 350001, People's Republic of China. [3]Medical Technology and Engineering College, Fujian Medical University, Fuzhou 350004, Fujian, People's Republic of China.

References

1. Chea N, Bulens SN, Kongphet-Tran T, Lynfield R, Shaw KM, Vagnone PS, et al. Improved phenotype-based definition for identifying Carbapenemase producers among Carbapenem-resistant Enterobacteriaceae. Emerg Infect Dis. 2015;21:1611–6.
2. Potter RF, D'Souza AW, Dantas G. The rapid spread of carbapenem-resistant Enterobacteriaceae. Drug Resist Updat. 2016;29:30–46.
3. Logan LK, Weinstein RA. The epidemiology of Carbapenem-resistant Enterobacteriaceae: the impact and evolution of a global menace. J Infect Dis. 2017;215:S28–36.
4. Esterly JS, Wagner J, McLaughlin MM, Postelnick MJ, Qi C, Scheetz MH. Evaluation of clinical outcomes in patients with bloodstream infections due to gram-negative bacteria according to carbapenem MIC stratification. Antimicrob Agents Chemother. 2012;56:4885–90.
5. Skurnik D, Roux D, Pons S, Guillard T, Lu X, Cywes-Bentley C, et al. Extended-spectrum antibodies protective against carbapenemase-producing Enterobacteriaceae. J Antimicrob Chemother. 2016;71:927–35.
6. Friedman ND, Carmeli Y, Walton AL, Schwaber MJ. Carbapenem-resistant Enterobacteriaceae: a strategic roadmap for infection control. Infect Control Hosp Epidemiol. 2017;38:580–94.
7. Morrill HJ, Pogue JM, Kaye KS, KL LP. Treatment options for Carbapenem-resistant Enterobacteriaceae infections. Open Forum Infect Dis. 2015;2: ofv050.
8. Ni W, Wei C, Zhou C, Zhao J, Liang B, Cui J, Wang R, et al. Tigecycline-Amikacin combination effectively suppresses the selection of resistance in clinical isolates of KPC-producing Klebsiella Pneumoniae. Front Microbiol. 2016;7:1304.
9. van Duin D, Kaye KS, Neuner EA, Bonomo RA. Carbapenem-resistant Enterobacteriaceae: a review of treatment and outcomes. Diagn Microbiol Infect Dis. 2013;75:115–20.
10. Perez F, El Chakhtoura NG, Papp-Wallace KM, Wilson BM, Bonomo RA. Treatment options for infections caused by carbapenem-resistant Enterobacteriaceae: can we apply "precision medicine" to antimicrobial chemotherapy? Expert Opin Pharmacother. 2016;17:761–81.
11. Hsu AJ, Tamma PD. Treatment of multidrug-resistant gram-negative infections in children. Clin Infect Dis. 2014;58:1439–48.
12. Paterson DL. Impact of antibiotic resistance in gram-negative bacilli on empirical and definitive antibiotic therapy. Clin Infect Dis. 2008;47:S14–20.
13. Hu FP, Guo Y, Zhu DM, Wang F, Jiang XF, Xu YC, et al. Resistance trends among clinical isolates in China reported from CHINET surveillance of bacterial resistance, 2005-2014. Clin Microbiol Infect. 2016;22(Suppl 1):S9–14.
14. He Q, Chen W, Huang L, Lin Q, Zhang J, Liu R, et al. Performance evaluation of three automated identification systems in detecting carbapenem-resistant Enterobacteriaceae. Ann Clin Microbiol Antimicrob. 2016;15:40.
15. CLSI. Performance Standards for Antimicrobial Susceptibility Testing. 27th ed. CLSI supplement M100. Wayne, PA: Clinical and Laboratory Standards Institute; 2017.
16. Doi Y, Arakawa Y. 16S ribosomal RNA methylation: emerging resistance mechanism against aminoglycosides. Clin Infect Dis. 2007;45:88–94.
17. Chen X, Zhang W, Pan W, Yin J, Pan Z, Gao S, et al. Prevalence of qnr, aac(6')-Ib-cr, qepA, and oqxAB in Escherichia Coli isolates from humans, animals, and the environment. Antimicrob Agents Chemother. 2012;56:3423–7.
18. Wang Q, Zhang Y, Yao X, Xian H, Liu Y, Li H, et al. Risk factors and clinical outcomes for carbapenem-resistant Enterobacteriaceae nosocomial infections. Eur J Clin Microbiol Infect Dis. 2016;35:1679–89.
19. Vergara-Lopez S, Dominguez MC, Conejo MC, Pascual A, Rodriguez-Bano J. Lessons from an outbreak of metallo-beta-lactamase-producing Klebsiella oxytoca in an intensive care unit: the importance of time at risk and combination therapy. J Hosp Infect. 2015;89:123–31.
20. Trecarichi EM, Tumbarello M. Therapeutic options for carbapenem-resistant Enterobacteriaceae infections. Virulence. 2017;8:470–84.

21. Lesho EP, Clifford RJ, Chukwuma U, Kwak YI, Maneval M, Neumann C, et al. Carbapenem-resistant Enterobacteriaceae and the correlation between carbapenem and fluoroquinolone usage and resistance in the US military health system. Diagn Microbiol Infect Dis. 2015;81:119–25.
22. Zavascki AP, Klee BO, Bulitta JB. Aminoglycosides against carbapenem-resistant Enterobacteriaceae in the critically ill: the pitfalls of aminoglycoside susceptibility. Expert Rev Anti-Infect Ther. 2017;15:519–26.
23. Dai W, Sun S, Yang P, Huang S, Zhang X, Zhang L. Characterization of carbapenemases, extended spectrum beta-lactamases and molecular epidemiology of carbapenem-non-susceptible Enterobacter Cloacae in a Chinese hospital in Chongqing. Infect Genet Evol. 2013;14:1–7.
24. Hu L, Zhong Q, Shang Y, Wang H, Ning C, Li Y, et al. The prevalence of carbapenemase genes and plasmid-mediated quinolone resistance determinants in carbapenem-resistant Enterobacteriaceae from five teaching hospitals in central China. Epidemiol Infect. 2014;142:1972–7.
25. Rahman M, Shukla SK, Prasad KN, Ovejero CM, Pati BK, Tripathi A, et al. Prevalence and molecular characterisation of New Delhi metallo-beta-lactamases NDM-1, NDM-5, NDM-6 and NDM-7 in multidrug-resistant Enterobacteriaceae from India. Int J Antimicrob Agents. 2014;44:30–7.
26. Cheng L, Cao XL, Zhang ZF, Ning MZ, Xu XJ, Zhou W, et al. Clonal dissemination of KPC-2 producing Klebsiella Pneumoniae ST11 clone with high prevalence of oqxAB and rmtB in a tertiary hospital in China: results from a 3-year period. Ann Clin Microbiol Antimicrob. 2016;15:1.
27. Xu A, Zheng B, Xu YC, Huang ZG, Zhong NS, Zhuo C. National epidemiology of carbapenem-resistant and extensively drug-resistant gram-negative bacteria isolated from blood samples in China in 2013. Clin Microbiol Infect. 2016;22:S1–8.
28. Snyder JW, Munier GK, Johnson CL. Direct comparison of the BD phoenix system with the MicroScan WalkAway system for identification and antimicrobial susceptibility testing of Enterobacteriaceae and nonfermentative gram-negative organisms. J Clin Microbiol. 2008;46:2327–33.
29. Calvo J, Cano ME, Pitart C, Marco F, Rodriguez-Martinez JM, Pascual A, et al. Evaluation of three automated systems for susceptibility testing of enterobacteria containing qnrB, qnrS, and/or aac(6')-Ib-cr. J Clin Microbiol. 2011;49:3343–5.
30. U.S.Food and Drug Administration. Class II specail controls guidance document antimicrobial susceptibility test (AST) systems; guidance for industry and FDA. Rockville. MD: U.S. Food and Drug Administration; 2007.

Prevalence and characteristics of ST131 clone among unselected clinical *Escherichia coli* in a Chinese university hospital

Bin Li[1], Yanfang Lu[2], Fangjun Lan[1], Qingwen He[1], Chen Li[3] and Yingping Cao[1*]

Abstract

Background: *Escherichia coli* clinical sequence type 131 (ST131) has emerged as an extensively antimicrobial resistant *E. coli* clonal group in recent years throughout the world. The aim of this study was to investigate the prevalence and molecular characteristics of ST131 among unselected *E. coli* clinical isolates in a Chinese university hospital.

Methods: Seven hundred consecutive *E. coli* isolates were collected at a Chinese university hospital between 2014 and 2015. Isolates belonging to ST131 were identified by PCR and multilocus sequence typing (MLST), and then characterized for antibiotic resistance, CTX-M-type extended-spectrum β-lactamase genes, fluoroquinolone resistance genes, O types, phylogenetic groups, virulence factors and PFGE patterns.

Results: Overall, 83 (11.6%) isolates were identified as ST131 group. The *H*30 lineage accounted for 53 (63.9%) of the ST131 isolates, including 13 *H*30-Rx and 40 *H*30 non-Rx. The remaining 30 isolates belonged to *H41* lineage. Two O types were identified in this study: O25b (66.3%) and O16 (33.7%). Compared with O25b-B2-ST131 isolates, O16-B2-ST131 isolates harbored less virulence factors of adhesins. ST131 *H*30 Rx isolates had significantly higher virulence score than those of other isolates. O16-B2-ST131 isolates were shown to have a lower resistance to quinolones than O25b-B2-ST131 isolates. 5 nonsynonymous mutations (GyrA S83 L, D87N, ParC S80I, E84V and ParE I529L) were strongly associated with ST131 *H30* and O25b isolates. Results of PFGE demonstrated that these isolates were classified into 68 pulsotypes and these subtypes were grouped into 23 different PFGE clusters using 70% similarity cut-off value.

Conclusions: This is the first study to reveal the prevalence and molecular characteristic of ST131 clonal group among consecutive clinical *E. coli* isolates in China. Our findings demonstrated that ST131 lineage accounts for a small proportion of clinical *E. coli* isolates in China, which included two major groups: O25b-B2-ST131 and O16-B2-ST131. Our results implies that O16-B2-ST131 subclone may be an important type of *E. coli* ST 131 in China, which suggests that future studies should not ignore such clone in this country.

Keywords: *E. coli*, ST131, Phylogenetic group, O25*b*, O16, *H*30

Background

Escherichia coli sequence type 131 (*E. coli* ST131) was identified among extended-spectrum *β*-lactamases (ESBL)-producing isolates in Asia, Europe and North America in 2008, and has rapidly emerged globally to become an important pathogen causing various infections in humans [1, 2]. *E. coli* ST131 is becoming the predominant extraintestinal pathogenic *E. coli* clone which drives multidrug resistance [1].

Although some of *E. coli* ST131 isolates are nontypeable for O antigen, most of these strains are of serotypes O25b and O16 [1, 2]. All *E. coli* ST131 isolates contain the *fimH* gene with high level of allelic diversity and *fimH*30 is the most common one [1]. *H*30 lineage of ST131 is named after *fimH*30 allele and includes two important sublineages (*H*30-R and *H*30-Rx) [1–3]. *E. coli* ST131 isolates are often resistant to fluoroquinolones and produce ESBL [4–6]. The *H*30 subclone comprises most of the fluoroquinolone-resistant ST131 isolates [4].

* Correspondence: caoyingping918@hotmail.com
[1]Department of Clinical Laboratory, Fujian Medical University Union Hospital, 29 Xinquan Rd, Fuzhou, Fujian 350001, People's Republic of China
Full list of author information is available at the end of the article

The main mechanism of fluoroquinolones resistance in *E. coli* ST131 isolates is aminoacid substitutions in the quinolone-resistance determining region (QRDR) of *gyrA*, *parC* and *parE* [1, 2, 6]. Within the *H*30 subclone, the *H*30-Rx subset is strongly associated with CTX-M β-lactamases [1, 2].

Regarding the spread of *E. coli* ST131, most investigations have focused on antimicrobial-resistant isolates, especially those resistant to fluoroquinolones and cephalosporins [1, 2]. *E. coli* ST131 has been detected among extended-spectrum *β*-lactamase-producing or fluoroquinolone-resistant isolates in China [7–9]. However, the prevalence of ST131 among unselected *E. coli* isolates remains unknown. The aim of this study was to investigate the prevalence and molecular characteristics of ST131 in a collection of 700 unselected clinical *E. coli* isolates collected at a university hospital in Southern China.

Methods

Bacterial isolates and screening for ST131

A total of 700 non-duplicate *E. coli* clinical isolates were consecutively collected at a Chinese university hospital (Fujian Medical University Union Hospital, Fuzhou, Fujian province, China) between August 2014 and August 2015. These isolates were obtained from urine (51.0%), blood (14.7%) and miscellaneous sources (34.3%). Isolates were identified by the Vitek-2 system GNI card (BioMèrieux, Missouri, France). All isolates were screened for ST131 by PCR-based method for ST131-associated SNPs in *mdh* and *gyrB* as previous described [10]. All the non-O25b, non-O16 and non-phylogenetic group B2 ST131 strains would be confirmed by multilocus sequence typing (MLST) to be ST131 according to the Achtman scheme using seven housekeeping genes (*adk, fumC, gyrB, icd, mdh, purA* and *recA*) (http://mlst.ucc.ie/mlst/dbs/Ecoli). All ST131 isolates detected were further tested by PCR using specific primers for the *fimH*30 allele for identification of the *H*30 subclone [11]. The *H*30-Rx subclone was identified using allele-specific PCR as previously described [11]. All the *H30*-PCR negative isolates underwent direct sequenceing of *fimH* as previously described [3].

Susceptibility testing

Antimicrobial susceptibility of *E. coli* ST131 isolates was determined by disk diffusion [12]. Drugs tested included aztreonam (ATM), cefotaxime (CTX), ceftazidime (CAZ), cefepime (FEP), ertapenem (ETP), imipenem (IPM), piperacillin-tazobactam (TZP), ciprofloxacin (CIP), levofloxacin (LEV), amikacin (AMK), and trimethoprim-sulfamethoxazole (SXT). The results were interpreted according to the breakpoints of the 2016 CLSI criteria [12]. *E. coli* ATCC 25922 was used for routine quality control.

Molecular characterization of ST131

Phylogenetic groups were determined using PCR method described by Clermont et al. previously [13]. Molecular O types were performed on all ST131 isolates by PCR with primers as described previously [14]. The ST131-associated O25b *rfb* variant was detected by a separated PCR assay [15]. The presence of 26 virulence factors (VFs) genes was evaluated by a multiplex PCR method [16].

The virulence score (VF score) was calculated for each isolate as the sum of all virulence-associated genes detected in this study [17]. The sum of all the VF scores of the isolates was then calculated, and finally this sum was divided by the number of isolates to give the mean VF score. *Pap* and *sfa-foc* were counted only once regardless of the number of elements or subunits identified [17].

Detection of $bla_{CTX\text{-}M}$ gene and fluoroquinolone resistance genes

Isolates nonsusceptible to cefotaxime or ceftazidime underwent detection of $bla_{CTX\text{-}M}$ using PCR [18]. As to CIP-resistant isolates, mutations in quinolone-resistance determining region (QRDR) of *gyrA*, *parC* and *parE* were determined by PCR and sequencing [19]. Regarding CIP-nonsusceptible or $bla_{CTX\text{-}M}$ producing isolates, the presence of plasmid mediated quinolone resistance determinants (PMQRs; *qnrA*, *qnrB*, *qnrC*, *qnrD*, *qnrS*, and *aac(6')-Ib-cr*) were detected by PCR as previously described [20, 21].

Pulsed-field gel electrophoresis analysis (PFGE) and dendrogram construction

ST131 isolates were subjected to PFGE analysis using XbaI digestion [18]. A PFGE dendrogram was constructed with BioNumerics software (Applied Maths, Sint-Martens-Latem, Belgium) according to the unweighted pair group method based on Dice coefficients. Isolates with a Dice similarity index ≥70% were considered to belong to the same PFGE cluster.

Statistical analysis

Data were analyzed using the SPSS 19.0. Comparisons of proportions were performed using χ^2 or Fisher's exact test (two tailed) or Mann-Whitney test. For each comparison, $p < 0.05$ was considered to be statistically significant.

Results

Prevalence of ST131 and its subclones

In total, 83 (11.6%) of the 700 clinical *E. coli* isolates were identified as ST131. ST131 accounted for 15.4% (55/357) of the urinary *E. coli* isolates and 11.7% (12/103) of the bloodstream isolates. *E. coli* ST131 strains were isolated from patients from 23 different wards. Females accounted for 60.2% (50/83) of the ST1193

Table 1 Characteristics of *E. coli* ST131 isolates by *fimH* subtyping

Characteristics	Total	ST131 subclones, number of isolates (%)			P[a]		
		H30Rx	H30 non-Rx	H41	H41 vs H30 non -Rx	H41 vs H30-Rx	H30 Rx vs H30 non-Rx
	N = 83 (%)	*n* = 13	*n* = 40	*n* = 30			
PCR O type							
O25b	55(66.3%)	12(92.3%)	40(100%)	3(10.0%)	< 0.001	< 0.001	
O16	28(33.7%)	1(7.7%)	0	27(90.0%)			
Antimicrobial resistance							
ATM	30(36.1%)	12(92.3%)	11(27.5%)	7(23.3%)		< 0.001	< 0.001
CAZ	22(26.5%)	10(76.9%)	5(12.5%)	7(23.3%)		0.002	< 0.001
CTX	59(71.1%)	12(92.3%)	28(70%)	19(63.3%)			
FEP	26(31.3%)	11(84.6%)	10(25.0%)	5(16.7%)		< 0.001	< 0.001
TZP	1(1.2%)	0	0	1(3.3%)			
CIP	58(69.9%)	13(100%)	40(100%)	5(16.7%)	< 0.001	< 0.001	
LEV	58(69.9%)	13(100%)	40(100%)	5(16.7%)	< 0.001	< 0.001	
AMK	7(8.4%)	3(23.1%)	1(2.50%)	3(10.0%)			0.042
SXT	56(67.5%)	10(76.9%)	24(60.0%)	22(73.3%)			
$bla_{CTX\text{-}M}$ type							
CTX-M-14	37(44.6%)	0	22(55.0%)	15(50.0%)		0.001	< 0.001
CTX-M-15	22(26.5%)	12(92.3%)	7(17.5%)	3(10.0%)		< 0.001	< 0.001
CTX-M-14,15	2(2.40%)	0	2(5.0%)	0			
CTX-M-123	1(1.2%)	0	0	1(3.3%)			
No ESBL[b]	21(25.3%)	1(7.7%)	11(27.5%)	9(30.0%)			
FQ^R genes[c]							
5 *gyrA, parC and parE* mutations[d]	51(61.4%)	13(100%)	35(87.5%)	3(10.0%)	< 0.001	< 0.001	
aac(6')-Ib-cr	14(16.9%)	10(76.9%)	0	4(13.3%)	0.012	< 0.001	< 0.001
qnr	4(4.8%)	0	2(5.0%)	2(6.70%)			
Adhesins							
papAH	22 (26.5%)	12(92.3%)	6 (15.0%)	4(13.3%)		< 0.001	< 0.001
papC	23 (27.7%)	13(100%)	6 (15.0%)	4(13.3%)		< 0.001	< 0.001
papEF	22 (26.5%)	12(92.3%)	7(17.5%)	3(10.0%)		< 0.001	< 0.001
papG allele I	0	0	0	0			
papG allele II	21 (25.3%)	12(92.3%)	6 (15.0%)	3(10.0%)		< 0.001	< 0.001
sfa/focDE	1 (1.2%)	0	1(2.50%)	0			
focG	0	0	0	0			
afa/draBC	7 (8.4%)	0	2(5.0%)	5(16.7%)			
fimH	82 (98.8%)	13(100%)	39(97.5%)	30(100%)			
gafD	0	0	0	0			
sfaS	7 (8.4%)	3(23.1%)	3(7.5%)	1(3.3%)			
Toxins							
hlyA	14 (16.9%)	11(84.6%)	1(2.50%)	2(6.70%)		< 0.001	< 0.001
cnf1	10 (12.0%)	8(61.5%)	1(2.50%)	1(3.3%)		0.002	< 0.001
cdtB	0	0	0	0			
cvaC	3 (3.6%)	0	0	3(10.0%)	0.042		

Table 1 Characteristics of *E. coli* ST131 isolates by *fimH* subtyping *(Continued)*

Characteristics	Total	ST131 subclones, number of isolates (%)			P^a		
	Total	H30Rx	H30 non-Rx	H41	H41 vs H30 non -Rx	H41 vs H30-Rx	H30 Rx vs H30 non-Rx
	N = 83 (%)	*n* = 13	*n* = 40	*n* = 30			
Siderophores							
fyuA	81 (97.6%)	13(100%)	38(95.0%)	30(100%)			
iutA	77 (92.8%)	13(100%)	38(95.0%)	26(86.7%)			
Capsules							
kpsMT II	62 (74.7%)	9(69.2%)	33(82.5%)	20(66.7%)			
kpsMT III	0	0	0	0			
kpsMT K1	10 (12.0%)	2(15.4%)	5(12.5%)	3(10.0%)			
kpsMT K5	47 (56.6%)	11(84.6%)	29(72.5%)	7(23.3%)	< 0.001	0.001	
Miscellaneous							
nfaE	0	0	0	0			
rfc	0	0	0	0			
malX	76 (91.6%)	13(100%)	37(92.5%)	26(86.7%)			
traT	73 (88.0%)	13(100%)	32(80.0%.)	28(93.3%)			
Virulence scores[e]	7	9	7	6		0.001	0.001

[a]*P* values, by either χ^2 or Fisher's exact test or Mann-Whitney test, are shown where $P < 0.05$
[b]ESBL, CTX-M-type extended-spectrum-β-lactamase genes
[c]FQ^R, fluoroquinolone resistance
[d]GyrA S83 L, D87N, ParC S80I, E84V, and ParE I529L
[e]median number of virulence factors (range)

isolates, and the median age was 62 years (range, 5 years to 89 years).

The results of O typing revealed that ST131 isolates belonged to two types (O25b and O16). All the 83 ST131 isolates were O-antigen typeable. O25b (66.3%) was the most prevalent type, followed by O16 (33.7%) (Table 1). The majority (52/55, 94.5%) of O25b ST131 isolates belonged to *fimH30*, while 96.4% (27/28) of O16 ST131 isolates were *fimH41*subclone. The distribution of O types was not significantly associated with specimen type or source (Table 2).

Subclone typing showed that *H*30 lineage comprised 63.9% (53/83) of the ST131 isolates, including 13 (15.7%) *H*30-Rx and 40 (48.2%) *H*30 non-Rx (Table 1). The remaining 30 isolates belonged to *fimH41* subclone. Among ciprofloxacin-resistant ST131 isolates, 84.5% (49/58) belonged to the *H*30 lineage.

Antimicrobial susceptibility

Among the 83 ST131 isolates, the highest rates of resistance were to CTX (71.7%), CIP (69.9%), LEV (69.9%) and SXT (67.5%). On the contrary, resistance rates were low to ATM (36.1%), FEP (31.3%), CAZ (26.5%), AMK (8.4%) and TZP (1.2%). None of the isolates was resistant to imipenem or ertapenem. These findings are summarized in Table 1.

Compared with O25b-ST131 isolates, O16-ST131 isolates were shown to have a lower resistance to fluoroquinolones (CIP and LEV) and FEP, and had a similar resistance to third generation cephalosporins (CTX and CAZ) (Table 2).

CTX-M ESBL and fluoroquinolone resistance mechanisms

bla_{CTX-M} genes were harbored by 62 (74.7%) *E. coli* ST131 isolates. Of these, 37 isolates carried $bla_{CTX-M-14}$, 22 isolates carried $bla_{CTX-M-15}$ and 1 isolates carried $bla_{CTX-M-123}$. The remaining 2 isolates co-produced $bla_{CTX-M-14}$ and $bla_{CTX-M-15}$.

All CTX-M-14 producers were *H*30 non-Rx and *H41*, whereas most ST131 *H30*-Rx subclones were CTX-M-15 producers (92.3%, 12/13; Table 1).

All 58 ciprofloxacin-resistant ST131 isolates contained 4 or 5 nonsynonymous mutations in *gyrA*, *parC* and *parE*. All these ST131 isolates had a set of 3 conserved QRDR amino acid substitutions (GyrA S83 L, D87N and ParC S80I). The presence of 5 mutations (GyrA S83 L, D87N, ParC S80I, E84V and ParE I529L) was significantly more prevalent among *H*30 isolates than *H41* ($P < 0.001$). These findings are summarized in Table 1. Meanwhile, these 5 mutations were strongly associated with O25b subclones (Table 3).

Three types of PMQR determinants were found in 16 ST131 isolates, including *aac(6')-Ib-cr* ($n = 14$), *qnrS1* ($n = 2$) and *qnrB1* (n = 2). Two ST131 isolates coproduced *qnrB1* and *aac(6')-Ib-cr*. *aac(6')-Ib-cr* were significantly concentrated in *H30*-Rx isolates than non H30-Rx isolates ($P < 0.001$) (Table 1).

Table 2 The sample sources and distribution of virulence factors among different O-serotype of *E. coli* ST131 isolates

Characteristics	Clonal groups, number of isolates (%)			P^{a}
	All isolates ($n = 83$)	O25b ($n = 55$)	O16 ($n = 28$)	O25b vs O16
Source				
Urine	55 (66.3%)	36 (65.5%)	19 (67.9%)	
Blood	12 (14.5%)	10 (18.2%)	2 (7.1%)	
Other	16 (19.3%)	9 (16.4%)	7 (25.0%)	
Antimicrobial resistance				
ATM	30 (36.1%)	24 (43.6%)	6 (21.4%)	
CAZ	22 (26.5%)	16 (29.1%)	6 (21.4%)	
CTX	59 (71.1%)	41 (74.5%)	18 (64.3%)	
FEP	26 (31.3%)	22 (40.0%)	4 (14.3%)	0.024
TZP	1 (1.2%)	0	1 (3.6%)	
CIP	58 (69.9%)	49 (89.1%)	9 (32.1%)	< 0.001
LEV	58 (69.9%)	49 (89.1%)	9 (32.1%)	< 0.001
AMK	7 (8.4%)	4 (7.3%)	3 (10.7%)	
SXT	56 (67.5%)	36 (65.5%)	20 (71.4%)	
Adhesins				
papAH	22 (26.5%)	19 (34.5%)	3 (10.7%)	0.034
papC	23 (27.7%)	21 (38.2%)	2 (7.1%)	0.004
papEF	22 (26.5%)	19 (34.5%)	3 (10.7%)	0.034
papG allele I	0	0	0	
papG allele II	21 (25.3%)	18 (32.7%)	3 (10.7%)	0.034
sfa/focDE	1 (1.2%)	1 (1.8%)	0	
focG	0	0	0	
afa/draBC	7 (8.4%)	2 (3.6%)	5 (17.9%)	0.040
fimH	82 (98.8%)	54 (98.2%)	28 (100%)	
gafD	0	0	0	
sfaS	7 (8.4%)	6 (10.9%)	1 (3.6%)	
Toxins				
hlyA	14 (16.9%)	11 (20.0%)	3 (10.7%)	
cnf1	10 (12.0%)	8 (14.5%)	2 (7.1%)	
cdtB	0	0	0	
cvaC	3 (3.6%)	1 (1.8%)	2 (7.1%)	
Siderophores				
fyuA	81 (97.6%)	53 (96.4%)	28 (100%)	
iutA	77 (92.8%)	52 (94.5%)	25 (89.3%)	
Capsules				
kpsMTII	62 (74.7%)	43 (78.2%)	19 (67.9%)	
kpsMTIII	0	0	0	
kpsMT K1	10 (12.0%)	8 (14.5%)	2 (7.1%)	
kpsMT K5	47 (56.6%)	40 (72.7%)	7 (25.0%)	< 0.001
Miscellaneous				
nfaE	0	0	0	
rfc	0	0	0	

Table 2 The sample sources and distribution of virulence factors among different O-serotype of *E. coli* ST131 isolates *(Continued)*

Characteristics	Clonal groups, number of isolates (%)			P^a
	All isolates (n = 83)	O25b (n = 55)	O16 (n = 28)	O25b vs O16
malX	76 (91.6%)	51 (92.7%)	25 (89.3%)	
traT	73 (88.0%)	46 (83.6%)	27 (96.4%)	
Virulence scores[b]	7 (3 to 11)	7 (3 to 11)	6 (4 to 10)	

[a]P values, by either χ^2 or Fisher's exact test, are shown where $P < 0.05$
[b]median number of virulence factors (range)

Virulence factors

The most frequent VF genes were *fimH* (type 1 fimbriae), *fyuA* (yersiniabactin), *iutA* (iron uptake gene), *malX* (pathogenicity-associated island marker), *kpsMT II* (group II capsule), and *traT* (outer membrane lipoprotein), each of which was detected in ≥60% of the isolates. In contrast, 8 genes were each identified in less than 10% of isolates, including cvaC, *sfa/focDE, sfaS, afa/draBC, focG, papG* allele I, *gafD, cdtB, kpsMTIII, nfaE* and *rfc*. The median virulence score was 7 (range, 3 to 11). Among the two O groups, the median virulence scores (ranges) were 7 (3 to 11) for O25b-ST131 and 6 (4 to 10) for O16-ST131, respectively.

ST131 *H30*-Rx isolates possessed the highest virulence score (mean, 9; range, 7 to11). ST131 *H30* non-Rx and *H41* isolates showed similar virulence scores and ranges of VFs (mean scores, 7 [range, 4 to 9] and 6 [range, 3 to 9], respectively). ST131 *H30*-Rx isolates had significantly higher virulence score than *H30* non-Rx and *H41* isolates (Table 1). Four adhesins (*papAH, papC, papEF* and *papG allele II*) and two toxins (*hlyA* and *cnf1*) were significantly more frequent among ST131 H30-Rx isolates (Table 1).

Bacterial clonal relatedness

PFGE analysis of the 83 *E. coli* ST131 isolates demonstrated that these isolates were classified into 68 pulsotypes (named 1–68, Fig. 1) and these subtypes were grouped into 23 different PFGE clusters (named A-W, in Fig. 1) using 70% similarity cut-off value. Two PFGE clusters (C and D) were predominant, grouping 13 and 14 isolates, respectively, whereas the other 21 PFGE clusters contained up to 9 ST131 isolates each (Fig. 1). Cluster C contained 92.3% (12/13) of *H30*-Rx isolates. The majority of O16 ST131 isolates belonged to two clusters (H and I), grouping 5 and 9 isolates. As shown in Fig. 1, at 63% similarity level, O25b-ST131 isolates were clustered into six major clonal groups, while 92.9% of the O16 isolates were clustered into two clonal groups (group one contained clusters H, I, J and K, and group two contained clusters O, P, Q, R and S).

Discussion

To our knowledge, this is the first molecular survey reporting the prevalence and characteristics of *E. coli* ST131 and its subclones among unselected clinical isolates in China. We found *E. coli* ST131 accounted for 11.6% of all *E. coli* isolates, which is similar to rates reported previously [1, 22, 23]. In addition, there was a similar distribution of ST131 among urine and blood samples. Meanwhile, the PFGE study indicated that ST131 isolates in this study were highly diverse at the pulsotype level and there was no predominated clone (Fig. 1).

O25b was previously considered the predominant ST131 clone type, while O16 isolates accounted for a small percentage [1, 2, 24]. Similar to previous studies [23, 24],

Table 3 Fluoroquinolone resistance mechanisms, O types and *fimH* subclone among 83 ST131 *E. coli* isolates

CIP[a]	*fim*H type (n)	O type (n)	N	gyrA	parC	parE	aac(6')-Ib-cr	qnr (n)
R	H30	O25b	48	S83 L, D87N	S80I, E84V	I529L	9	*qnrS1*(1)
R	H41	O16	3	S83 L, D87N	S80I, E84V	I529L	1	*qnrB1*(1)
R	H30	O25b	1	S83 L, D87N	S80I	P415L	–	–
R	H41	O16	1	S83 L, D87N	S80I	I529L	–	–
R	H41	O16	1	S83 L, D87N	S80I	S458A	1	–
R	H41	O16	3	S83 L, D87N	S80I	L445H	1	–
R	H41	O25b	1	S83 L, D87N	S80I	L445H	–	–
I	H41	O25b	1	ND[b]	ND	ND	1	*qnrB1*(1)
S	H41	O16	19	ND	ND	ND	1	–
S	H41	O25b	2	ND	ND	ND		*qnrS1*(1)[c]
S	H30	O25b	3	ND	ND	ND	–	–

[a]R, resistant; I, intermediate; S, susceptible
[b]ND, not detected
[c]In this isolate, $bla_{CTX\text{-}M\text{-}15}$ was positive

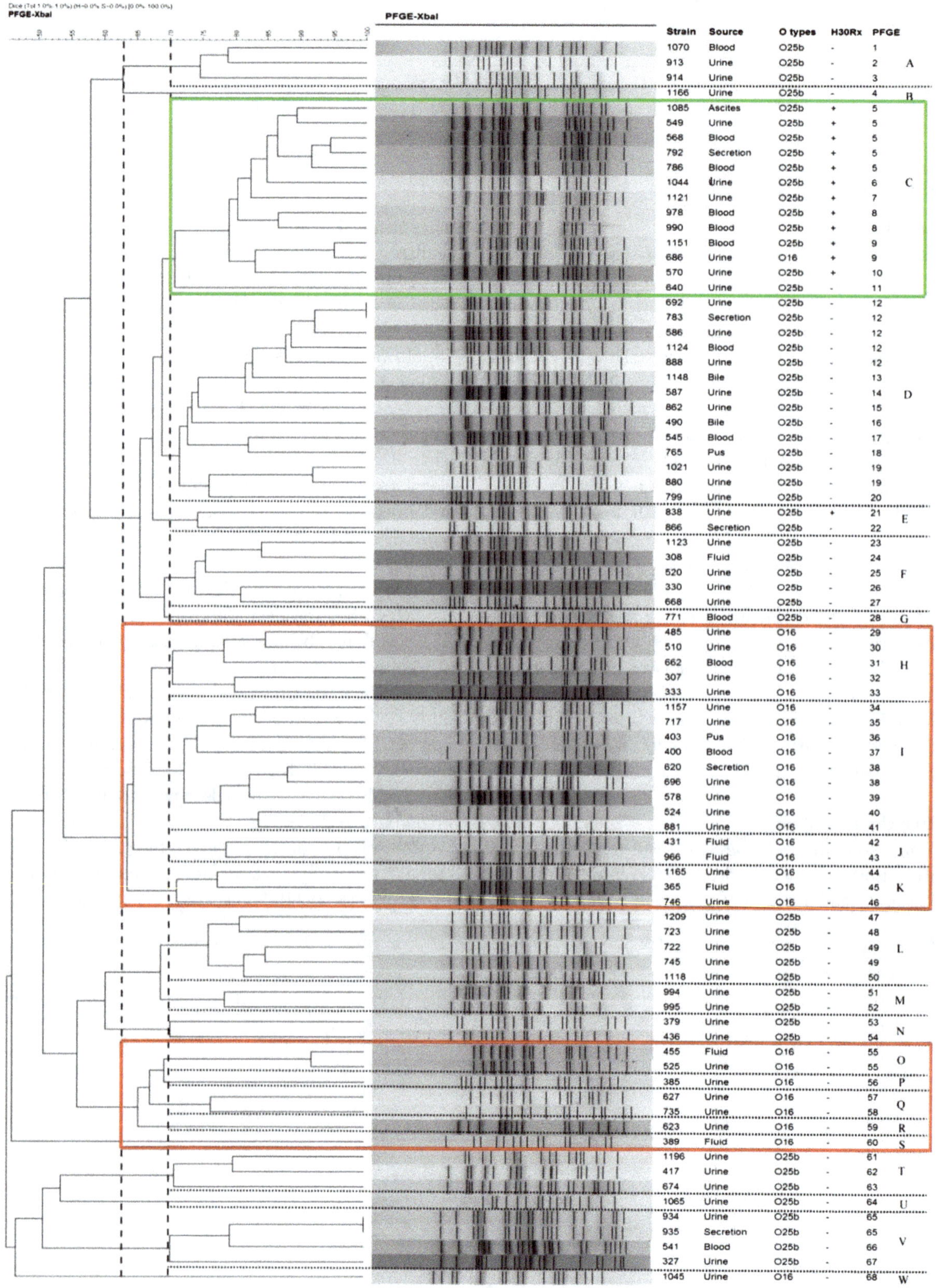

Fig. 1 Pulsed-field gel electrophoresis (PFGE) of XbaI-digested DNA from 83 ST131 *E. coli* isolates. Strain designation, Sample source, O serotype, *H*30 Rx and PFGE patterns are shown. Green box indicated the main cluster of ST131 *H*30 Rx isolates using 70% similarity cut-off value. Red box showed the two main clusters of O16 ST131 isolates at 63% similarity level

O25b-B2-ST131 in this study was the predominant clone among clinical *E. coli* isolates. Notably, a high percentage (33.6%) of O16-B2-ST131 was found in the present study. In China, a recent study found that O16-B2-ST131 accounted for the predominant subset among ST131 fecal *E. coli* isolates [25]. However, among *E. coli* clinical isolates, all other researches focused on O25b-B2-ST131 in our country and no data are available on the prevalence of O16-B2-ST131 among *E. coli* clinical isolates till now, the present study is the first to show the presence of O16-B2-ST131 in this country. Taken together with the previous study [25], these findings suggest that O16-B2-ST131 may emerge as an important type of *E. coli* ST131 in China. The rate of O25b-B2-ST131 was not striking in this study. However, the O16-B2-ST131 may need special attention for the high percentages found in our results and previous study [25]. As discussed before, the clonal group should be investigated in the future study in other geographical regions in China [25, 26].

The *H*30 lineage was a very important ST131 subclone, which firstly appeared in the year of 2000 and expanded rapidly to become the most dominant and extensively distributed multidrug-resistant lineage of *E. coli* worldwide [1, 2]. Within the *H*30 subclone, the *H*30-Rx subset is a major drug-resistant pathogen among fluoroquinolone-resistant *E. coli* isolates and is associated with $bla_{CTX-M-15}$ [1, 2]. In this study, we also explored the prevalence of *H*30 lineage and *H*30-Rx sublineage among *E. coli* ST131 isolates. *H*30 lineage accounted for the majority of ST131 isolates in our study, which is similar to those in previous studies [22, 23]. However, the prevalence of *H*30-Rx ST131 was obviously lower than those reported in other researches [23, 27]. Meanwhile, the great majority of *H*30-Rx isolates harbored $bla_{CTX-M-15}$ in this study. Resistances to 11 most commonly used antimicrobials were evaluated in this study. Our findings support the strong association of *H*30-Rx sublineage with multidrug resistance and the presence of $bla_{CTX-M-15}$ (Table 1). We also identified the *H*30-Rx with the presence of *aac(6')-Ib-cr* (Table 1). Resistance of fluoroquinolones is mainly due to chromosomal mutations in the QRDR regions, especially in gyrA and parC [28, 29]. In this study, A set of 3 conserved mutations in QRDR regions (GyrA S83 L, D87N, and ParC S80I) could be found in all the CIP-resistant ST131 isolates. These chromosomal mutations have been previously linked to fluoroquinolone resistance [23, 30]. Meanwhile, 5 mutations (GyrA S83 L, D87N, ParC S80I, E84V and ParE I529L) were strongly associated with *H30* ST131 isolates, which is similar to the previous studies [23, 31].

Regarding virulence factors, *fimH*, *fyuA*, *iutA*, *kpsMTII* and *traT* were the most prevalent virulence factors found in this study, which have been associated with *E. coli* ST131 isolates in previous studies [1, 32]. There was a similar prevalence rate for these five virulence factors within different O types ST131 isolates (Table 2). O16-B2-ST131 isolates harbored similar number of virulence genes than O25b-ST131 isolates. Compared with O25b-B2-ST131 isolates, O16-B2-ST131 isolates harbored less virulence factors of adhesins (*papAH*, *papC*, *papEF* and *papG alleleII*).The *pap* adhesion genes probably played an important role in the pathophysiology of pyelonephritis caused by *E. coli* [33, 34]. This property probably suggests that O16-B2-ST131 isolates have a lower adhesive ability and pathogenicity than O25b-B2-ST131. Meanwhile, O25b-B2-ST131 isolates were significantly more likely to possess *kpsMT K5* than O16-B2-ST131 isolates. *kpsMT K5* is a capsule synthesis gene [16]. The possession of the gene may enhance the pathogenesis of O25b-B2-ST131 isolates due to the evasion of phagocytosis (capsule encoded by *kpsMT K5*).

In conclusion, to our knowledge, this is the first report on the prevalence and molecular characteristic of ST131 clonal group among consecutive clinical *E. coli* isolates in China. Our findings demonstrated that ST131 lineage accounts for a small proportion of clinical *E. coli* isolates in China, which included two major groups: O25b-B2-ST131 and O16-B2-ST131. Our results implies that O16-B2-ST131 subclone may be an important type of *E. coli* ST 131 in China, which suggests that future studies should not ignore such clone in this country.

Abbreviations

E. coli: *Escherichia coli*; ESBL: Extended-spectrum β-lactamases; MLST: multilocus sequence typing; QRDR: Quinolone-resistance determining region; PFGE: Pulsed-field gel electrophoresis analysis; ST: Sequence type; VF: Virulence score

Acknowledgements

The authors thank Prof. Yohei Doi, University of Pittsburgh School of Medicine (USA) for his useful discussion and for his critical review of the manuscript.We also thank Prof. Hu Fupin, Institute of Antibiotics, Huashan Hospital, for his kindly help in performing PFGE experiment.

Funding

This study was supported by the Fujian Provincial Funds for Distinguished Young Scientists in Colleges and Universities, China (grant no. JA13134), and the Medical Elite Cultivation Program of Fujian, China (grant no. 2015-ZQN-ZD-15).

Authors' contributions

BL and YC designed the experiment, BL wrote the manuscript. YL, FL and QH performed the experiments. CL participated in data analysis. YC reviewed the draft. All authors read and approved the final manuscript.

Consent for publication

Not applicable.

Competing interests

The authors declare that they have no competing interests.

Author details
[1]Department of Clinical Laboratory, Fujian Medical University Union Hospital, 29 Xinquan Rd, Fuzhou, Fujian 350001, People's Republic of China. [2]Department of Clinical Laboratory, Maternal and Children's Health Hospital of Fujian Province, Fuzhou, Fujian 350001, China. [3]Department of Infectious Disease, Fujian Medical University Union Hospital, Fuzhou, Fujian 350001, China.

References

1. Nicolas-Chanoine MH, Bertrand X, Madec JY. Escherichia Coli ST131, an intriguing clonal group. Clin Microbiol Rev. 2014;27:543–74.
2. Mathers AJ, Peirano G, Pitout JD. The role of epidemic resistance plasmids and international high-risk clones in the spread of multidrug-resistant Enterobacteriaceae. Clin MicrobioRev. 2015;28:565–91.
3. Johnson JR, Tchesnokova V, Johnston B, Clabots C, Roberts PL, Billig M, et al. Abrupt emergence of single dominant multidrug-resistant strain of Escherichia Coli. J Infect Dis. 2013;207:919–28.
4. Sauget M, Cholley P, Vannier A, Thouverez M, Nicolas-Chanoine MH, Hocquet D, et al. Trends of extended-spectrum β-lactamase-producing Escherichia Coli sequence type 131 and its H30 subclone in a French hospital over a 15-year period. Int J Antimicrob Agents. 2016;48:744–7.
5. Matsumura Y, Johnson JR, Yamamoto M, Nagao M, Tanaka M, Takakura S, et al. CTX-M-27- and CTX-M-14-producing, ciprofloxacin-resistant Escherichia Coli of the H30 subclonal group within ST131 drive a Japanese regional ESBL epidemic. J Antimicrob Chemother. 2015;70:1639–49.
6. Ben Zakour NL, Alsheikh-Hussain AS, Ashcroft MM, Khanh Nhu NT, Roberts LW, Stanton-Cook M, et al. Sequential Acquisition of Virulence and Fluoroquinolone Resistance has Shaped the evolution of Escherichia Coli ST131. MBio. 2016;7:e00347–16.
7. Wang LH, Liu PP, Wei DD, Liu Y, Wan LG, Xiang TX, et al. Clinical isolates of uropathogenic Escherichia Coli ST131 producing NDM-7 metallo-β-lactamase inChina. Int J Antimicrob Agents. 2016;48:41–5.
8. Zhang F, Zhu D, Xie L, Guo X, Ni Y, Sun J. Molecular epidemiology of carbapenemase-producing Escherichia Coli and the prevalence of ST131 subclone H30 in shanghai, China. Eur J Clin Microbiol Infect Dis. 2015;34:1263–9.
9. Wang S, Zhao SY, Xiao SZ, FF G, Liu QZ, Tang J, et al. Antimicrobial resistance and molecular epidemiology of Escherichia Coli causing bloodstream infections in three hospitals in shanghai, China. PLoS One. 2016;11:e0147740.
10. Johnson JR, Menard M, Johnston B, Kuskowski MA, Nichol K, Zhanel GG. Epidemic clonal groups of Escherichia Coli as a cause of antimicrobial-resistant urinary tract infections in Canada, 2002 to 2004. Antimicrob Agents Chemother. 2009;53:2733–9.
11. Colpan A, Johnston B, Porter S, Clabots C, Anway R, Thao L, et al. *Escherichia coli* sequence type 131 (ST131) subclone *H30* as an emergent multidrug-resistant pathogen among US veterans. Clin Infect Dis. 2013;57:1256–65.
12. Clinical and Laboratory Standards Institute. Performance Standards for Antimicrobial Susceptibility Testing; 24th Informational Supplement, M100-S26. PA: Wayne; 2016.
13. Clermont O, Christenson JK, Denamur E, Gordon DM. The Clermont *Escherichia coli* phylo-typing method revisited: improvement of specificity anddetection of new phylo-groups. Environ Microbiol Rep. 2013;5:58–65.
14. Li D, Liu B, Chen M, Guo D, Guo X, Liu F, et al. A multiplex PCR method to detect 14 *Escherichia coli* serogroups associated with urinary tract infections. J Microbiol Methods. 2010;82:71–7.
15. Clermont O, Dhanji H, Upton M, Gibreel T, Fox A, Boyd D, et al. Rapid detection of the O25b-ST131 clone of *Escherichia coli* encompassing the CTX-M-15-producing strains. J Antimicrob Chemother. 2009;64:274–7.
16. Johnson JR, Stell AL. Extended virulence genotypes of *Escherichia coli* strains from patients with urosepsis in relation to phylogeny and host compromise. J Infect Dis. 2000;181:261–72.
17. Oteo J, Gonzalez-Lopez JJ, Ortega A, Quintero-Zarate JN, Bou G, Cercenada E, et al. Inhibitor-resistant TEM- and OXA-1- producing Escherichia Coli isolates resistant to amoxicillin-clavulanate are more clonal and possess lower virulence gene content than susceptible clinical isolates. Antimicrob Agents Chemother. 2014;58:3874–81.
18. Li B, Sun JY, Liu QZ, Han LZ, Huang XH, Ni YX. High prevalence of CTX-M β-lactamases in faecal *Escherichia coli* strains from healthy humans in Fuzhou, China. Scand J Infect Dis. 2011;43:170–4.
19. Komp Lindgren P, Karlsson A, Hughes D. Mutation rate and evolution of fluoroquinolone resistance in Escherichia Coli isolates from patients with urinary tract infections. Antimicrob Agents Chemother. 2003;47:3222–32.
20. Robicsek A, Strahilevitz J, Jacoby GA, Macielag M, Abbanat D, Park CH, et al. Fluoroquinolone-modifying enzyme: a new adaptation of a common aminoglycoside acetyltransferase. Nat Med. 2006;12:83–8.
21. Yamane K, Wachino J, Suzuki S, Kimura K, Shibata N, Kato H, et al. New plasmid-mediated fluoroquinolone efflux pump, QepA, found in an *Escherichia coli* clinical isolate. Antimicrob Agents Chemother. 2007;51:3354–60.
22. Lafolie J, Nicolas-Chanoine MH, Grenouillet F, Hocquet D, Bertrand X. Prevalence of *Escherichia coli* sequence type 131 and its *H30* subclone among *E. coli* isolates in a French hospital. Int J Antimicrob Agents. 2014;44:466–8.
23. Kim SY, Park YJ, Johnson JR, JK Y, Kim YK, Kim YS. Prevalence and characteristics of *Escherichia coli* sequence type 131 and its *H30* and *H30*Rx subclones: a multicenter study from Korea. Diagn Microbiol Infect Dis. 2016;84:97–101.
24. Banerjee R, Johnson JRA. New clone sweeps clean: the enigmatic emergence of *Escherichia coli* sequence type 131. Antimicrob Agents Chemother. 2014;58: 4997–5004.
25. Zhong YM, Liu WE, Liang XH, Li YM, Jian ZJ, Hawkey PM. Emergence and spread of O16-ST131 and O25b-ST131 clones among faecal CTX-M-producing Escherichia Coli in healthy individuals in Hunan Province, China. J Antimicrob Chemother. 2015;70:2223–7.
26. Matsumura Y, Yamamoto M, Nagao M, Hotta G, Matsushima A, Ito Y, et al. Emergence and spread of B2-ST131-O25b, B2-ST131-O16 and D-ST405 clonal groups among extended-spectrum-β-lactamase-producing *Escherichia coli* in Japan. J Antimicrob Chemother. 2012;67:2612–20.
27. Peirano G, van der Bij AK, Freeman JL, Poirel L, Nordmann P, Costello M, et al. Characheristics of Escherichia Coli sequence type 131 isolates that produce extended-spectrum β-lactamases: global distribution of the H30-Rx sublineage. Antimicrob Agents Chemother. 2014;58:3762–7.
28. Hooper DC, Jacoby GA. Mechanisms of drug resistance: quinolone resistance. Ann N Y Acad Sci. 2015;1354:12–31.
29. Aldred KJ, Kerns RJ, Osheroff N. Mechanism of quinolone action and resistance. Biochemistry. 2014;53:1565–74.
30. Johnning A, Kristiansson E, Angelin M, Marathe N, Shouche YS, Johansson A, et al. Quinolone resistance mutations in the faecal microbiota of Swedish travellers to India. BMC Microbiol. 2015;15:235.
31. Johnson JR, Johnston B, Kuskowski MA, Sokurenko EV, Tchesnokova V. Intensity and mechanisms of fluoroquinolone resistance within the H30 and H30Rx subclones of Escherichia Coli sequence type 131 compared with other fluoroquinolone-resistant E. Coli. Antimicrob Agents Chemother. 2015;59:4471–80.
32. Olesen B, Frimodt-Møller J, Leihof RF, Struve C, Johnston B, Hansen DS, et al. Temporal trends in antimicrobial resistance and virulence-associated traits within the Escherichia Coli sequence type 131 clonal group and its H30 and H30-Rx subclones, 1968 to 2012. Antimicrob Agents Chemother. 2014;58:6886–95.
33. Farrell DJ, Morrissey I, De Rubeis D, Robbins M, Felmingham DAUK. Multicentre study and the antimicrobial susceptibility of bacterial pathogens causing urinary tract infection. J Inf Secur. 2003;46:94–100.
34. Tarchouna M, Ferjani A, Ben-Selma W, Boukadida J. Distribution of uropathogenic virulence genes in *Escherichia coli* isolated from patients with urinary tract infection. Int J InfectDis. 2013;17:e450–3.

10

Fecal carriage of extended-spectrum β-lactamase- and carbapenemase-producing Enterobacteriaceae in Egyptian patients with community-onset gastrointestinal complaints

H.M. Abdallah[1,3*], N. Alnaiemi[1,2,3], E.A. Reuland[1], B.B. Wintermans[1], A. Koek[1], A.M. Abdelwahab[3], A. Samy[4], K.W. Abdelsalam[5] and C.M.J.E. Vandenbroucke-Grauls[1]

Abstract

Objectives: The aim of this study was to determine the prevalence of extended-spectrum β-lactamase (ESBL) and carbapenemase production among Enterobacteriaceae isolated from ambulatory patients with gastrointestinal complaints admitted to El-Ahrar General Hospital, Zagazig, Egypt in the period between January 2013 and May 2013.

Methods: One hundred and thirteen Enterobacteriaceae isolates were recovered from 100 consecutive Egyptian patients with community–onset gastrointestinal complaints. The fecal samples were plated directly on selective EbSA-ESBL Screening Agar and on MacConkey agar. Isolate identification was performed with matrix-assisted laser desorption ionization time-of-flight mass spectrometry (MALDI-TOF-MS). Screening for ESBLs and carbapenemases production was done by both the automated VITEK®2 system with AST N198 and by disk diffusion method. Real-time PCR and sequencing were used to characterize the resistance genes. Phylogroups of the *E. coli* isolates were determined by a triplex PCR-based method.

(Continued on next page)

* Correspondence: hmmuhamed@vet.zu.edu.eg
[1]Medical Microbiology and Infection Control, VU University Medical Center, Amsterdam, The Netherlands
[3]Department of Microbiology, Faculty of Veterinary Medicine, Zagazig University, Zagazig, Egypt
Full list of author information is available at the end of the article

(Continued from previous page)

Results: Of 100 patients screened for fecal colonization with extended-spectrum β-lactamase -producing Enterobacteriaceae (ESBL-E) and carbapenemase- producing Enterobacteriaceae (CPE), 68 were colonized with ESBL-E whereas five patients were positive for CPE. One hundred and thirteen Enterobacterceae isolates were recovered from 100 fecal samples, they belonged to *E. coli* (n = 72), *Klebsiella pneumoniae* (n = 23), *Enterobacter cloacae*(n = 3), *Salmonella* spp. (n = 1) and other Enterobacterceae isolates (n = 14). The bla_{CTX-M} gene was detected in 89.04% (65/73) of the ESBL-producing Enterobacteriaceae, whereas bla_{SHV} and bla_{TEM} were detected in 30.14% (22/73) and 19.18% (14/73) respectively. Three out of 5 carbapenem-resistant isolates harbored New Delhi metallo-beta-lactamase (NDM) and 2 produced Verona integron-encoded metallo- beta -lactamase (VIM). Twenty-two (47.83%) of the ESBL positive isolates were multidrug resistant (MDR). Phylogenetic analysis showed that, of the 51 ESBL-EC isolates, 17 belonged to group B2, 13 to group D, 11 to group A and 10 to group B1.

Conclusions: Nearly two-thirds of the Enterobacteriaceae isolates recovered from feces of ambulatory patients with community–onset gastrointestinal complaints admitted to El-Ahrar General Hospital, Zagazig, Egypt were ESBL producers and one in every 20 patients included in our study was colonized by carbapenemase-producing Enterobacteriaceae. These high colonization rates are worrying, therefore prudent antimicrobial use should be adopted in Egyptian community settings.

Keywords: Carbapenemase-ESBL-Egypt-resistance-Enterobacteriaceae

Background

Infections due to extended-spectrum beta-lactamase–and carbapenemase-producing Enterobacteriaceae represent a major global health threat [1] since such bacteria are usually resistant to multiple antimicrobial agents and carbapenems are expensive and not always available, especially in less wealthy countries. Infections with these resistant strains are associated with treatment failure, high mortality, and increased healthcare costs [2–4].

ESBL-producing Enterobacteriaceae (ESBL-E) and carbapenemase-producing Enterobacteriaceae (CPE) are incriminated in both nosocomial and community-acquired infection [5, 6]. The fecal carriage rate of ESBL-E has mainly been investigated during nosocomial outbreaks, whilst few studies were conducted in community settings [5, 7]. High community carriage rates were reported in Thailand (69.3%) and China (50.5%) [8, 9]. Lower rates were demonstrated in most European countries (not more than 12%) and North America (less than 2%) [10–13]. In Egypt, data on the prevalence of ESBL-E in the community remain scarce. A study performed in Cairo (urban population) reported high fecal carriage rate (63.3%) of ESBL-E among healthy individuals [14]. To the best of our knowledge, no previous research has been carried out to determine the fecal carriage rate of CPE in the community. In this study, we aimed to assess the prevalence of ESBL-E and CPE among ambulatory patients with community–onset gastrointestinal complaints admitted to El-Ahrar General Hospital, Zagazig (semi-urban population, 65 km from Cairo), Egypt.

Methods

Bacterial isolates

This study was performed in the period between January 2013 and May 2013, at El-Ahrar General Hospital, Zagazig, Egypt, a 608-bed hospital affiliated to the Egyptian health ministry. Approximately 1.5 g of feces was collected aseptically from 100 consecutive patients admitted to the hospital with community–onset gastrointestinal complaints (one sample per patient). Fecal samples were obtained for routine diagnosis of the gastrointestinal complaints and in addition to routine testing for gastrointestinal pathogens. The patients had no past history of travel to the Indian subcontinent or to South-Eastern Asia, nor relatives that had recently traveled to those regions. Fecal samples were suspended in 5 mL of saline (0.9%) and 100 ul of each sample was plated directly on selective EbSA-ESBL Screening Agar [15] for the isolation of bacteria resistant to broad-spectrum cephalosporins and on MacConkey agar for the characterization of the dominant isolates. At least one and up to five colonies per agar plate were investigated. Bacteria were identified by the automated Vitek® MS system (BioMérieux, Marcy l'Étoile, France).

Phenotypic screening and confirmation of ESBL-E and CPE

Antibiotic susceptibility testing was performed by both the automated VITEK®2 system with AST card N198 (BioMérieux, Marcy l'Étoile, France) and by disk diffusion on Mueller-Hinton agar using ceftazidime (30 μg), cefotaxime (30 μg), meropenem (10 μg), and imipenem (10 μg) disks. The AST card antimicrobial agents panel were ampicillin, amoxicillin-clavulanic acid, piperacillin, piperacillin-tazobactam, cefuroxime, cefoxitin, cefepime, ceftazidime, cefotaxime, meropenem, imipenem, ciprofloxacin, norfloxacin, gentamicin, tobramycin, nitrofurantoin, and trimethoprim-sulfamethoxazole. The results of antibiotic susceptibility tests were interpreted according to the clinical breakpoints recommended by Clinical and

Laboratory Standards Institute (CLSI) and the Dutch Society of Medical Microbiology [16, 17]. ESBL production was confirmed with the ESBL combination disks (Rosco, Taastrup, Denmark) according to the guidelines of the Dutch Society of Medical Microbiology [17].

Carbapenemases production was confirmed by carbapenemases double disk synergy test [18]. Enhancement of the inhibition zone in the area between the inhibitor-containing disk (boronic acid and/or dipicolinic acid) and any one of the two carbapenems discs used (meropenem and /or imipenem) was regarded as a positive result [17, 19].

Characterization of β-lactamase-encoding genes

ESBL phenotypes were analyzed for the presence of genes encoding bla_{TEM}, bla_{SHV} and $bla_{CTX\text{-}M}$ by real-time PCR using primers described before [20–22]. Carbapenem-resistant isolates were tested for the presence of genes encoding bla_{KPC}, bla_{NDM}, $bla_{OXA\text{-}48}$, bla_{IMP}, and bla_{VIM} by multiplex PCRs as previously described [23]. DNA extraction was done by a boiling lysis method as described [24]. The PCR Amplification conditions were described elsewhere [25, 26].

DNA sequencing analysis

The Purified PCR products of ESBL producers were sequenced with the Sanger ABI 3730 XL automated DNA sequencer by a commercial company (BaseClear, Leiden, The Netherlands). Nucleotide sequences were aligned by the Codon Code Aligner software (Version 5.0.2) and compared to sequences available at the National Center for Biotechnology Information website (www.ncbi.nlm.nih.gov).

E-coli Phylogroups

E. coli isolates were segregated into phylogroups (A, B1, B2 or D) by a triplex PCR targeting *chuA*, *yjaA* and the *TspE4.C2* DNA fragment, as developed by Clermont et al. [27].

Statistical analysis

All statistical analyses were performed according to Newcombe, Robert G [28].

Results

Sixty-eight out of 100 feces samples yielded ESBL-E while CPE was identified in 5% of theses samples. Some samples demonstrated the growth of more than one species of Enterobacteriaceae, resulting in 113 isolates available for analysis. ESBLs were identified in 64.61% (73/113) (with 95% confidence interval (CI): 55.44–72.80) of the isolates and five (4.42%) (95% CI: 1.9–9.94) isolates showed carbapenemase activity. The prevalence of different ESBL types among the different Enterobacteriaceae species is shown in Table 1. It was highest in *Klebsiella pneumoniae.* Because only one *Salmonella* strain isolated, which produced CTX-M, we could not estimate the prevalence of ESBL-production in this species. All five carbapenem-resistant Enterobacteriaceae isolates were *K. pneumoniae.*CTX-M enzymes were detected in 89.04% (65/73) of the ESBL-producing Enterobacteriaceae, whereas SHV and TEM were detected in 30.14% (22/73) and 19.18% (14/73) respectively. The simultaneous presence of CTX-M, SHV, and TEM was identified in 9 isolates, 12 isolates coproduced CTX-M and SHV, 4 harbored CTX-M and TEM genes, one expressed SHV and TEM genes and 40 produced CTX-M genes only. Seven *E.coli* isolate expressed ESBL phenotype but no TEM, SHV or CTX-M were detected by PCR.

A summary of the distribution of different ß-lactamase-encoding genes among different Enterobacteriaceae is shown in Table 1.

Three out of 5 carbapenem-resistant *K. pneumoniae* harbored *blaNDM* and 2 produced *blaVIM*. No isolate expressed a combination of carbapenemase resistance genes.Of the 65 CTX-M – producing Enterobacteriaceae isolates, 52 (80%) produced CTX-M-15, five (7.7%) produced CTX-M-3, four (6.2%) produced CTX-M-14, one produced CTX-M-27, one produced CTX-M-32, and two, which belonged to CTX-M group 9, remained unidentified.

Antimicrobial susceptibility testing revealed that of the 73 ESBL-positive isolates, 58 (79.45%) expressed co-resistance to trimethoprim/sulfamethoxazole, 48 (65.75%) to quinolones (ciprofloxacin and /or norfloxacin), 33 (45.21%) to aminoglycosides (gentamicin and/or

Table 1 Prevalence of the different types of ß-lactamase-encoding genes among different Enterobacteriaceae species

Species	No. of isolates	No. of ESBL positive isolates (%)	CTX-M alone	CTX-M + TEM	CTX-M + SHV	TEM + SHV	CTX-M + TEM + SHV
E.coli	72	51 (70.83)	38	3	2	0	1
Klebsiella pneumoniae	23	19 (82.61)	0	0	10	1	8
Enterobacter spp	3	2 (66.66)	1	1	0	0	0
Salmonella spp	1	1 (100)	1	0	0	0	0
Other species	14	0(0)	0	0	0	0	0
Total	113	73 (64.61)	40	4	12	1	9

Table 2 The antimicrobial resistance pattern of CPE

Sample No.	Gentamicin	Tobramycin	Ciprofloxacin	Norfloxacin	Nitrofurantoin	Cotrimoxazole
1	R[a]	R	S	S	S	R
2	R	R	S	S	S	R
3	R	R	I	R	S	R
4	S[a]	R	R	R	R	R
5	R	R	R	R	S	R

[a]*R* resistant, *S* sensitive

tobramycin) and only one to nitrofurantoin. Twenty-two (30.14%) of the ESBL-positive isolates were multidrug resistant (MDR) (i.e. resistant to at least one agent in three or more classes of antimicrobials (aminoglycosides, quinolones and cotrimoxazole) [29].The antimicrobial resistance pattern of CPE is provided in Table 2

Phylogenetic analysis of *E.coli* isolate revealed that, ESBL-positive isolates were evenly distributed over the different phylogroups, while phylogroup A was under-represented among ESBL-negative *E. coli* (Table 3).

Discussion

This study was conducted to determine the prevalence of extended-spectrum β-lactamase and carbapenemase production among Enterobacteriaceae isolates recovered from the feces of ambulatory patients with community–onset gastrointestinal complaints admitted to El-Ahrar General Hospital, Zagazig, Egypt.

Our findings showed that almost two in every three Egyptian patients with community–onset gastrointestinal complaints are carriers of ESBL-E. Furthermore, nearly 5% of these patients were colonized with CPE. This high rate of colonization with ESBL-E and CPE is most likely due to imprudent antimicrobial use, as in Egypt and other developing countries, antimicrobial agents are readily available and can be purchased as a commodity. What is more, many Egyptian patients receive antimicrobial treatment without the advice or prescription of a physician or other trained health care provider. Also, even when the antimicrobial treatment is officially prescribed, it is almost entirely empirical and not based on individual susceptibility data nor on surveillance data [30].

Table 3 Phylogenetic groups of *E-coli* isolates

Phylogroups	No. of ESBL positive *E.coli*	No. of ESBL-negative *E.coli*
A	11	2
B1	10	8
B2	17	5
D	13	6
Total	51	21

Overall, the rate of fecal ESBL-E demonstrated in our study is higher than reported from many other countries in Africa, Asia, Europe and North America, but lower than what has been described for Thailand [9–13, 31–34].

The prevalence of fecal ESBL-E found in a study conducted in Cairo by Abdul Rahman and El-Sherif in 2011, was similar to what we observed [14]. In that study, ESBL-E were detected phenotypically, without genotypic confirmation and the prevalence of CPE was not determined.

CTX-M enzymes were the most common ß-lactamases among the Enterobacteriaceae isolates, followed by SHV and TEM. These results are consistent with those of previous studies from other countries around the world [11–13, 35, 36] that reported the dominance of CTX-M over other types of ESBLs. Which CTX-M alleles are dominant may differ by geographical region; we found that CTX-M-15 was the most frequently identified genotype among CTX-M–producing Enterobacteriaceae isolates. These findings confirm the reports of the worldwide spread and predominance of CTX-M-15 [37, 38].

Approximately one in every 20 patients included in our study, was colonized with CPE. This high frequency of carriage of CPE has not been described before in any African country and is quite alarming. It raises public health concern about the efficacy of carbapenems, which are the last resort for treatment of multidrug-resistant enterobacterial infections [39].

The bla_{NDM} gene was identified in three of the five *Klebsiella pneumoniae* isolates which showed a carbapenem–resistant phenotype while the other two isolates expressed a bla_{VIM} gene.

Our findings of NDM–producing isolates among patients who had no identified epidemiological link with the Indian subcontinent, the main reservoir of these isolates, along with the recent reports of NDM-producing Enterobacteriaceae derived from Egyptian septicemic patients and from retail chicken meat in Zagazig, Egypt [40, 41], support the hypothesis of the presence of autochthonous NDM-producing strains in the Middle East region [42].

The presence of Enterobacteriaceae producing NDM or VIM has been documented recently in several countries in the Middle East and North Africa [41, 43–45]. All reports, however, are case reports, describing the molecular characteristics of a few strains isolated from clinical specimens in hospitalized patients. Our study is the first that documents the prevalence, hence the size of the problem, in community-dwelling persons.

The antibiotic susceptibility testing revealed that four-fifths of ESBL-positive isolates were also resistant to trimethoprim/sulfamethoxazole, nearly two-thirds also to quinolones, and one-third also to aminoglycosides. Approximately half of the isolates were multidrug resistant, which stresses the public health threat by these isolates, which leave few options for treatment. Nitrofurantoin still had good activity against ESBL-E and CPE.

ESBL- *E. coli* isolates mainly belonged to the virulent groups B2/D, whereas ESBL- negative *E. coli* isolates were nearly equally distributed over the commensal groups A/B1 and the virulent groups B2/D. This finding suggests that there may be a relationship between virulence and resistance determinants, in contrast to the previously suggested trade-off between virulence and resistance [46].

Conclusion

In conclusion, nearly two third of the Enterobacteriaceae isolates recovered from feces of Egyptian patients in Zagazig region with community–onset gastrointestinal complaints were ESBL producers and one in every 20 patients included in our study was colonized with CPE. These high rates call for better surveillance of resistance in Egypt, and for a more prudent antimicrobial use. Regulation of sales of antimicrobial agents, as recently introduced in India would be a large step forward [47].

Abbreviations

CLSI: Clinical and laboratory standards institute; CPE: Carbapenemase-producing Enterobacteriaceae.; ESBL: Extended-spectrum β-lactamase.; ESBL-E: Extended-spectrum β-lactamase -producing Enterobacteriaceae.; MALDI-TOF-MS: Matrix-assisted laser desorption ionization time-of-flight mass spectrometry.; MDR: Multidrug- resistant.; NDM: New Delhi metallo-beta-lactamase.; VIM: Verona integron-encoded metallo- beta -lactamase.

Acknowledgements

We would like to express our gratitude to the staff of the microbiology department, El-Ahrar General Hospital, Zagazig, Egypt, for collecting the feces samples.

Funding

The research is funded by the joint supervision mission between Egyptian high education ministry and VU medical center, the Netherlands.

Authors' contributions

CV, NA, HA, AK Substantial contributions to the conception or design of the work; or the acquisition, analysis, or interpretation of data for the work; and HA, NA, CV, BW, KA, ER: Drafting the work or revising it critically for important intellectual content; and HA, NA, CV, AM, AS Final approval of the version to be published; and HA, CV. Agreement to be accountable for all aspects of the work in ensuring that questions related to the accuracy or integrity of any part of the work are appropriately investigated and resolved. All authors read and approved the final manuscript.

Competing interests

The authors declare that they have no competing interests.

Consent for publication

Not applicable

Author details

[1]Medical Microbiology and Infection Control, VU University Medical Center, Amsterdam, The Netherlands. [2]Laboratory for Medical Microbiology and Public Health, Hengelo, The Netherlands. [3]Department of Microbiology, Faculty of Veterinary Medicine, Zagazig University, Zagazig, Egypt. [4]National Laboratory for Veterinary Quality Control on Poultry Production, Animal Health Research Institute, Dokki, Giza, Egypt. [5]Department of Virology, Faculty of Veterinary Medicine, Zagazig University, Zagazig, Egypt.

References

1. Shaikh S, Fatima J, Shakil S, Rizvi SMD, Kamal MA. Antibiotic resistance and extended-spectrum beta-lactamases: types, epidemiology and treatment. Saudi J Biol Sci. 2015;22:90–101. [cited 2016 Mar 31]. Available from: http://www.pubmedcentral.nih.gov/articlerender.fcgi?artid=4281622&tool=pmcentrez&rendertype=abstract
2. Bradford PA. Extended-spectrum beta-lactamases in the 21st century: characterization, epidemiology, and detection of this important resistance threat. Clin Microbiol Rev. 2001;14:933–51. [cited 2014 Dec 27], table of contents. Available from: http://cmr.asm.org/content/14/4/933.abstract?ijkey=ee4d374e9991270b273bab1b470247e510edb106&keytype2=tf_ipsecsha
3. de Kraker MEA, Jarlier V, Monen JCM, Heuer OE, van de Sande N, Grundmann H. The changing epidemiology of bacteraemias in Europe: trends from the European antimicrobial resistance surveillance system. Clin Microbiol Infect. 2013;19:860–8. [cited 2015 Jan 26]. Available from: http://www.ncbi.nlm.nih.gov/pubmed/23039210
4. Schwaber MJ, Navon-Venezia S, Kaye KS, Ben-Ami R, Schwartz D, Carmeli Y. Clinical and economic impact of bacteremia with extended- spectrum-beta-lactamase-producing obacteriaceae. Antimicrob Agents Chemother. 2006;50:1257–62. [cited 2015 Feb 11]. Available from: http://aac.asm.org/content/50/4/1257.abstract?ijkey=89ea06a2b38fe1368a38aae72d8b7525105143258&keytype2=tf_ipsecsha
5. Lukac PJ, Bonomo RA, Logan LK. Extended-spectrum β-lactamase-producing Enterobacteriaceae in children: Old Foe, Emerging Threat. Clin. Infect. Dis. 2015 [cited 2015 Feb 5];civ020-. Available from: http://cid.oxfordjournals.org/content/early/2015/01/15/cid.civ020.short
6. Girlich D, Bouihat N, Poirel L, Benouda A, Nordmann P. High rate of faecal carriage of extended-spectrum β-lactamase and OXA-48 carbapenemase-producing Enterobacteriaceae at a university hospital in Morocco. Clin Microbiol Infect. 2014;20:350–4. [cited 2015 Feb 10]. Available from: http://www.ncbi.nlm.nih.gov/pubmed/23927757
7. Mirelis B, Navarro F, Miró E, Mesa RJ, Coll P, Prats G. Community transmission of extended-spectrum beta-lactamase. Emerg Infect Dis. 2003;9:1024–5. [cited 2015 Mar 2]. Available from: http://www.pubmedcentral.nih.gov/articlerender.fcgi?artid=3020612&tool=pmcentrez&rendertype=abstract
8. Luvsansharav U-O, Hirai I, Nakata A, Imura K, Yamauchi K, Niki M, et al. Prevalence of and risk factors associated with faecal carriage of CTX-M β-lactamase-producing Enterobacteriaceae in rural Thai communities. J Antimicrob Chemother. 2012;67:1769–74. [cited 2015 Mar 2]. Available from: http://jac.oxfordjournals.org/content/67/7/1769.abstract?ijkey=4534e73fe311b5ddc7a4110a60de8e0f71f35b83&keytype2=tf_ipsecsha
9. Li B, Sun J-Y, Liu Q-Z, Han L-Z, Huang X-H, Ni Y-X. High prevalence of CTX-M β-lactamases in faecal Escherichia Coli strains from healthy humans in Fuzhou, China. Scand J Infect Dis. 2011;43:170–4. [cited 2015 Mar 23]. Available from: http://www.ncbi.nlm.nih.gov/pubmed/21128708
10. Valverde A, Coque TM, Sánchez-Moreno MP, Rollán A, Baquero F, Cantón R. Dramatic increase in prevalence of fecal carriage of extended-spectrum

beta-lactamase-producing Enterobacteriaceae during nonoutbreak situations in Spain. J Clin Microbiol. 2004;42:4769–75. [cited 2015 Mar 2]. Available from: http://www.pubmedcentral.nih.gov/articlerender.fcgi?artid=522353&tool=pmcentrez&rendertype=abstract

11. Valenza G, Nickel S, Pfeifer Y, Eller C, Krupa E, Lehner-Reindl V, et al. Extended-spectrum-β-lactamase-producing Escherichia Coli as intestinal colonizers in the German community. Antimicrob Agents Chemother. 2014;58:1228–30. [cited 2015 Mar 2]. Available from: http://www.pubmedcentral.nih.gov/articlerender.fcgi?artid=3910888&tool=pmcentrez&rendertype=abstract
12. Reuland EA, Overdevest ITMA, Al Naiemi N, Kalpoe JS, Rijnsburger MC, Raadsen SA, et al. High prevalence of ESBL-producing Enterobacteriaceae carriage in Dutch community patients with gastrointestinal complaints. Clin Microbiol Infect. 2013;19:542–9. [cited 2014 Jun 25]. Available from: http://www.ncbi.nlm.nih.gov/pubmed/22757622
13. Weisenberg SA, Mediavilla JR, Chen L, Alexander EL, Rhee KY, Kreiswirth BN, et al. Extended spectrum beta-lactamase-producing Enterobacteriaceae in international travelers and non-travelers in New York City. PLoS One. 2012;7: e45141. [cited 2015 Mar 2]. Available from: http://journals.plos.org/plosone/article?id=10.1371/journal.pone.0045141
14. Abdul Rahman EM, El-Sherif RH. High rates of intestinal colonization with extended-spectrum lactamase-producing Enterobacteriaceae among healthy individuals. J Investig Med. 2011;59:1284–6. [cited 2015 Mar 19]. Available from: http://www.ncbi.nlm.nih.gov/pubmed/22068018
15. Al Naiemi N, Murk JL, Savelkoul PHM, Vandenbroucke-Grauls CMJ, Debets-Ossenkopp YJ. Extended-spectrum beta-lactamases screening agar with AmpC inhibition. Eur J Clin Microbiol Infect Dis. 2009;28:989–90. [cited 2014 Aug 11]. Available from: http://www.pubmedcentral.nih.gov/articlerender.fcgi?artid=2723665&tool=pmcentrez&rendertype=abstract
16. CLSI. Performance standards for antimicrobial 2014.
17. al Naiemi N, Cohen Stuart J, Leverstein van Hall M. NVMM guideline laboratory detection of highly resistant microorganisms (HRMO) ,version 2.0. 2012; Available from: http://www.nvmm.nl/richtlijnen/hrmo-laboratory-detection-highly-resistant-microorganisms.
18. Pasteran F, Mendez T, Guerriero L, Rapoport M, Corso A. Sensitive screening tests for suspected class a carbapenemase production in species of Enterobacteriaceae. J Clin Microbiol. 2009;47:1631–9. [cited 2014 Nov 19]. Available from: http://www.pubmedcentral.nih.gov/articlerender.fcgi?artid=2691115&tool=pmcentrez&rendertype=abstract
19. Tsakris A, Kristo I, Poulou A, Themeli-Digalaki K, Ikonomidis A, Petropoulou D, et al. Evaluation of boronic acid disk tests for differentiating KPC-possessing Klebsiella Pneumoniae isolates in the clinical laboratory. J Clin Microbiol. 2009; 47:362–7. [cited 2014 Dec 24]. Available from: http://www.pubmedcentral.nih.gov/articlerender.fcgi?artid=2643660&tool=pmcentrez&rendertype=abstract
20. Olesen I, Hasman H, Aarestrup FM. Prevalence of beta-lactamases among ampicillin-resistant Escherichia Coli and salmonella isolated from food animals in Denmark. Microb Drug Resist. 2004;10:334–40. [cited 2014 Sep 8]. Available from: http://www.ncbi.nlm.nih.gov/pubmed/15650379
21. Weill F-X, Demartin M, Tandé D, Espié E, Rakotoarivony I. Grimont PAD. SHV-12-like extended-spectrum-beta-lactamase-producing strains of salmonella enterica serotypes Babelsberg and Enteritidis isolated in France among infants adopted from Mali. J Clin Microbiol. 2004;42: 2432–7. [cited 2014 Sep 8]. Available from: http://www.pubmedcentral.nih.gov/articlerender.fcgi?artid=427894&tool=pmcentrez&rendertype=abstract
22. Mulvey MR, Soule G, Boyd D, Demczuk W, Ahmed R. Characterization of the first extended-spectrum beta-lactamase-producing salmonella isolate identified in Canada. J Clin Microbiol. 2003;41:460–2. [cited 2014 Sep 11]. Available from: http://www.pubmedcentral.nih.gov/articlerender.fcgi?artid=149628&tool=pmcentrez&rendertype=abstract
23. Poirel L, Walsh TR, Cuvillier V, Nordmann P. Multiplex PCR for detection of acquired carbapenemase genes. Diagn Microbiol Infect Dis. 2011;70:119–23. [cited 2014 Aug 5]. Available from: http://www.sciencedirect.com/science/article/pii/S0732889310005559
24. De Medici D, Croci L, Delibato E, Di Pasquale S, Filetici E, Toti L. Evaluation of DNA extraction methods for use in combination with SYBR green I real-time PCR to detect salmonella enterica serotype Enteritidis in poultry. Appl Environ Microbiol. 2003;69:3456–61. [cited 2014 Sep 24]. Available from: http://aem.asm.org/content/69/6/3456.full
25. Naas T, Oxacelay C, Nordmann P. Identification of CTX-M-type extended-spectrum-beta-lactamase genes using real-time PCR and pyrosequencing. Antimicrob Agents Chemother. 2007;51:223–30. [cited 2014 Nov 28]. Available from: http://www.pubmedcentral.nih.gov/articlerender.fcgi?artid=1797662&tool=pmcentrez&rendertype=abstract
26. Wang L, Gu H, Lu X. A rapid low-cost real-time PCR for the detection of Klebsiella pneumonia carbapenemase genes. Ann Clin Microbiol Antimicrob. 2012;11:9. [cited 2014 Nov 28]. Available from: http://www.pubmedcentral.nih.gov/articlerender.fcgi?artid=3377543&tool=pmcentrez&rendertype=abstract
27. Clermont O, Bonacorsi S, Bingen E. Rapid and simple determination of the Escherichia Coli phylogenetic group. Appl Environ Microbiol. 2000; 66:4555–8. [cited 2014 Nov 27] Available from: http://www.pubmedcentral.nih.gov/articlerender.fcgi?artid=92342&tool=pmcentrez&rendertype=abstract
28. Newcombe RG. Two-sided confidence intervals for the single proportion: comparison of seven methods. Stat Med. 1998;17:857–72. [cited 2016 May 18]. Available from: http://www.ncbi.nlm.nih.gov/pubmed/9595616
29. Epstein S. Small Animal Critical Care Medicine. Small Anim. Crit. Care Med. Elsevier; 2015 [cited 2014 Oct 13]. Available from: http://www.sciencedirect.com/science/article/pii/B9781455703067001033
30. Knobler SL, Lemon SM, Najafi M, Burroughs T. Factors Contributing to the Emergence of Resistance [Internet]. National Academies Press (US); 2003 [cited 2015 Mar 23]. Available from: http://www.ncbi.nlm.nih.gov/books/NBK97126/
31. Ahmed SF, MMM A, Mohamed ZK, Moussa TA, Klena JD. Fecal carriage of extended-spectrum β-lactamases and AmpC-producing Escherichia Coli in a Libyan community. Ann Clin Microbiol Antimicrob. 2014;13:22. [cited 2015 Feb 9]. Available from: http://www.ann-clinmicrob.com/content/13/1/22
32. Ben Sallem R, Ben Slama K, Estepa V, Jouini A, Gharsa H, Klibi N, et al. Prevalence and characterisation of extended-spectrum beta-lactamase (ESBL)-producing Escherichia Coli isolates in healthy volunteers in Tunisia. Eur J Clin Microbiol Infect Dis. 2012;31:1511–6. [cited 2015 Feb 20]. Available from: http://www.ncbi.nlm.nih.gov/pubmed/22065280
33. Luvsansharav U-O, Hirai I, Niki M, Nakata A, Yoshinaga A, Moriyama T, et al. Prevalence of fecal carriage of extended-spectrum β-lactamase-producing Enterobacteriaceae among healthy adult people in Japan. J Infect Chemother. 2011;17:722–5. [cited 2015 Apr 1]. Available from: http://www.ncbi.nlm.nih.gov/pubmed/21359543
34. Kader AA, Kumar A, Kamath KA. Fecal carriage of extended-spectrum beta-lactamase-producing Escherichia Coli and Klebsiella Pneumoniae in patients and asymptomatic healthy individuals. Infect Control Hosp Epidemiol. 2007; 28:1114–6. [cited 2015 Mar 23]. Available from: http://www.ncbi.nlm.nih.gov/pubmed/17932839
35. Zhang J, Zheng B, Zhao L, Wei Z, Ji J, Li L, et al. Nationwide high prevalence of CTX-M and an increase of CTX-M-55 in Escherichia Coli isolated from patients with community-onset infections in Chinese county hospitals. BMC Infect Dis. 2014;14:659. [cited 2015 Apr 9]. Available from: http://www.biomedcentral.com/1471-2334/14/659
36. Pournaras S, Ikonomidis A, Kristo I, Tsakris A, Maniatis AN. CTX-M enzymes are the most common extended-spectrum beta-lactamases among Escherichia Coli in a tertiary Greek hospital. J Antimicrob Chemother. 2004; 54:574–5. [cited 2015 Apr 9]. Available from: http://jac.oxfordjournals.org/content/54/2/574.full
37. Rossolini GM, D'Andrea MM, Mugnaioli C. The spread of CTX-M-type extended-spectrum beta-lactamases. Clin Microbiol. 2008;14(Suppl 1):33–41. [cited 2014 Jun 10]. Available from: http://www.ncbi.nlm.nih.gov/pubmed/18154526
38. Cantón R, Coque TM. The CTX-M beta-lactamase pandemic. Curr Opin Microbiol. 2006;9:466–75. [cited 2015 Apr 10]. Available from: http://www.ncbi.nlm.nih.gov/pubmed/16942899
39. Vardakas KZ, Tansarli GS, Rafailidis PI, Falagas ME. Carbapenems versus alternative antibiotics for the treatment of bacteraemia due to Enterobacteriaceae producing extended-spectrum β-lactamases: a systematic review and meta-analysis. J Antimicrob Chemother. 2012;67: 2793–803. [cited 2015 Apr 9]. Available from: http://jac.oxfordjournals.org/content/67/12/2793.abstract?ijkey=d56e6b71d2644189b8663c79402a480aa6b02f3d&keytype2=tf_ipsecsha
40. Abdallah HM, Reuland EA, Wintermans BB, Al Naiemi N, Koek A, Abdelwahab AM, et al. Extended-Spectrum β-Lactamases and/or Carbapenemases-Producing Enterobacteriaceae Isolated from Retail Chicken Meat in Zagazig, Egypt. PLoS One. Public Library of Science; 2015 [cited 2015 Nov 12];10:e0136052. Available from: http://www.plosone.org/article/Metrics/info:doi/10.1371/journal.pone.0136052

41. Abdallah HM, Wintermans BB, Reuland EA, Koek A, al Naiemi N, Ammar AM, et al. Extended-Spectrum β-Lactamase- and Carbapenemase-Producing Enterobacteriaceae Isolated from Egyptian Patients with Suspected Blood Stream Infection. PLoS One [Internet]. Public Library of Science; 2015 [cited 2015 Nov 12];10:e0128120. Available from: http://journals.plos.org/plosone/article?id=10.1371/journal.pone.0128120
42. Nordmann P, Poirel L, Walsh TR, Livermore DM. The emerging NDM carbapenemases. Trends Microbiol. [Internet]. 2011;19:588–595 [cited 2015 Mar 24]. Available from: http://www.ncbi.nlm.nih.gov/pubmed/22078325.
43. Sonnevend A, Al Baloushi A, Ghazawi A, Hashmey R, Girgis S, Hamadeh MB, et al. Emergence and spread of NDM-1 producer Enterobacteriaceae with contribution of IncX3 plasmids in the United Arab Emirates. J Med Microbiol. 2013;62:1044–50. [cited 2014 Oct 14]. Available from: http://www.ncbi.nlm.nih.gov/pubmed/23579399
44. Shahcheraghi F, Nobari S, Rahmati Ghezelgeh F, Nasiri S, Owlia P, Nikbin VS, et al. First report of New Delhi metallo-beta-lactamase-1-producing Klebsiella Pneumoniae in Iran. Microb Drug Resist. 2013;19:30–6. [cited 2014 Oct 14]. Available from: http://www.ncbi.nlm.nih.gov/pubmed/22984942
45. Nordmann P, Naas T, Poirel L, Carbapenemases CA. Global spread of Carbapenemase- producing Enterobacteriaceae. Emerg Infect Dis. 2011;17:1791–8.
46. Clermont O, Lavollay M, Vimont S, Deschamps C, Forestier C, Branger C, et al. The CTX-M-15-producing Escherichia Coli diffusing clone belongs to a highly virulent B2 phylogenetic subgroup. J Antimicrob Chemother. 2008; 61:1024–8. [cited 2015 Apr 13]. Available from: http://jac.oxfordjournals.org/content/61/5/1024.abstract?ijkey=bbb28712027050a89bd7bd8255b3666af11a677e&keytype2=tf_ipsecsha
47. Ghafur A. Perseverance, persistence, and the Chennai declaration. Lancet. Infect. Dis. [Internet]. Elsevier; 2013 [cited 2015 Nov 17];13:1007–8. Available from: http://www.thelancet.com/article/S1473309913703141/fulltext

11

Implementation of short incubation MALDI-TOF MS identification from positive blood cultures in routine diagnostics and effects on empiric antimicrobial therapy

Robin Köck[1,2*], Jörg Wüllenweber[1], Dagmar Horn[3], Christian Lanckohr[4], Karsten Becker[1] and Evgeny A. Idelevich[1]

Abstract

Background: Results of blood culture (BC) diagnostics should be swiftly available to guide treatment of critically ill patients. Conventional BC diagnostics usually performs species identification of microorganisms from mature solid medium colonies. Species identification might be speed up by using matrix-assisted laser desorption ionization time-of-flight (MALDI-TOF) mass spectrometry (MS) of biomass from shortly incubated solid media.

Methods: This single-center analysis compared the applicability of MALDI-TOF-based species identification from shortly incubated cultures in laboratory routine vs. conventional diagnostics and assessed its effects of on empiric antibiotic therapy.

Results: Median time between detection of BCs as "positive" by incubators and further processing (e.g. microscopy) was 6 h 21 min. Median time between microscopy and result reporting to the ward was 15 min. Including 193 BCs, MALDI-TOF from shortly incubated biomass resulted in significantly faster ($p > 0.001$) species identification. Species results became available for clinicians after a median of 188 min (231 min for Gram-positive bacteria, 151 min for Gram-negative bacteria) compared to 909 min ($n = 192$ BCs) when conventional diagnostics was used. For 152/179 bacteremia episodes (85%) empiric antibiotic therapy had already been started when the microscopy result was reported to the ward; microscopy led to changes of therapies in 14/179 (8%). In contrast, reporting the bacterial species (without antibiogram) resulted in therapeutic adjustments in 36/179 (20%). Evaluating these changes revealed improved therapies in 26/36 cases (72%).

Conclusions: Species identification by MALDI-TOF MS from shortly incubated subcultures resulted in adjustments of empiric antibiotic therapies and might improve the clinical outcome of septic patients.

Keywords: Antibiotic stewardship, MALDI-TOF MS, Sepsis, Diagnostics, Blood culture

Background

Taking blood cultures (BC) is one of the most important components of diagnostics performed for critically ill patients. As the mortality of septic patients is highly dependent on an accurate therapeutic approach during the early phase of the infection, treatment follows the general principle *"frapper fort et frapper vite"* (as postulated by Paul Ehrlich in 1913) [1]. This means that empiric therapy is initiated immediately using adequate doses of antibiotics covering the expected spectrum of pathogens [2]. Hence, the results of BC diagnostics will usually not be used to start treatment, but rather to reassess whether initial empiric therapy was accurate and to adjust it, if necessary. This makes BC diagnostics a key issue of antibiotic stewardship programs aiming to de-escalate empiric broad-spectrum antibiotics and improve the rational use of antimicrobials [3].

* Correspondence: koeck.robin@klinikum-oldenburg.de
[1]Institute of Medical Microbiology, University Hospital Münster, Domagkstr. 10, 48149 Münster, Germany
[2]Present address: Institute of Hospital Hygiene, University of Oldenburg, European Medical School Oldenburg-Groningen, Rahel-Straus-Str. 10, 26133 Oldenburg, Germany
Full list of author information is available at the end of the article

However, a disadvantage associated with culture-based BC diagnostics is that it follows the "biological" clock rate of microbial growth but not the clock speed determined by the clinical progress of a severe infection. This hampers early adjustment of empiric antimicrobial therapies to diagnostic findings and leads to, first, increased morbidity or mortality of severely ill patients, and second, an extended empiric use of broad-spectrum antibiotics [4].

As a result, many recent studies have assessed the technical effectiveness of culture-independent BC diagnostic methods with the aim of identifying DNA of the causative species in the blood sample more rapidly [5–10]. However, PCR approaches are still expensive and have drawbacks regarding sensitivity and specificity [11, 12]. An alternative is to conventionally incubate BC bottles in an automated system and use matrix-assisted laser desorption ionization time-of-flight mass-spectrometry (MALDI-TOF MS) directly from BC bottles in which microbial growth was indicated by the automated system [13]. This approach is also valuable, but requires more laborious and costly processing of the BC in the microbiological laboratory.

Therefore, Idelevich et al. recently evaluated a simple alternative method for species identification: it was demonstrated that MALDI-TOF performed from "immature" biomass growing on solid media shortly (2–4 h) after inoculation with broth from a positive BC bottle, successfully identified the growing microorganisms [14]. This can be done in all laboratories where MALDI-TOF MS is available and does not increase consumable costs compared with conventional BC diagnostics (as species diagnostics has to be done anyway) [15].

While Idelevich et al. assessed the "technical" accuracy of this method, its feasibility in clinical, microbiological lab-routine has not been described. Moreover, it is unclear to what extent clinicians use the faster species information provided by MALDI-TOF MS from shortly incubated cultures for adjustments of empiric antibiotic therapy, because species information is initially provided without antibiograms. Therefore, we assessed these two issues in this retrospective study. The results shall allow for conclusions whether implementing MALDI-TOF based species identification from shortly incubated biomass has effects on empiric antimicrobial therapy.

Methods

This analysis retrospectively assessed the effects of a change in microbiological BC diagnostics. The study was performed at the Institute of Medical Microbiology, University Hospital Münster (UHM), Germany. The laboratory offers microbiological service routinely from 7:30 a.m. to 6:30 p.m. (Monday through Friday), 7:30 a.m. through 1:00 p.m. (Saturday) and 9:00 a.m. through noon (Sunday). The institute provides service almost exclusively for the UHM, which is a maximum care university hospital with about 1400 beds in Northwestern Germany. The facilities of the institute are located on the UHM campus, i.e. the distance of the microbiological laboratory to all clinics, wards and other facilities of the hospital does not exceed one kilometer.

Conventional BC diagnostics

Conventional BC diagnostics comprised the following routine procedures:

a.) BC bottles (BD BACTEC™ PLUS media) were transported from the wards to the microbiological laboratory. After arrival in the laboratory they were placed in an automated BC incubation system (BD BACTEC™ 9240). If growth in a BC bottle was indicated by the automated system, the bottle was immediately processed and streaked onto solid media (Columbia and chocolate blood agar, Schaedler agar additionally for anaerobic culture bottles). Solid media were immediately placed in an incubator and a Gram-stain was performed. The result of the Gram stain was immediately communicated to a physician on the respective ward (by phone call) and was reported to the ward as a preliminary finding electronically.

b.) Further routine diagnostic procedures were as follows: species identification was done via MALDI-TOF MS and antibiotic susceptibility testing (mostly) via VITEK 2 automated system. Susceptibility testing was initiated from "mature" colonies growing on solid media in the afternoon (for BC bottles detected before 9 h in the morning) or the next day (for all BC bottles detected after 9 h); species identification was done from mature colonies the next day for all BCs.

Diagnostic changes

MALDI-TOF MS based species identification from immature biomass growing on solid media was implemented as follows: Step a.) described for conventional diagnostics remained unchanged. In step b.) the solid media inoculated with material from the positive BC bottle were visually evaluated for the first time approximately 2-3 h after start of incubation. As soon as growth of biomass (rather mature "colonies") was visible on the agar plates, species identification was performed from these "young" cultures using MALDI-TOF MS. As soon as the species identification result was available (criteria for reliability as mentioned in [14]), it was reported to the ward. If no growth was visible, or no successful identification was achieved, the next visual evaluation was performed after further 2-3 h of incubation, followed by MALDI-TOF MS in case of visible growth. Further identification attempts after longer incubation were only performed in individual cases at the discretion of technologist or clinical microbiologist. In addition, standardized susceptibility testing (using VITEK-2) was initiated.

Data assessment

We assessed all positive BCs from 01.01.2013–30.06.2013 (before diagnostic change) and 01.01.2014–30.06.2014 (after diagnostic change). We considered all BC bottles (filled with blood, other body fluids were excluded). BCs fulfilling the following criteria were then removed from the dataset: i.) mixed cultures (i.e. >1 pathogen in one bottle, removed due to uncomplete or unreliable MALDI-TOF results), ii.) detection of fungi and anaerobic bacteria (removed due to slow growth), iii.) detection of coagulase-negative staphylococci, corynebacteria and propionibacteria (as we aimed to assess and evaluate the effects of MALDI-TOF on empiric therapy, the BCs were removed due to unclear clinical relevance and unclear effects on empiric therapy), iv.) consecutive cultures of the same patient (i.e. if the same pathogen was detected in more than one BC of the same patient, only the culture which was first indicated as "positive" by the BC incubator remained in the dataset).

For all BCs remaining in the final dataset, the following parameters were assessed from the laboratory software (OpusL, OSM, Essen, Germany) and the electronic patient record (Orbis, AGFA Healthcare, Bonn, Germany), where they are routinely recorded:

1. Date and time of a documented Gram stain result (i.e. the time is recorded when the result is entered in the computer system),
2. Date and time of the first report of a microscopic result to the ward (i.e. the time of the phone call is actively recorded by the person communicating the result),
3. Date and time of successful species identification (i.e. the time is recorded when the species name is entered in the lab software),
4. Date and time of the species available on the ward (i.e. the time when the finding appears in the electronic patient record, which is after entering it in the lab software (see point 3 and after electronic validation).
5. For all cultures after implementation of MALDI-TOF MS from shortly incubated cultures, we additionally assessed antibiotic therapy of the patient for a time period starting two days before the BC became positive and ending after reporting the species result to the ward. The quality of therapeutic adjustments attributable to the intervention was evaluated within a local antibiotic stewardship team, including an intensive care clinician, microbiologists and a pharmacist. An adjustment was considered rational when the new therapy was more likely to target or more efficient to treat the detected microorganism than the previous therapy.

Statistical differences were assessed using Chi-Square or t-test (Epi Info™, version 7.2, CDC Atlanta, USA); $p < 0.05$ was considered significant.

Results

Infrastructural parameters

In the half-year period before the diagnostic change 1185 BC sets with microbial growth from 544 patients were retrieved compared with 1132 BC sets from 540 patients after implementation of MALDI-TOF MS from shortly incubated cultures. After clearing the dataset (with respect to criteria i. to iv. see Methods), we analyzed data for 192 BCs before and 193 BCs after the diagnostic change, respectively ($p = 0.62$). Of all 385 BCs, 117 (30%) were indicated as "positive" by the BC incubator during routine service times of the microbiological laboratory and 268 (70%) outside service hours. Overall, the median time between bacterial growth reported by the BC incubation system and microscopy was 381 min (mean 410 min, range 6 min-1188 min). There was a major difference depending on whether the BC bottle was flagged "positive" during the service time of the laboratory or not; during service time: median 48 min (mean 65 min, range 6 min-1123 min) vs. outside service time: median 547 min (mean 561 min, range 18 min-1188 min), $p < 0.001$). The median time (mean, range) between microscopy and report of the result to the ward was 15 min (44 min, 0–1386 min).

Species identification time using conventional diagnostics vs. MALDI-TOF MS from shortly incubated cultures in clinical microbiological lab-routine

After implementation of the new concept for processing BCs in the laboratory, the time needed to report a species identification result (after initial microscopy) was significantly reduced (Table 1), even though this study partly included BCs for which MALDI-TOF MS was not carried out the same day. This effect was more prominent for Gram-negative (median 2.5 h) than for Gram-positive microorganisms (median about 4 h, Table 1).

Effects of species report on antimicrobial therapy

For the time after implementation of MALDI-TOF MS from shortly incubated cultures we analyzed antibiotic therapies for the patients with bacteremia (Fig. 1). The species distribution for microorganisms detected in the 193 BCs included in the intervention phase is shown in Fig. 2. The 193 BCs were derived from patients on nephrology wards ($n = 35$, including patients in an emergency department), hemato-oncology wards ($n = 35$), cardiology

Table 1 Time until species identification before and after implementation of MALDI-TOF MS from shortly incubated cultures

Bacterial pathogen	Before[a] (in minutes; median (mean; range))	After[a] (in minutes; median (mean; range))	P
All bacteria	909 (776; 2–1439)	188 (342; 0–1439)	<0.001
Gram-negative	811 (942; 9–1438)	151 (277; 36–1433)	<0.001
Gram-positive	849 (742; 2–1439)	231 (400; 0–1439)	<0.001

[a]time between microscopy and availability of species identification result before and after implementation of MALDI-TOF MS from shortly incubated cultures in laboratory routine

wards ($n = 20$), gastroenterology wards ($n = 19$), surgical intensive care units (ICU) ($n = 26$), pediatric wards ($n = 18$), general-, heart- and trauma-surgical wards ($n = 15$), neurology wards ($n = 9$), transplantation wards ($n = 7$), urology wards ($n = 4$), orthopedic wards ($n = 3$), wards for radiotherapy ($n = 2$), dermatology and ENT wards (each $n = 1$). The 193 BCs were taken from 172 different patients. If patients were included more than once, this was not due to consecutive cultures (see methods), but due to more than one bacteremia episode of this patient in which different bacteria were identified. For 179 of the BCs (from 158 patients), we were able to analyze the antibiotic prescriptions initiated for the respective patients (Fig. 1). The remaining patients were discharged or had died when the BC was detected positive. For 152 of the 179 bacteremia episodes (85%) an empiric antibiotic therapy was already initiated at the time of the initial contact with the ward (i.e. report of microscopy result).

Overall, after reporting the microscopy results antibiotic therapies were changed in 14/179 (8%) patients (Fig. 1). For none of these 14 cases the antimicrobial therapy was later adjusted again after the species identification result became available (before results of susceptibility tests were ready).

Overall, rapid reporting of the species identification result (without antibiogram) caused adjustments in empiric therapies of 36/179 (20%) bacteremia episodes. The mean time between reporting of species results to the ward and documented change of antibiotic therapy was 168 min (median 186 min, range 0–434 min).

Evaluating these 36 bacteremia episodes showed that the adjustments led to a better therapy in 26/36 cases (72%). Criterion for evaluating an adjustment as reasonable was that the identified species was more likely targeted with the antibiotic used than the previously used therapy (evaluations for single cases are shown in the supplementary material, Additional file 1: Table S1). Among the 36 cases in which adjustments of antibiotic treatment were performed after species identification, therapeutic changes were more often performed, if *S. aureus* was reported, as compared to all other pathogens (13/41 vs. 23/152, $p = 0.03$).

Discussion

The major aim of this study was to compare species identification times for microorganisms from BCs using a conventional diagnostic approach versus MALDI-TOF MS based species identification from shortly incubated

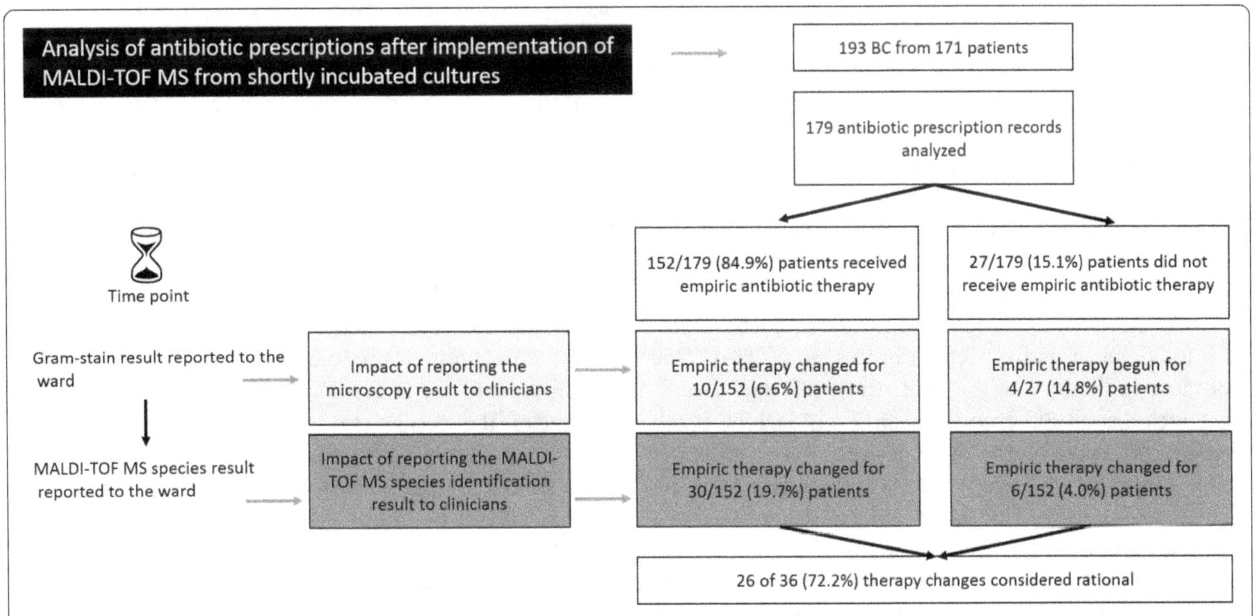

Fig. 1 Effects of MALDI-TOF MS species identification on empiric antimicrobial therapy

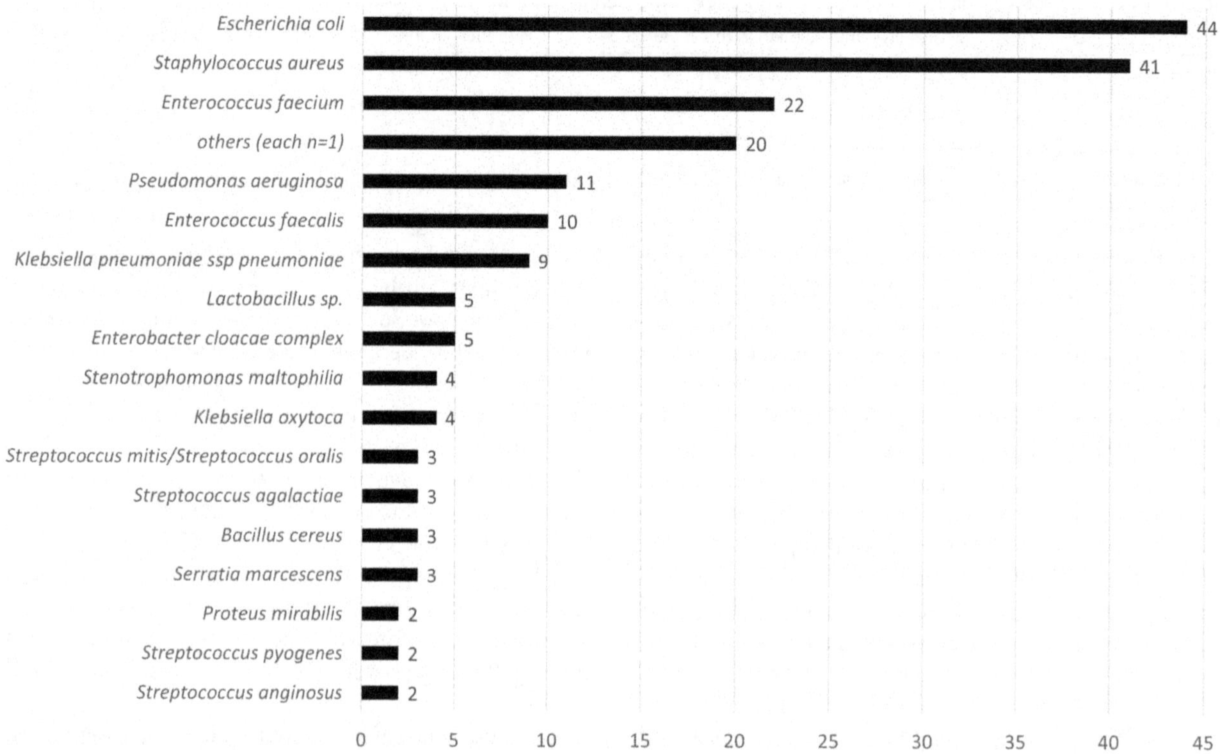

Fig. 2 Pathogens in blood cultures included ($n = 193$). Microorganisms summarized under "others (each $n = 1$)": *Haemophilus influenzae, Lactobacillus gasseri, Citrobacter freundii, Acinetobacter baumannii, Brevibacterium casei, Bacillus licheniformis, Salmonella* serovar Typhi, *Proteus vulgaris group, Enterococcus casseliflavus, Bacillus simplex, Streptococcus gallolyticus, Raoultella ornithinolytica, Streptococcus dysgalactiae subsp. equisimilis, Rothia dentocariosa, Rothia mucilaginosa, Streptococcus pneumoniae, Listeria monocytogenes, Streptococcus sanguinis, Moraxella osloensis, Pantoea agglomerans*

biomass. Technically, the applicability, validity and microbiological accuracy of this method has been demonstrated before in a pilot study [14]. In this study, we found that the results of the pilot study held true in daily routine. Performing MALDI-TOF MS of immature cultures resulted in a significant reduction of the median time until species identification for bacteria from BCs. Particularly for fast growing Gram-negative microorganisms, the median time until species identification was reduced to less than three hours. However, compared with our pilot studies the mean time until availability of species results was slightly higher (5.9 h for Gram-positive cocci and 2 h for Gram-negative rods in the study by Idelevich et al. vs. 6.7 h for Gram-positive bacteria and 4.6 h for Gram-negative bacteria in this study) [14]. This is because in contrast to the pilot study, this data assessment includes all BC cultures even if MALDI-TOF MS was not performed on the same day (e.g. for cultures detected in the late afternoon or on weekends where the service hours of the laboratory were restricted). These results are important as they show that the pilot studies do not markedly overestimate the benefits of MALDI-TOF MS of shortly incubated cultures when this technique is applied in microbiological routine diagnostics.

The application of PCR-based BC diagnostic tests has also resulted in a significant reduction of the time until species identification [16] and, partly, results were available even faster. However, major advantages of the diagnostic approach evaluated here are that it can be done without any additional consumable costs and that it leads to cultivated microorganisms ready for further characterization, in particular susceptibility testing. The efforts regarding re-organizing workflows of technical personnel and additional hands-on time was limited in our hands and the intervention was easy to implement in diagnostic routine. However, it should be noted that this study was done in a microbiological laboratory serving a single university hospital. This limited the daily number of BC bottles, which had to be processed and facilitated communication of the results to the wards. In regional labs with larger catchment areas and service for several facilities, the implementation of this diagnostic approach might be more challenging. However, recent and future developments in the field of laboratory automation including "smart" incubators and automated growth detection may facilitate the approach reported here.

Besides the positive effects of performing MALDI-TOF MS from immature biomass on the speed of diagnostics, we also found that our lab infrastructure limits the achievements made [5, 17, 18]. As the majority of BC bottles were reported "positive" by the automated incubator outside the service hours of the laboratory, the median time until further processing of a BC bottle (i.e. microscopy and plating on solid media) was >6 h. Besides offering longer service hours, another option to solve this problem might be the installation of BC incubators in areas of the hospital available for clinical personnel so that BC bottles can be continuously loaded into the systems [19]. The second infrastructural parameter assessed in this study was the time between performing microscopy and report of this result to ward. We are convinced that the 15 min interval observed is a reasonable. Outliers (>1000 min for reporting the microscopy results) were due to cases in which initial microscopy failed to identify bacteria in the Gram stain where they were actually present [20].

Besides evaluating the applicability of MALDI-TOF MS-based diagnostics in laboratory routine, we aimed to assess whether knowledge of the species (even without an antibiogram) led to adjustments of antibiotic therapies. We found that the clinicians changed empiric antibiotic therapies in 20% of all cases after communication of the species test result. This was more frequent than adjustments made based on microscopy results alone (8%). Hence, MALDI-TOF MS had an important clinical effect. On the other hand, a majority of antibiotic therapies remained unchanged. This could be explained by, first, adherence to well-designed guidelines for empiric therapies covering the reported species, second, difficulties of the treating physicians to correctly interpret the species report (without an antibiogram) with respect to how to adjust empiric therapies in a way that they are more accurate and sophisticated, or third, disregarding the diagnostic finding. Detailed evaluations of the quality of single therapeutic adjustments were difficult, as other diagnostic findings than BC results, such as allergies to antibiotics, data for organ insufficiencies and the overall prognosis of the clinical case must be considered. This is a major limitation of the retrospective study design. However, assessing the quality of adjustments after species identification in a local antibiotic stewardship team revealed that the majority of adjustments was appropriate. Clinicians particularly made adjustments for *S. aureus* bacteremia (32%), even if at this stage, antibiograms were not yet available. This might be due to the fact that at the UHM all patients are screened at admission for nasopharyngeal carriage of MRSA and, hence, MRSA bacteremia, which is mostly caused by strains colonizing the nares prior to infection [21], is rather unlikely, if a negative screening result from the nares is available. Moreover, the proportion of MRSA on all *S. aureus* isolates from BCs at our institutions followed the nationally declining trend in Germany and was <15% in 2014 (EARS-net, http://ecdc.europa.eu/, own data not shown). Interestingly, we found that in 11/13 *S. aureus* bacteremia cases (and 72% of all cases in which adjustments of antibiotic therapies were made) the modified therapy included the microorganism better the initial empiric regimen. Delport et al. recently reported positive clinical effects of performing MALDI-TOF MS from shortly incubated colonies. They observed in a pediatric patient collective that antibiotics were earlier optimized and the patients even had a favorable outcome and a shorter length of stay [22].

Conclusions

Overall, more rapid species diagnostics led to adjustments of empiric therapies in 20% and these adjustments improved calculated therapies in 72%. Therefore, the local antibiotic stewardship program shall focus on improved communication of the more rapid species results, maybe starting with a special emphasis of *S. aureus* bacteremia cases.

Acknowledgement
Not applicable.

Funding
This study was supported by the EU-funded project EurHealth-1Health [EU/INTERREG VA-681377].

Authors' contributions
RK and EAI wrote the manuscript. JW, EAI and KB implemented MALDI-TOF MS from shortly incubated cultures. RK, DH, CL, JW, KB and EAI evaluated the antibiotic prescriptions within the local antibiotic stewardship team. All authors read and approved the final manuscript.

Competing interests
The authors declare that they have no competing interests.

Consent for publication
Not applicable.

Author details
[1]Institute of Medical Microbiology, University Hospital Münster, Domagkstr. 10, 48149 Münster, Germany. [2]Present address: Institute of Hospital Hygiene, University of Oldenburg, European Medical School Oldenburg-Groningen, Rahel-Straus-Str. 10, 26133 Oldenburg, Germany. [3]Pharmacy Department, University Hospital Münster, Albert-Schweitzer-Campus 1, 48149 Münster, Germany. [4]Department for Anaesthesiology, Intensive Care Medicine and Pain Therapy, University Hospital Münster, Albert-Schweitzer-Campus 1, 48149 Münster, Germany.

References

1. Ehrlich P. Address in Pathology, ON CHEMIOTHERAPY: Delivered before the Seventeenth International Congress of Medicine. Br Med J. 1913;2:353–9.
2. Dellinger RP, Levy MM, Rhodes A, Annane D, Gerlach H, Opal SM, et al. Surviving sepsis campaign: international guidelines for management of severe sepsis and septic shock: 2012. Crit Care Med. 2013;41:580–637.
3. Köck R, Kipp F, Ellger B. Blood culture diagnostic–challenge or routine standard of care? Anästhesiol Intensivmed Notfallmedizin Schmerzther. 2015;50:124–31.
4. Ferrer R, Martin-Loeches I, Phillips G, Osborn TM, Townsend S, Dellinger RP, et al. Empiric antibiotic treatment reduces mortality in severe sepsis and septic shock from the first hour: results from a guideline-based performance improvement program. Crit Care Med. 2014;42:1749–55.
5. Idelevich EA, Silling G, Niederbracht Y, Penner H, Sauerland MC, Tafelski S, et al. Impact of multiplex PCR on antimicrobial treatment in febrile neutropenia: a randomized controlled study. Med Microbiol Immunol (Berl). 2015;204:585–92.
6. Reers Y, Idelevich EA, Pätkau H, Sauerland MC, Tafelski S, Nachtigall I, et al. Multiplex PCR assay underreports true bloodstream infections with coagulase-negative staphylococci in hematological patients with febrile neutropenia. Diagn Microbiol Infect Dis. 2016;85:413–5.
7. Tafelski S, Nachtigall I, Adam T, Bereswill S, Faust J, Tamarkin A, et al. Randomized controlled clinical trial evaluating multiplex polymerase chain reaction for pathogen identification and therapy adaptation in critical care patients with pulmonary or abdominal sepsis. J Int Med Res. 2015;43:364–77.
8. Lucignano B, Ranno S, Liesenfeld O, Pizzorno B, Putignani L, Bernaschi P, et al. Multiplex PCR allows rapid and accurate diagnosis of bloodstream infections in newborns and children with suspected sepsis. J Clin Microbiol. 2011;49:2252–8.
9. Lamoth F, Jaton K, Prod'hom G, Senn L, Bille J, Calandra T, et al. Multiplex blood PCR in combination with blood cultures for improvement of microbiological documentation of infection in febrile neutropenia. J Clin Microbiol. 2010;48:3510–6.
10. Rath P-M, Saner F, Paul A, Lehmann N, Steinmann E, Buer J, et al. Multiplex PCR for rapid and improved diagnosis of bloodstream infections in liver transplant recipients. J Clin Microbiol. 2012;50:2069–71.
11. Pletz MW, Wellinghausen N, Welte T. Will polymerase chain reaction (PCR)-based diagnostics improve outcome in septic patients? A clinical view. Intensive Care Med. 2011;37:1069–76.
12. Liesenfeld O, Lehman L, Hunfeld K-P, Kost G. Molecular diagnosis of sepsis: New aspects and recent developments. Eur J Microbiol Immunol. 2014;4:1–25.
13. Clerc O, Prod'hom G, Vogne C, Bizzini A, Calandra T, Greub G. Impact of matrix-assisted laser desorption ionization time-of-flight mass spectrometry on the clinical management of patients with Gram-negative bacteremia: a prospective observational study. Clin Infect Dis. 2013;56:1101–7.
14. Idelevich EA, Schüle I, Grünastel B, Wüllenweber J, Peters G, Becker K. Rapid identification of microorganisms from positive blood cultures by MALDI-TOF mass spectrometry subsequent to very short-term incubation on solid medium. Clin Microbiol Infect. 2014;20:1001–6.
15. Idelevich EA, Becker K. Identification and Susceptibility Testing From Shortly Incubated Cultures Accelerate Blood Culture Diagnostics at No Cost. Clin Infect Dis. 2016;62:268–9.
16. Banerjee R, Teng CB, Cunningham SA, Ihde SM, Steckelberg JM, Moriarty JP, et al. Randomized Trial of Rapid Multiplex Polymerase Chain Reaction-Based Blood Culture Identification and Susceptibility Testing. Clin Infect Dis. 2015; 61:1071–80.
17. Schmitz RPH, Keller PM, Baier M, Hagel S, Pletz MW, Brunkhorst FM. Quality of blood culture testing - a survey in intensive care units and microbiological laboratories across four European countries. Crit Care Lond Engl. 2013;17:R248.
18. Rönnberg C, Mildh M, Ullberg M, Özenci V. Transport time for blood culture bottles: underlying factors and its consequences. Diagn Microbiol Infect Dis. 2013;76:286–90.
19. Kerremans JJ, van der Bij AK, Goessens W, Verbrugh HA, Vos MC. Immediate incubation of blood cultures outside routine laboratory hours of operation accelerates antibiotic switching. J Clin Microbiol. 2009;47:3520–3.
20. Peretz A, Isakovich N, Pastukh N, Koifman A, Glyatman T, Brodsky D. Performance of Gram staining on blood cultures flagged negative by an automated blood culture system. Eur J Clin Microbiol Infect Dis. 2015;34:1539–41.
21. von Eiff C, Becker K, Machka K, Stammer H, Peters G. Nasal carriage as a source of *Staphylococcus aureus* bacteremia. Study Group. N Engl J Med. 2001;344:11–6.
22. Delport JA, Strikwerda A, Armstrong A, Schaus D, John M. Quality of Care Is Improved by Rapid Short Incubation MALDI-ToF Identification from Blood Cultures as Measured by Reduced Length of Stay and Patient Outcomes as Part of a Multi-Disciplinary Approach to Bacteremia in Pediatric Patients. PLoS One. 2016;11:e0160618.

12

Evaluation of a *Stenotrophomonas maltophilia* bacteremia cluster in hematopoietic stem cell transplantation recipients using whole genome sequencing

Stefanie Kampmeier[1*], Mike H. Pillukat[1], Aleksandra Pettke[2,3], Annelene Kossow[1], Evgeny A. Idelevich[2] and Alexander Mellmann[1]

Abstract

Background: *Stenotrophomonas maltophilia* ubiquitously occurs in the hospital environment. This opportunistic pathogen can cause severe infections in immunocompromised hosts such as hematopoietic stem cell transplantation (HSCT) recipients. Between February and July 2016, a cluster of four patients on the HSCT unit suffered from *S. maltophilia* bloodstream infections (BSI).

Methods: For epidemiological investigation we retrospectively identified the colonization status of patients admitted to the ward during this time period and performed environmental monitoring of shower heads, shower outlets, washbasins and toilets in patient rooms. We tested antibiotic susceptibility of detected *S. maltophilia* isolates. Environmental and blood culture samples were subjected to whole genome sequence (WGS)-based typing.

Results: Of four patients with *S. maltophlilia* BSI, three were found to be colonized previously. In addition, retrospective investigations revealed two patients being colonized in anal swab samples but not infected. Environmental monitoring revealed one shower outlet contaminated with *S. maltophilia*. Antibiotic susceptibility testing of seven *S. maltophlia* strains resulted in two trimethoprim/sulfamethoxazole resistant and five susceptible isolates, however, not excluding an outbreak scenario. WGS-based typing did not result in any close genotypic relationship among the patients' isolates. In contrast, one environmental isolate from a shower outlet was closely related to a single patient's isolate.

Conclusion: WGS-based typing successfully refuted an outbreak of *S. maltophilia* on a HSCT ward but uncoverd that sanitary installations can be an actual source of *S. maltophilia* transmissions.

Keywords: *Stenotrophomonas maltophilia*, Outbreak investigation, Whole genome sequence-based typing, Immunocompromised hosts

Background

Stenotrophomonas maltophilia, an intrinsically multidrug resistant gram negative pathogen, is widely distributed in aqueous habitats such as, sink drains, endoscopes and hemodialysis water within clinical settings [1, 2]. Usually, this pathogen is not highly virulent in immunocompetent individuals but can cause severe infections including bacteremia, peritonitis and meningitis in immunocompromised hosts resulting in complications, e.g. septic shock, respiratory failure, tissue necrosis and septic thrombophlebitis [3]. Recipients of hematopoietic stem cell transplantations (HSCT) are especially at risk and suffer from pulmonary hemorrhage resulting in higher mortality rates compared to non-HSCT patients [4].

In recent years, an increasing incidence of *S. maltophilia* is reported on oncologic wards [5]. Moreover, several outbreaks and pseudo-outbreaks caused by this pathogen have been reported [6, 7]. In addition to epidemiological

* Correspondence: Stefanie.Kampmeier@ukmuenster.de
[1]Institute of Hygiene, University Hospital Münster, Robert–Koch–Strasse 41, 48149 Münster, Germany
Full list of author information is available at the end of the article

investigations, different typing methods, e.g. pulse field gel electrophoresis (PFGE) and multi locus sequence typing (MLST) are used to identify the genetical relationship among different *S. maltophilia* isolates [8–11]. These techniques are useful in excluding outbreak scenarios, if MLST sequence types (ST) or PFGE patterns of isolated pathogens differ. In case of identical STs or highly similar PFGE patterns both methods reach their discriminatory limits. In these cases an outbreak is assumed, although more precise methods uncover and accidental cluster. Additionally, inter-laboratory comparability is limited using PFGE. Therefore, whole genome sequence-based typing (WGS) approaches are increasingly seen as gold standard method for highly discriminatory typing [12] and the superiority of WGS in comparison to other typing methods was already demonstrated for several bacterial pathogens [13–17]. Moreover, we could recently demonstrate the high reproducibility of WGS, which is another prerequisite for the applicability in clinical routine [18].

Here we evaluated a cluster of *S. maltophilia* bacteremia in recipients of allogeneic stem cell grafts using WGS-based typing.

Methods

Cluster detection, epidemiological investigations and infection control measures

The 1500-bed University Hospital Münster includes two HSCT-units each comprising 10 patient rooms, which are all HEPA-filtered and equipped with separated bathrooms for each patient (Fig. 1). In total, 193 patients were admitted to the HSCT-units during 2016. Patients usually receive an allogenic HSCT.

S. maltophilia bloodstream infections (BSI) were defined as one or more blood cultures positive for *S. maltophilia* obtained from patients with clinical signs of infection (fever >38 °C, chills, hypotension) according to the critieria given by the European Centre for Disease Prevention and Control [19]. Four *S. maltophilia* BSI were detected in patients (P1, P3, P4, P6) in the HSCT ward between February and July 2016. As this number exceeds the average baseline of 0.5 *S. maltophilia* BSI per year detected during 2011–2015, an epidemiological investigation was initiated. Routine environmental screening of aqueous habitats (shower heads, shower outlets, washbasins and toilets) within patients' rooms in the HSCT unit, normally focusing on multidrug resistant

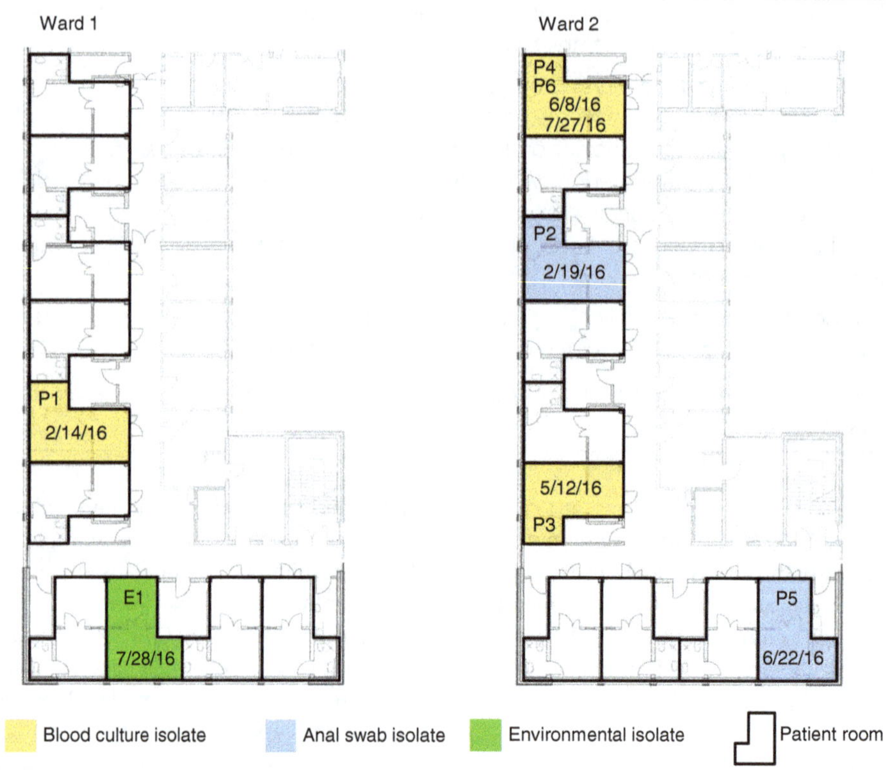

Fig. 1 Distribution and isolation dates of *S. maltophilia* on the HSCT-unit. Distribution of blood culture (yellow), anal swab (blue) and environmental (green) isolates detected during February and July 2016 on both HSCT wards. Patient rooms on wards are highlighted by black edges. Dates of *S. maltophilia* detection are assigned to the according patient room

Pseudomonas aeruginosa, was expanded to *S. maltophilia*. Patients colonized with *S. maltophilia*, coincidentally detected in anal/rectal swabs or stool samples (as screening of HSCT-patients concentrates on multidrug resistant *Pseudomonas aeruginosa*), were retrospectively identified. Moreover, hand hygiene and surface disinfection measures were intensified.

Identification and susceptibility testing

Positive blood culture samples were detected using an automated blood culture system (BACTEC™ 9240, Becton Dickinson GmbH, Heidelberg, Germany). Environmental samples were plated on Columbia sheep blood agar (Oxoid, Wesel, Germany) and MacConkey agar (Becton Dickinson, Heidelberg, Germany) after enrichment in Tryptic Soy Broth (Becton Dickinson) for 24 h at 36 °C. Subsequent species identification was performed by Matrix-Assisted Laser Desorption/Ionization-Time of Flight-Mass Spectrometry (MALDI-TOF MS; Bruker, Bremen, Germany). Susceptibility testing for trimethoprim-sulfamethoxazole (TMP-SMX) was performed using disk diffusion method in accordance with the European Committee on Antimicrobial Susceptibility Testing (EUCAST) standards and interpreted using EUCAST clinical breakpoints (version 6).

Whole genome sequencing (WGS) based typing

To determine the clonal relationship of *S. maltophilia* strains isolated from blood cultures, the isolates were subjected to WGS using the Illumina MiSeq platform (Illumina Inc., San Diego, USA) as described previously [13]. Retrospectively identified colonization isolates were not subjected to WGS as they were no longer available in contrast to BSI isolates, that are stored for a longer time period. Using SeqSphere+ software version 2.0 beta (Ridom GmbH, Münster, Germany), all coding regions were extracted and compared in a gene-by-gene approach (core genome multilocus sequence typing, cgMLST) using *S. maltophilia* K279a strain (GenBank accession number AM743169.1) as a reference sequence. Instead of a published cgMLST scheme, which is not yet available, this ad hoc scheme was used to differentiate the cluster. SeqSphere+ software was used to display the clonal relationship in a minimum-spanning tree (MST). For backwards compatibility with classical molecular typing, i. e. MLST, the MLST sequence types (ST) were extracted from the WGS data in silico.

Results

Epidemiological investigation and susceptibility testing

Chronological order and spacial distribution of isolated *S. maltophilia* is displayed in Fig. 1. Isolates were obtained from blood culture samples of patients on both wards. Two of the four isolates (isolated from P4 and P6) were detected within short intervals in two patients both admitted to room 1 on ward 2. Of the four patients suffering from *S. maltophilia* bacteremia, three (P1, P4 and P6) were previously tested positive for *S. maltophilia* in stool samples or anal swabs. Additionally, two colonized patients (anal swabs; P2, P5) admitted to ward 2 were uncovered by the retrospective analysis (Table 1). One environmental isolate (E1) could be detected in a shower outlet of a patient room that was a patient with *S. maltophilia* infection. Susceptibility testing revealed all patient isolates to be susceptible to TMP-SMX, except isolate P3. The environmental isolate was resistant to TMP-SMX (Table 1).

Clinical characteristics and outcome of patients with *S. maltophilia* bacteremia

All patients with *S. maltophilia* BSI suffered from acute myeloid leukemia as the underlying disease. P2 and P5, who were only colonized by *S. maltophilia*, suffered from chronic lymphatic leukemia and myeloproliferative neoplasm. Except P1, all patients had already received allogenic SCT at the time of *S. maltophilia* detection. P1 and P6 developed an acute respiratory distress syndrome. P1, P3, and P6 died due to *S. maltophilia* bacteremia.

WGS-based typing

We analyzed four bloodstream isolates and the environmental isolate by WGS. Comparison via cgMLST, based on 1876 genes present in all isolates, revealed no genetical relationship among isolates originating from patients (Fig. 2). In contrast, *S. maltophilia* strains isolated from P3 and E1 showed a similar genotype with only four alleles difference, suggesting a relationship between these two isolates. P3 and E1 harbored the MLST ST 94. All other isolates harbored new MLST STs.

Discussion

S. maltophilia has emerged as an important nosocomial pathogen associated with increased mortality rates in patients suffering from hematological malignancies and receiving hematopoietic stem cell transplantations [20, 21]. In this study, WGS was used to evaluate a cluster of four *S. maltophilia* BSI in patients partially suffering from pulmonary dysfunction associated with the infection due to this

Table 1 Patients with *S. maltophilia* colonizations and blood stream infections during February and July 2016

Patient no.	Anal colonization	Blood stream infection	Strain susceptibility to TMP-SMX	WGS performed
P1	+	+	S	+
P2	+	–	S	–
P3	–	+	R	+
P4	+	+	S	+
P5	+	–	S	–
P6	+	+	S	+

TMP-SMX – trimethoprim-sulfamethoxazole, WGS – whole genome sequencing

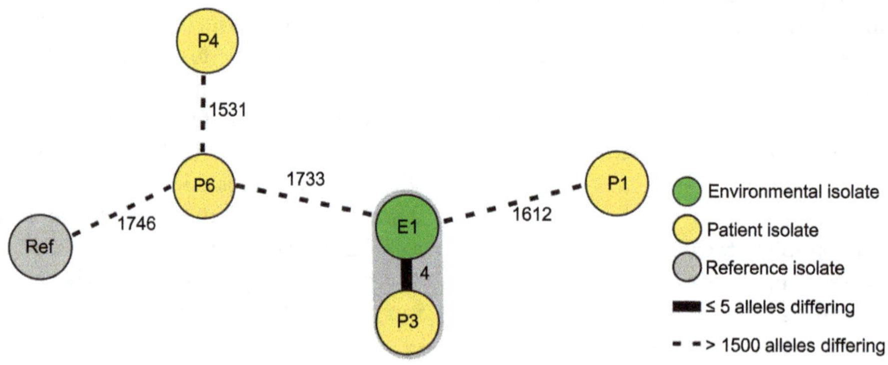

Fig. 2 Minimum spanning tree of *S. maltophilia* isolates. Minimum spanning tree of four blood culture isolates (P, *yellow*), one environmental isolate (E, *green*) from the HSCT unit and one outgroup isolate (Ref, non-HSCT unit, isolated in May 2016, *grey*) based on up to 1876 target genes, pairwise ignoring missing values. Genotypes are consecutively numbered, starting with P1 (isolated in February 2016). Each dot represents one genotype and is colored according to its origin. Different connecting lines and numbers on these lines show the number of alleles differing between two genotypes

pathogen [4]. Susceptibility testing, normally used as a first indication of nosocomial transmission of bacterial strains, could not exclude a spread of one single clone. WGS and subsequent cgMLST analysis, methods that have shown to provide detailed information in evaluating the epidemiology in nosocomial clusters of other pathogens [22], excluded a genetical relation and therefore an outbreak scenario.

A number of different sources are possibly responsible for the increasing number of *S. maltophilia* BSI. Due to its multidrug resistant nature, selection of this pathogen can easily occur in patients after receiving broad-spectrum antibiotics [23]. Moreover, *S. maltophilia* infections occur frequently in combination with the distinct immunocompromised status of HSCT recipients [24]. On the other hand, several environmental sites such as sink drains could be detected as sources of *S. maltophilia* within hospital settings [25].

To what extent these habitats are origins for hospital-acquired colonizations or infections of *S. maltophilia* could not yet be shown in detail. In this study we documented a genetical relation between an environmental and a patient blood stream infection isolate by analyzing WGS data. Although there was no local proximity, *S. maltophilia* could be transmitted from the environment to a patient or vice versa, at least giving the possibility of further spread via aqueous habitats in the HSCT unit.

Conclusion

WGS- analysis can be used to precisely refute an outbreak of *S. maltophilia*. Additionally, WGS- based typing documented sanitary installations in HSCT units to be an actual source or result of transmission between environmental and human habitats. Hence, in addition to classical infection control strategies, monitoring of aqueous habitats has to be established within the rooms of HSCT recipients in order to prevent transmission of these multidrug resistant organisms, as recently also shown for *P. aeruginosa* [26].

Abbreviations

BSI: Blood stream infection; cgMLST: Core genome multilocus sequence typing; HSCT: Hematopoietic stem cell transplantation; MST: Minimum spanning tree; PFGE: Pulsed field gel electrophoresis; ST: Sequence type; WGS: Whole genome sequencing

Acknowledgements

Not applicable.

Funding

None.

Authors' contributions

SK, AP, EAI were responsible for all data collection. SK, MHP, AK and AM were involved in data analysis and interpretation. All authors contributed to and approved the final draft of manuscript.

Consent for publication

Not applicable.

Competing interests

The authors declare that they have no competing interests.

Author details

[1]Institute of Hygiene, University Hospital Münster, Robert-Koch-Strasse 41, 48149 Münster, Germany. [2]Institute of Medical Microbiology, University Hospital Münster, Münster, Germany. [3]Science for Life Laboratory, Division of Translational Medicine and Chemical Biology, Department of Medical Biochemistry and Biophysics, Karolinska Institute, Stockholm, Sweden.

References

1. Abbott IJ, Peleg AY. Stenotrophomonas, Achromobacter, and nonmelioid Burkholderia species: antimicrobial resistance and therapeutic strategies. Semin Respir Crit Care Med. 2015;36:99–110.
2. Brooke JS. *Stenotrophomonas maltophilia*: an emerging global opportunistic pathogen. Clin Microbiol Rev. 2012;25:2–41.
3. Al-Anazi KA, Al-Jasser AM. Infections caused by *Stenotrophomonas maltophilia* in recipients of hematopoietic stem cell transplantation. Front Oncol. 2014;4:232.
4. Tada K, Kurosawa S, Hiramoto N, et al. *Stenotrophomonas maltophilia* infection in hematopoietic SCT recipients: high mortality due to pulmonary hemorrhage. Bone Marrow Transplant. 2013;48:74–9.

5. Safdar A, Rolston KV. *Stenotrophomonas maltophilia*: changing spectrum of a serious bacterial pathogen in patients with cancer. Clin Infect Dis. 2007;45:1602–9.
6. Guyot A, Turton JF, Garner D. Outbreak of *Stenotrophomonas maltophilia* on an intensive care unit. J Hosp Infect. 2013;85:303–7.
7. Waite TD, Georgiou A, Abrishami M, et al. Pseudo-outbreaks of *Stenotrophomonas maltophilia* on an intensive care unit in England. J Hosp Infect. 2016;92:392–6.
8. Corlouer C, Lamy B, Desroches M, et al. *Stenotrophomonas maltophilia* healthcare-associated infections: identification of two main pathogenic genetic backgrounds. J Hosp Infect. 2017;96:183–8.
9. Crispino M, Boccia MC, Bagattini M, et al. Molecular epidemiology of *Stenotrophomonas maltophilia* in a university hospital. J Hosp Infect. 2002;52:88–92.
10. Gherardi G, Creti R, Pompilio A, et al. An overview of various typing methods for clinical epidemiology of the emerging pathogen *Stenotrophomonas maltophilia*. Diagn Microbiol Infect Dis. 2015;81:219–26.
11. Tanimoto K. *Stenotrophomonas maltophilia* strains isolated from a university hospital in Japan: genomic variability and antibiotic resistance. J Med Microbiol. 2013;62:565–70.
12. Salipante SJ, SenGupta DJ, Cummings LA, et al. Application of whole-genome sequencing for bacterial strain typing in molecular epidemiology. J Clin Microbiol. 2015;53:1072–9.
13. Mellmann A, Bletz S, Boking T, et al. Real-time genome sequencing of resistant bacteria provides precision infection control in an institutional setting. J Clin Microbiol. 2016;54:2874–81.
14. Joensen KG, Scheutz F, Lund O, et al. Real-time whole-genome sequencing for routine typing, surveillance, and outbreak detection of verotoxigenic *Escherichia coli*. J Clin Microbiol. 2014;52:1501–10.
15. Davis RJ, Jensen SO, Van Hal S, et al. Whole genome sequencing in real-time investigation and Management of a *Pseudomonas aeruginosa* outbreak on a neonatal intensive care unit. Infect Control Hosp Epidemiol. 2015;36:1058–64.
16. Kwong JC, Mercoulia K, Tomita T, et al. Prospective whole-genome sequencing enhances National Surveillance of *Listeria monocytogenes*. J Clin Microbiol. 2016;54:333–42.
17. Fitzpatrick MA, Ozer EA, Hauser AR. Utility of whole-genome sequencing in characterizing Acinetobacter epidemiology and analyzing hospital outbreaks. J Clin Microbiol. 2016;54:593–612.
18. Mellmann A, Andersen PS, Bletz S, et al. High Interlaboratory reproducibility and accuracy of next-generation-sequencing-based bacterial genotyping in a ring trial. J Clin Microbiol. 2017;55:908–13.
19. European Centre for Disease Prevention and Control. Annual Epidemiological Report - Healthcare-associated infections acquired in intensive care units. 2016. https://ecdc.europa.eu/en/publications-data/healthcare-associated-infections-acquired-intensive-care-units-annual. Accessed 05 Nov 2017.
20. Micozzi A, Venditti M, Monaco M, et al. Bacteremia due to *Stenotrophomonas maltophilia* in patients with hematologic malignancies. Clin Infect Dis. 2000;31:705–11.
21. Labarca JA, Leber AL, Kern VL, et al. Outbreak of *Stenotrophomonas maltophilia* bacteremia in allogenic bone marrow transplant patients: role of severe neutropenia and mucositis. Clin Infect Dis. 2000;30:195–7.
22. Willems S, Kampmeier S, Bletz S, et al. Whole-genome sequencing elucidates epidemiology of nosocomial clusters of *Acinetobacter baumannii*. J Clin Microbiol. 2016;54:2391–4.
23. Chang YT, Lin CY, Chen YH, et al. Update on infections caused by *Stenotrophomonas maltophilia* with particular attention to resistance mechanisms and therapeutic options. Front Microbiol. 2015;6:893.
24. Paez JI, Costa SF. Risk factors associated with mortality of infections caused by *Stenotrophomonas maltophilia*: a systematic review. J Hosp Infect. 2008;70:101–8.
25. Brooke JS. Pathogenic bacteria in sink exit drains. J Hosp Infect. 2008;70:198–9.
26. Kossow A, Kampmeier S, Willems S, et al. Control of multidrug-resistant *Pseudomonas aeruginosa* in allogeneic hematopoietic stem cell transplant recipients by a novel bundle including remodeling of sanitary and water supply systems. Clin Infect Dis. 2017;65:935–42.

Comparison of subsequent infection in methicillin-resistant *Staphylococcus aureus* nasal carriers between ST72 community-genotype and hospital genotypes

So Yeon Park[1,4], Doo Ryeon Chung[1,2,3*], Yu Ri Kang[1,3], So Hyun Kim[1,3], Sun Young Cho[1,2], Young Eun Ha[1], Cheol-In Kang[1], Kyong Ran Peck[1] and Jae-Hoon Song[1,3]

Abstract

Background: Carriage of methicillin-resistant *Staphylococcus aureus* (MRSA) is an important risk factor of subsequent infection. The purpose of our study was to compare the rates of subsequent infection among newly-admitted patients carrying MRSA between community-genotype and hospital-genotypes

Methods: In this retrospective cohort study, we compared the rates of subsequent MRSA infection, time to subsequent infection and mortality in the following 6 months between the community-genotype ST72 MRSA cohort and the hospital-genotypes ST5 / ST239 MRSA cohort.

Results: We identified 198 patients carrying ST72 and 156 patients carrying ST5 or ST239. There was no difference in the rates of subsequent infection between ST72 cohort and ST5 / ST239 cohort (13.1% vs. 12.8%; $P = 0.931$). The median time to development of subsequent infection was not significantly different (27 days vs. 88 days; $P = 0.0877$). The Kaplan-Meier method showed no difference in the cumulative rate of being free of subsequent infection between the cohorts ($P = 0.9209$). Overall mortality rates at 6 months did not differ (1.5% vs. 1.9%; $P = 1.000$)

Conclusions: We found no evidence that rates of subsequent MRSA infection were different between newly-admitted patients carrying community-genotype ST72 MRSA and those whom carrying hospital-genotypes ST5 or ST239 MRSA.

Keywords: Genotype, Kaplan-meier estimate, Methicillin-resistant *Staphylococcus aureus*, Cohort study, Carrier state

Background

Methicillin-resistant *Staphylococcus aureus* (MRSA) infections have imposed a high burden on healthcare resources as well as significant morbidity and mortality, and a recent emergence of community-associated MRSA (CA-MRSA) worldwide has added another concern. MRSA carriage has been identified as a strong risk factor for subsequent infection [1, 2]. Approximately 11% - 25% of patients who newly acquired MRSA were reported to develop subsequent infection during hospitalization [3, 4]. Although several CA-MRSA clones have emerged as important pathogens both in the community and the hospitals worldwide [5–7] and have shown different characteristics in the pattern of colonization and infection from the hospital-genotype MRSA clones [7, 8], there has been no study comparing the rates of subsequent MRSA infection in hospitalized patients carrying MRSA between the community-genotype and hospital-genotype strains.

In Korea, dominant MRSA clones endemic in the hospitals have been sequence type 5 (ST5) and ST239 clones, while ST72 clone has emerged in the community

* Correspondence: iddrchung@gmail.com
[1]Division of Infectious Diseases, Department of Internal Medicine, Samsung Medical Center, Sungkyunkwan University School of Medicine, 81 Irwon-ro, Gangnam-gu, Seoul 06351, Republic of Korea
[2]Center for Infection Prevention and Control, Samsung Medical Center, Seoul, South Korea
Full list of author information is available at the end of the article

and has spread into the hospitals [9–11]. A recent single center study from Korea showed that the most frequent genotype in newly-admitted patients carrying MRSA was ST72, followed by ST5 and ST239 [12]. In this study, we compared the rates of subsequent MRSA infection among newly-detected hospitalized patients carrying MRSA between the community-genotype and the hospital-genotype cohort.

Methods

Study design and study participants

A retrospective cohort study was performed at Samsung Medical Center (Seoul, Republic of Korea), a university-affiliated tertiary care hospital with 1983 patient beds. We identified patients who were newly-detected MRSA nasal carriers between January 1, 2007 and March 31, 2010 from the previous study [12]. MRSA nasal screening was performed in selected newly-admitted patients according to the active surveillance policy for infection prevention purpose of the hospital. The indications for screening included the referral patients from the other hospitals or the chronic care facilities, the patients scheduled for operations in the departments of orthopedic surgery, neurosurgery, thoracic surgery and general surgery, the patients receiving hemodialysis or peritoneal dialysis, MRSA isolation from clinical specimens and carriage of vancomycin-resistant *Enterococcus* (VRE). Conventional culture methods were used for screening and confirmation of nasal carrier status of MRSA. The MRSA isolates were collected and stocked in the Asian Bacterial Bank (Seoul, Republic of Korea). Patients were excluded from the study if nasal MRSA carriage had been already known prior to the study period.

The patients carrying MRSA belonging to the sequence types other than ST72, ST5 and ST239 were excluded. We also excluded the patients who could not be followed up at least 6 months and had not developed subsequent MRSA infection until that time point (Fig. 1). Cohort 1 included the patients carrying MRSA with community-genotype, ST72, and cohort 2 included those who carried MRSA with hospital-genotypes, ST5 or ST239. If the patients developed MRSA infection multiple times, the first episode was only included in the analysis. This study was approved by the Institute Review Board of Samsung Medical Center.

Data collection

Demographic and clinical characteristics, laboratory data, and outcome data were collected from the electronic medical records. The McCabe classification was used to categorize the severity of the underlying medical condition as non-fatal, ultimately fatal, or rapidly fatal [13]. Outcome variables included the rates of subsequent MRSA infection within six months after new detection of MRSA nasal colonization, overall mortality rates at six months, and time to development of subsequent MRSA infection. The type of infections was also described.

Microbiological and molecular characterization

The Vitek 2 automated system (bioMerieux, Marcy l'Etoile, France) was used for microbiological identification and antimicrobial susceptibility testing. The MICs

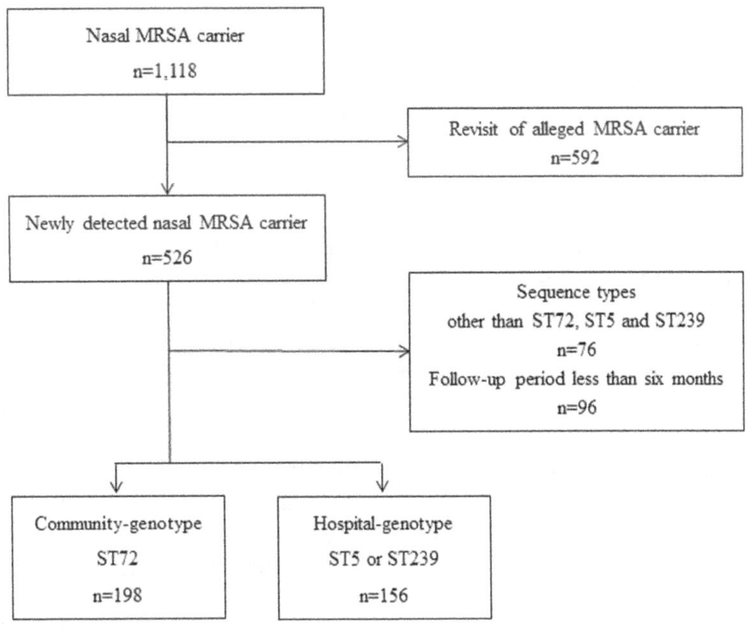

Fig. 1 Flow chart summarizing identification of study cohorts

were determined according to the standards established by the Clinical and Laboratory Standards Institute (CLSI) [14]. Multilocus sequence typing (MLST) was carried out using PCR amplification and sequencing of seven housekeeping genes (*arcC, aroE, glpF, gmk, pta, tpi,* and *yqiL*), as previously described [15]. The allelic profiles and sequence types (STs) were assigned according to the MLST web site (http//saureus.mlst.net/).

Statistical analysis

All tests of significance were two-tailed. *P*-values <0.05 were considered statistically significant. Categorical variables were compared between the groups using Chi-square test or Fisher's exact test. Continuous variables were compared using the Mann–Whitney *U* test. Multivariate logistic regression analysis was used to determine the risk factors of subsequent MRSA infection. Stepwise model comparison was used to determine the best model using the PASW version 18.0 (SPSS Inc., Chicago, IL, USA). Times to development of subsequent MRSA infection during the follow-up period were calculated by the Kaplan-Meier method and compared between the cohorts using the log-rank test. Stata version 11.2 (StataCorp, College Station, TX, USA) was used for this analysis.

Results

Study population

We identified 1118 patients with nasal MRSA colonization during the study period. Among those patients, 592 known MRSA carriers revisiting the hospital were excluded. The patients carrying MRSA strains belonging to ST72, ST5 or ST239 who were followed up for at least 6 months were included in this study. A total of 354 patients carrying MRSA were included (Fig. 1). Among those MRSA isolates, the most frequent sequence type was ST72 (55.9%). ST5 and ST239 accounted for 23.8% and 5.4%, respectively. The most frequent reasons for nasal MRSA screening were transfer from other hospital (36.2%) and pre-operative screening (33.6%). Other reasons included MRSA isolation from clinical specimens (9.0%), carriage of VRE (6.5%), and undergoing hemodialysis or continuous ambulatory peritoneal dialysis (CAPD) (4.2%). Among the MRSA isolates from nasal carriers who were screened for pre-operative screening, ST72 (67.2%) was more frequent than ST5 or ST239 (Table 1).

Comparison of characteristics of MRSA carriers between ST72 cohort and ST5 / ST239 cohort

The demographic and clinical characteristics of MRSA nasal carriers were compared between ST72 cohort and ST5 / ST239 cohort (Table 1). The most frequent comorbidity in ST72 cohort was solid tumor (24.2%), followed by cardiovascular disease, diabetes mellitus, liver disease, neurologic disease, and chronic kidney disease. Solid tumor was more frequent in ST72 cohort than in ST5 / ST239 cohort, whereas hematologic malignancy was more frequent in ST5 / ST239 cohort.

Subsequent MRSA infection

The median duration of follow-up after detection of nasal MRSA carriage was 1058 days (range 11–2441 days) in ST72 cohort and 774.5 days (range 13–2515 days) in ST5 / ST239 cohort (*P* = 0.555). Among MRSA carriers of ST72 cohort, 13.1% developed subsequent MRSA infection similar to the rate in ST5 / ST239 cohort (12.8%) (*P* = 0.931). The median time to development of subsequent MRSA infection following new detection of nasal carriage was 27 days in ST72 cohort, which was not a statistically significant difference compared to ST5 / ST239 cohort (88 days). The Kaplan-Meier method was used to calculate the cumulative rate of being free of subsequent MRSA infection, and no significant difference was observed between two cohorts (*P* = 0.9209) (Fig. 2). Overall mortality rates did not differ between two cohorts (1.5% vs. 1.9%) (*P* = 1.000).

The most frequent type of subsequent MRSA infections was pneumonia (50%), followed by urinary tract infection (13.0%), primary bacteremia (10.9%), surgical site infection (8.7%), intra-abdominal infection (8.7%), and skin and soft tissue infection (6.5%). There was no difference in distribution of infection types between two cohorts. Among 26 cases of subsequent MRSA infections in ST72 cohort, 19 (73.1%) were hospital-onset.

Risk factors for subsequent MRSA infection in MRSA nasal carrier cohorts

Multivariate analysis showed that the nasal carriers who also had MRSA isolated from culture of clinical specimens had 33-fold increased risk of subsequent MRSA infection (Table 2). Chronic lung disease and transfer from another hospital were also the risk factors for subsequent MRSA infection (O.R. 4.870 and O.R. 2.375, respectively).

Predictive factors for ST72 MRSA nasal carriage

Multivariate analysis showed that predictive factors for ST72 MRSA among MRSA nasal carriage were pre-operative screening for MRSA nasal carriage (odds ratio 1.828; 95% CI 1.127–2.967; *P* = 0.015) and solid tumor (odds ratio 1.747; 95% CI 1.004–3.040; *P* = 0.048).

Discussion

We found no evidence that rates of subsequent MRSA infection were different between community-genotype ST72 MRSA nasal carrier cohort and hospital-genotype ST5 / ST239 cohort. Comparison of the cumulative rates of being free of subsequent MRSA infection using the Kaplan-Meier method also revealed no significant

Table 1 Comparison of demographic and clinical characteristics of the patients colonized with methicillin-resistant *Staphylococcus aureus* between ST72 and ST5 / ST239 cohorts

Variable	No. (%)		*P* value
	Community-genotype ST72 MRSA cohort (*n* = 198)	Hospital-genotype ST5 / ST239 MRSA cohort (*n* = 156)	
Female gender	77 (38.9)	61 (39.1)	0.967
Age, median (IQR)	53.0 (4.0–65.0)	65.5 (52.8–71.8)	0.177
Reason for nasal MRSA screening			
Transfer from other hospital	68 (34.3)	60 (38.5)	0.423
Pre-operative screening	80 (40.4)	39 (25.0)	0.002
MRSA isolated from clinical specimens	22 (11.1)	10 (6.4)	0.139
Carriage of vancomycin-resistant *Enterococcus*	10 (5.1)	13 (8.3)	0.213
Undergoing HD or CAPD	9 (4.5)	6 (3.8)	0.746
Location before admission			0.520
Tertiary hospital	141 (71.2)	113 (72.4)	
Home	34 (17.2)	26 (16.7)	
General hospital	19 (9.6)	11 (7.1)	
Chronic care facility	4 (2.0)	6 (3.8)	
Admission due to infection other than MRSA infection	32 (16.2)	39 (25.0)	0.039
Comorbidity			
Solid tumor	48 (24.2)	24 (15.4)	0.040
Cardiovascular disease	40 (20.2)	33 (21.2)	0.826
Diabetes mellitus	26 (13.1)	32 (20.5)	0.062
Liver disease	21 (10.6)	14 (9.0)	0.610
Neurologic disease	20 (10.1)	24 (15.4)	0.135
Chronic kidney disease	19 (9.6)	21 (13.5)	0.254
Solid organ transplantation	7 (3.5)	3 (1.9)	0.522
Chronic lung disease	5 (2.5)	10 (6.4)	0.072
Hematologic malignancy	4 (2.0)	11 (7.1)	0.031
CAPD	0 (0.0)	3 (1.9)	0.085
HSCT	0 (0.0)	1 (0.6)	0.441
Severity of underlying disease			0.651
Rapidly fatal	9 (4.6)	5 (3.2)	
Ultimately fatal	102 (51.5)	76 (48.7)	
Nonfatal	87 (43.9)	75 (48.7)	

ST sequence type, *IQR* Interquartile range, *HD* hemodialysis, *CAPD* Continuous ambulatory peritoneal dialysis, *HSCT* hematopoietic stem cell transplantation

difference between two cohorts. In most previous reports studying subsequent MRSA infection rates among MRSA carriers, the difference of infection rates according to the genotype was not studied. Our study is unique in this regard because we compared the subsequent MRSA infection rates between hospital-endemic MRSA clones and CA-MRSA clone highly prevalent in Korea.

A retrospective cohort study in the US tertiary care medical center showed that 33% of MRSA carriers developed MRSA infections in the following year [16]. Another retrospective cohort study in the US hospitals showed that persistent MRSA colonizers had an increased risk of death (HR 2.58) and MRSA infection (HR 10.89) [17]. A retrospective cohort study conducted in Alaska aiming to determine if carriage of CA-MRSA increased the risk for subsequent soft tissue infection revealed nasal MRSA carriage to be a significant risk factor for skin infections in the first year when compared with MSSA and non–*S. aureus* carriers [18]. In contrast, the study from the Asian countries is sparse. The report

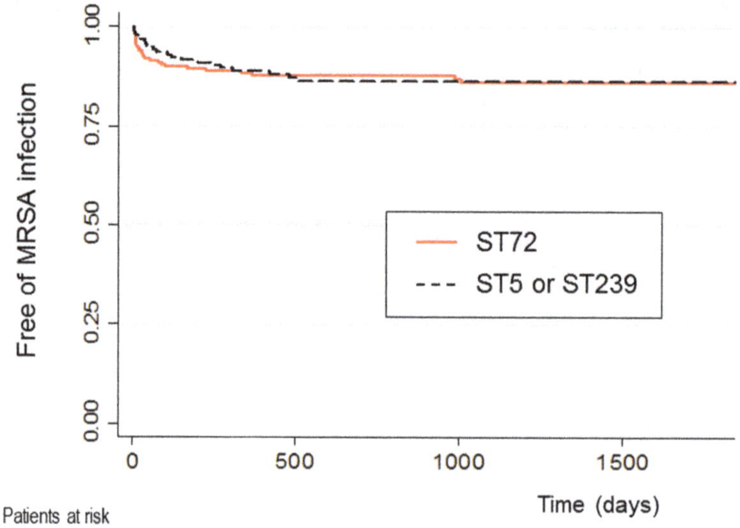

Patients at risk

Days		90	180	270	360	450	540	630	720	810	900	990	1080	1170	1260	1350	1440	1530	1620	1710	1800
ST72	198	179	173	162	149	135	126	118	113	108	100	97	92	84	79	77	73	63	54	44	35
ST5 or ST239	156	146	140	124	113	103	93	83	80	75	72	69	68	65	62	61	58	44	40	35	28

Fig. 2 Kaplan-Meier curves for the cumulative risk of subsequent MRSA infection

from the single center in Singapore showed that 14.4% of the MRSA carriers developed MRSA infection with median time to infection of 22 days [19].

It is interesting that ST72 MRSA cohort tended to have a shorter duration until developing subsequent MRSA infection compared to ST5 / ST239 cohort. A study from Singapore showed that risk of infection was much higher shortly after the initial acquisition; however the genotypes of MRSA were not determined [19]. In the retrospective cohort study from the US tertiary care medical center which also provided no information on genotypes showed that infection occurred a median of 56 days post-detection [16]. Higher virulence potential of CA-MRSA has been suggested in various community-genotype MRSA clones. USA300 clone is well known to be highly virulent [20]. Enhanced virulence of ST59 CA-MRSA over hospital-associated lineages was also demonstrated [21]. However, the virulence of ST72 MRSA needs to be more elucidated. Two studies comparing the virulence of ST72 MRSA with that of ST5 revealed lower virulence of ST72 MRSA strains [22, 23]. Several genes associated with adhesion and virulence were absent or rarely found in ST72 isolates.

Our study has demonstrated that isolation of MRSA from culture of clinical specimens was the most significant risk factor for subsequent MRSA infection in nasal carrier cohorts using the multivariate analysis. Although anterior nares are the most frequent carriage sites for *S. aureus*, multiple body sites can be colonized and CA-MRSA appears to be different in the distribution of colonization sites [7, 24]. As for USA300 strains, perirectal and inguinal area were common sites of colonization following the nares [25]. The frequencies of colonization in those areas were higher compared to non-USA300 strains.

There are some limitations in our study. First, this study focused on screening the nasal MRSA carriers according to the infection prevention and control policy of the hospital, and screening for the MRSA carriage at other body sites was not routinely performed. The MRSA surveillance study from the hospitals in Taiwan, in which majority of the isolates were clonotypes belonging to ST239, showed that nares cultures alone detected only 72.5% - 81.5% of all colonized patients [26]. As CA-MRSA strains are known to colonize various body sites rather than the nares frequently, the carriers who have a higher potential to develop subsequent MRSA infection could be excluded, affecting the results. Second, this was a retrospective design, and so many patients whose follow-up period less than 6 months were excluded from the analysis. It could affect the results. Third, the genotypes of MRSA isolates from subsequent infection were unknown, and so the relationship of MRSA isolates between the colonizing strains and the strains causing subsequent infection were not determined. Lastly, this is a single center study and caution should be exercised in generalizing our results.

Conclusions

In conclusion, we found no evidence that rates of subsequent MRSA infection were different between newly-

Table 2 Risk factors for subsequent MRSA infection in MRSA nasal carrier cohorts

Variable	No. (%)		*P*	Adjusted OR (95% CI)	*P*
	Patients with subsequent MRSA infection (*n* = 46)	Patients with no subsequent MRSA infection (*n* = 308)			
Female gender	16 (34.8)	122 (39.6)	0.531		
Age, median (IQR)	57.5 (41.0–67.0)	52.5 (5.5–66.0)	0.111		
ST72 MRSA	26 (56.5)	172 (55.8)	0.931		
Reason for nasal MRSA screening					
Transfer from other hospital	24 (52.2)	104 (33.8)	0.015	2.375 (1.094–5.157	0.029
Pre-operative screening	11 (23.9)	108 (35.1)	0.135		
MRSA isolated from clinical specimens	23 (50.0)	9 (2.9)	<0.001	33.235 (13.102–84.303)	<0.001
Carriage of VRE	2 (4.3)	21 (6.8)	0.752		
Undergoing HD or CAPD	3 (6.5)	12 (3.9)	0.425		
Admission due to infection other than MRSA infection	17 (37.0)	54 (17.5)	0.002	0.576 (0.240–1.387)	0.219
Comorbidity					
Solid tumor	9 (16.9)	63 (20.5)	0.889		
Cardiovascular	10 (21.7)	63 (20.5)	0.841		
Diabetes mellitus	11 (23.9)	47 (15.3)	0.198		
Liver disease	6 (13.0)	29 (9.4)	0.442		
Neurologic disease	4 (8.7)	40 (13.0)	0.631		
Chronic kidney disease	8 (17.4)	32 (10.4)	0.162		
Solid organ transplantation	2 (4.3)	8 (2.6)	0.625		
Chronic lung disease	7 (15.2)	8 (2.6)	0.001	4.870 (1.193–19.872)	0.027
Hematologic malignancy	3 (6.5)	12 (3.9)	0.425		
CAPD	0 (0.0)	3 (1.0)	1.000		
HSCT	0 (0.0)	1 (0.3)	1.000		
Severity of underlying disease			0.335		
Rapidly fatal	3 (6.5)	11 (3.6)			
Ultimately fatal	26 (56.5)	152 (49.4)			
Nonfatal	17 (37.0)	145 (47.1)			

MRSA methicillin-resistant *Staphylococcus aureus*, *OR* odds ratio, *IQR* Interquartile range, *ST* sequence type, *VRE* vancomycin-resistant *Enterococcus*, *HD* hemodialysis, *CAPD* continuous ambulatory peritoneal dialysis, *HSCT* hematopoietic stem cell transplantation

admitted patients carrying community-genotype ST72 MRSA and those whom carrying hospital-genotypes ST5 or ST239 MRSA in the following 6 months. This study also suggests the importance of post-discharge surveillance in determining the incidence of healthcare-associated infections due to MRSA, considering that infections occur after a considerable period of time after becoming a carrier.

Acknowledgements
Not applicable.

Funding
This work was supported by the Basic Science Research Program through the National Research Foundation of Korea (NRF) funded by the Ministry of Education, Science and Technology (NRF-2016M3A9B6918694) and by a grant from the Korean Health Technology R&D Project, Ministry of Health & Welfare, Republic of Korea (HI12C0756).

Authors' contributions
SYP performed the data collection. YRK and SHK performed the laboratory experiments. SYP, YRK, SYC, and DRC performed the analysis. SYP, YEH, CIK, KRP, JHS and DRC conceived the study, participated in its design and drafted the manuscript. All authors read and approved the final manuscript.

Competing interests
The authors declare that they have no competing interests.

Consent for publication
Not applicable.

Author details
[1]Division of Infectious Diseases, Department of Internal Medicine, Samsung Medical Center, Sungkyunkwan University School of Medicine, 81 Irwon-ro, Gangnam-gu, Seoul 06351, Republic of Korea. [2]Center for Infection Prevention and Control, Samsung Medical Center, Seoul, South Korea. [3]Asia Pacific Foundation for Infectious Diseases, Seoul, South Korea. [4]Present address: Division of Infectious Diseases, Kangdong Sacred Heart Hospital, Hallym University College of Medicine, Seoul, South Korea.

References

1. von Eiff C, Becker K, Machka K, Stammer H, Peters G. Nasal carriage as a source of *Staphylococcus aureus* bacteremia. Study group. N Engl J Med. 2001;344:11–6.
2. Wertheim HFL, Vos MC, Ott A, van Belkum A, Voss A, Kluytmans JAJW, et al. Risk and outcome of nosocomial *Staphylococcus aureus* bacteraemia in nasal carriers versus non-carriers. Lancet. 2004;364:703–5.
3. Coello R, Glynn JR, Gaspar C, Picazo JJ, Fereres J. Risk factors for developing clinical infection with methicillin-resistant *Staphylococcus aureus* (MRSA) amongst hospital patients initially only colonized with MRSA. J Hosp Infect. 1997;37:39–46.
4. Davis KA, Stewart JJ, Crouch HK, Florez CE, Hospenthal DR. Methicillin-resistant *Staphylococcus aureus* (MRSA) nares colonization at hospital admission and its effect on subsequent MRSA infection. Clin Infect Dis. 2004;39:776–82.
5. Moran GJ, Krishnadasan A, Gorwitz RJ, Fosheim GE, McDougal LK, Carey RB, Talan DA, Group EMINS. Methicillin-resistant S. *aureus* infections among patients in the emergency department. N Engl J Med. 2006;355:666-674.
6. Maree CL, Daum RS, Boyle-Vavra S, Matayoshi K, Miller LG. Community-associated methicillin-resistant *Staphylococcus aureus* isolates causing healthcare-associated infections. Emerg Infect Dis. 2007;13:236–42.
7. DeLeo FR, Otto M, Kreiswirth BN, Chambers HF. Community-associated meticillin-resistant *Staphylococcus aureus*. Lancet. 2010;375:1557–68.
8. Naimi TS, LeDell KH, Como-Sabetti K, Borchardt SM, Boxrud DJ, Etienne J, et al. Comparison of community- and health care-associated methicillin-resistant *Staphylococcus aureus* infection. JAMA. 2003;290:2976–84.
9. Kim ES, Song JS, Lee HJ, Choe PG, Park KH, Cho JH, et al. A survey of community-associated methicillin-resistant *Staphylococcus aureus* in Korea. J Antimicrob Chemother. 2007;60:1108–14.
10. Song JH, Hsueh PR, Chung DR, Ko KS, Kang CI, Peck KR, et al. Spread of methicillin-resistant *Staphylococcus aureus* between the community and the hospitals in Asian countries: an ANSORP study. J Antimicrob Chemother. 2011;66:1061–9.
11. Joo EJ, Chung DR, Ha YE, Park SY, Kang SJ, Kim SH, et al. Community-associated Panton-valentine leukocidin-negative meticillin-resistant *Staphylococcus aureus* clone (ST72-MRSA-IV) causing healthcare-associated pneumonia and surgical site infection in Korea. J Hosp Infect. 2012;81:149–55.
12. Park SY, Chung DR, Yoo JR, Baek JY, Kim SH, Ha YE, et al. Sequence type 72 community-associated meticillin-resistant *Staphylococcus aureus* emerged as a predominant clone of nasal colonization in newly admitted patients. J Hosp Infect. 2016;93:386–9.
13. McCabe W, Jackson G. Gram-negative bacteremia: I. Etiology and ecology. Arch Intern Med. 1962;110:847–55.
14. Clinical and Laboratory Standards Institute. Performance standards for antimicrobial susceptibility testing; Twenty-First Informational Supplement M100-S21. Wayne, PA; 2009.
15. Enright MC, Day NP, Davies CE, Peacock SJ, Spratt BG. Multilocus sequence typing for characterization of methicillin-resistant and methicillin-susceptible clones of *Staphylococcus aureus*. J Clin Microbiol. 2000;38:1008–15.
16. Huang SS, Hinrichsen VL, Datta R, Spurchise L, Miroshnik I, Nelson K, et al. Methicillin-resistant *Staphylococcus aureus* infection and hospitalization in high-risk patients in the year following detection. PLoS One. 2011;6:e24340.
17. Gupta K, Martinello RA, Young M, Strymish J, Cho K, Lawler E. MRSA nasal carriage patterns and the subsequent risk of conversion between patterns, infection, and death. PLoS One. 2013;8:e53674.
18. Stevens AM, Hennessy T, Baggett HC, Bruden D, Parks D, Klejka J. Methicillin-resistant *Staphylococcus aureus* carriage and risk factors for skin infections, southwestern Alaska. USA Emerg Infect Dis. 2010;16:797–803.
19. Balm MN, Lover AA, Salmon S, Tambyah PA, Fisher DA. Progression from new methicillin-resistant *Staphylococcus aureus* colonisation to infection: an observational study in a hospital cohort. BMC Infect Dis. 2013;13:491.
20. Li M, Diep BA, Villaruz AE, Braughton KR, Jiang X, DeLeo FR, et al. Evolution of virulence in epidemic community-associated methicillin-resistant *Staphylococcus aureus*. Proc Natl Acad Sci U S A. 2009;106:5883–8.
21. Li M, Dai Y, Zhu Y, Fu CL, Tan VY, Wang Y, et al. Virulence determinants associated with the Asian community-associated methicillin-resistant *Staphylococcus aureus* lineage ST59. Sci Rep. 2016;6:27899.
22. Joo EJ, Choi JY, Chung DR, Song JH, Ko KS. Characteristics of the community-genotype sequence type 72 methicillin-resistant *Staphylococcus aureus* isolates that underlie their persistence in hospitals. J Microbiol. 2016;54:445–50.
23. Park KH, Chong YP, Kim SH, Lee SO, Choi SH, Lee MS, et al. Community-associated MRSA strain ST72-SCC*mec*IV causing bloodstream infections: clinical outcomes and bacterial virulence factors. J Antimicrob Chemother. 2015;70:1185–92.
24. Wertheim HF, Melles DC, Vos MC, van Leeuwen W, van Belkum A, Verbrugh HA, et al. The role of nasal carriage in *Staphylococcus aureus* infections. Lancet Infect Dis. 2005;5:751–62.
25. Popovich KJ, Aroutcheva A, Hota B, Beavis KG, Hayden MK, Weinstein RA. Anatomic sites of colonization with community-associated methicillin-resistant *Staphylococcus aureus*. Infect Control Hosp Epidemiol. 2014l35:1192-1194.
26. Lauderdale TL, Wang JT, Lee WS, Huang JH, McDonald LC, Huang IW, et al. Carriage rates of methicillin-resistant *Staphylococcus aureus* (MRSA) depend on anatomic location, the number of sites cultured, culture methods, and the distribution of clonotypes. Eur J Clin Microbiol Infect Dis. 2010;29:1553–9.

14

Pervasive antibiotic misuse in the Cambodian community: antibiotic-seeking behaviour with unrestricted access

Chhorvoin Om[1], Frances Daily[2], Erika Vlieghe[3], James C. McLaughlin[2] and Mary-Louise McLaws[1*]

Abstract

Background: Antibiotic misuse is widespread in resource-limited countries such as Cambodia where the burden of infectious diseases is high and access to antibiotics is unrestricted. We explored healthcare seeking behaviour related to obtaining antibiotics and drivers of antibiotic misuse in the Cambodian community.

Methods: In-depth interviews were held with family members of patients being admitted in hospitals and private pharmacies termed pharmacy attendants in the catchment areas of the hospitals. Nurses who run community primary healthcare centres located within the hospital catchment areas were invited to attend focus group discussions. Nvivo version 10 was used to code and manage thematic data analysis.

Results: We conducted individual interviews with 35 family members, 7 untrained pharmacy attendants and 3 trained pharmacists and 6 focus group discussions with 30 nurses. Self-medication with a drug-cocktail was widespread and included broad-spectrum antibiotics for mild illness. Unrestricted access to antibiotics was facilitated by various community enablers including pharmacies or drug outlets, nurse suppliers and unofficial village medical providers referred to as "village Pett" whose healthcare training has historically been in the field and not at university. These enablers supplied the community with various types of antibiotics including broad spectrum fluoroquinolones and cephalosporins. When treatment was perceived to be ineffective patients would prescriber-shop various suppliers who would unfailingly provide them with antibiotics. The main driver of the community's demand for antibiotics was a mistaken belief in the benefits of antibiotics for a common cold, high temperature, pain, malaria and 'Roleak' which includes a broad catch-all for perceived inflammatory conditions. For severe illnesses, patients would attend a community healthcare centre, hospital, or when their finances permitted, a private prescriber.

Conclusions: Pervasive antibiotic misuse was driven by a habitual supplier-seeking behaviour that was enabled by unrestricted access and misconceptions about antibiotics for mild illnesses. Unofficial suppliers must be stopped by supporting existing regulations with tough new laws aimed at outlawing supplies outside registered pharmacies and fining registered pharmacist/owners of these pharmacies for supplying antibiotics without a prescription. Community primary healthcare centres must be strengthened to become the frontline antibiotic prescribers in the community thereby enabling the community's access to inexpensive and appropriate healthcare. Community-based education program should target appropriate health-seeking pathways and the serious consequences of antibiotic misuse.

Keywords: Antibiotic resistance, Behaviour, Unofficial prescriber, Self-medication, Nurse prescriber, Pharmacy, Drug outlet

* Correspondence: m.mclaws@unsw.edu.au
[1]School of Public Health and Community Medicine, UNSW Medicine, UNSW, Level 3 Samuels Building, Sydney 2052, NSW, Australia
Full list of author information is available at the end of the article

Background

Inappropriate antibiotic use is a global problem and contributes to the global crisis of antibiotic resistance [1, 2]. Global antibiotic resistance severely affects developing countries where infectious diseases are endemic [3, 4] and persistent inappropriate antibiotic use prevails [5–8]. Infectious diseases cause 58.6% of deaths and 63.6% of disability-adjusted life years (DALY) loss for the global poor which is in stark contrast in the global richer countries where deaths and DALY loss from infectious diseases account for just 7.7% and 10.9%, respectively [9]. A study of antibiotic use in 12 low-resourced countries found between 25 and 75% of patients received antibiotics inappropriately from primary healthcare [10]. Global community surveys reported that between 19 and 100% of antimicrobial use outside northern Europe and North America was non-prescribed [7].

In developing countries inappropriate antibiotic practice involves both the patient and the healthcare provider and is driven by the patient's socio-economic level and behavioural and cultural factors of both the patient and practitioner [8, 11–14]. Other contributing factors of inappropriate antibiotic use in low-resourced settings include cultural healthcare seeking preferences, beliefs that antibiotics are magic and strong drugs can cure and prevent many diseases [13]. A study in neighbouring Vietnam reported that mothers received antibiotics from community privately owned unofficial drug outlets for anticipated symptoms such as sore throat, cough, fever and diarrhoea [15].

Cambodia is not immune to multidrug-resistant microorganisms that cause common infections, such as bloodstream and urinary tract infections, in various locations around the country [16–19]. Not surprising, extended spectrum beta-lactamase resistance was found in 48% of *E. coli* isolates from adult bloodstream infection in Cambodia while the rate of methicillin-resistance *Staphylococcus aureus* was also high at 22% of *S. aureus* isolates [19]. Inappropriate prescribing is also common in Cambodia with estimates between 60 and 100% of all visits to primary healthcare providers receiving an antibiotic [20, 21]. Non-prescription antibiotic use is a common practice in the Cambodian community [22, 23] with respiratory tract infections and diarrhoea in children under five years of age being the most common indication for antibiotic use [23]. There are no studies that have explored the antibiotic-seeking behaviour in the community and we report here an exploration of this behaviour and drivers of antibiotic misuse in Cambodia.

Methods

Study design and setting

We used qualitative in-depth interviews with individuals and focus group discussions (FGDs) with nurses from primary healthcare centres to collect data between September 2013 and February 2014. Cambodia is a lower middle-income country located in Southeast Asia with a population in 2015 of 15.58 million [24] of whom 80% reside in rural areas [25]. Although poverty has declined it still prevails at a rate of 17.7% with 8.1 million Cambodians described as poor or near poor [24]. The majority (90%) of the Cambodian poor live in the countryside [24]. The Cambodian public healthcare system consists of 1236 healthcare facilities including 91 hospitals, 1024 healthcare centres that charge very low fees and 121 remote rural healthcare outposts that are staffed twice monthly [26]. Over half of all healthcare services are provided by the private sector [27].

Sampling and data collection

A purposeful sampling method [28] was used to select a sample of public hospitals for the participation in a cross-sectional survey of physicians' prescribing prior to this study [29]. A purposeful selection of family members of patients admitted to the selected public hospitals was used to enrol participants for individual interviews. Purposeful selection was used for pharmacy attendants from private pharmacies and nurses from community primary healthcare centres located within the catchment areas of the selected hospitals for interviews and FGDs, respectively. A Cambodian physician (CO) conducted all interviews and FGDs in Khmer. Data collection continued until data saturation was reached [30, 31]. Informed consent was collected from each participant and all interviews and FGDs were digitally recorded.

Data analysis

All digital audio records of interviews and FGDs were transcribed verbatim into Khmer language. The transcribed Khmer texts were checked and edited against the digital audio records for accuracy before being translated into English by a local translation consultant. All the English translations were checked and edited by two independent consultants: the physician who edited the Khmer text transcription and an independent English-Khmer speaking consultant who conducted overall checks of the translation. One author (CO) checked the translation against the transcribed Khmer text and edited any portions that were unclear. Data were analysed using thematic data analysis and presented as thematic syntheses [32, 33]. Data were inductively coded by two researchers separately (CO and MM) to insure validity [34]. Data were coded using Nvivo version 10 software program while another coder coded the text directly. The two coders compared the coding and checked for consistency and any discrepancies were addressed.

Results

We conducted 45 individual interviews with 35 family members of patients being hospitalized and 7 untrained pharmacy attendants and 3 trained pharmacists. Six FGDs were conducted with 30 nurses from 6 community primary healthcare centres within the catchment areas of the hospitals where family members were interviewed. The findings revealed a widespread misuse of antibiotics in the community that was facilitated by antibiotic-seeking behaviours, unrestricted access to antibiotics, and poor knowledge about antibiotics.

Healthcare and antibiotic-seeking behaviour

Participating family members spoke about the severity of illness and the factors that influenced their healthcare and antibiotic-seeking behaviour. Judgement of the severity of symptoms was a common practice used to determine what level of healthcare would be accessed. For a mild illness such as a common cold, mild diarrhoea or general unwell feeling patients would self-prescribe medication purchased and freely available from a nearby pharmacy or village drug outlet.

"When I have a minor headache, sore throat or fever I go to buy medicines from pharmacy." Family Member # 2-NMCH

"When I'm sick such as from headache, tiny ache, I always buy medicines in the village; 1 dose, 2 doses [something] like that." Family Member # 2-BT

In local terminology the words *Dambao Krapeas* (gastric ulcer), *Roleak Krapeas* (gastritis), *Dambao Posvean* (intestinal ulcer), or *roleak Posvean* (intestinitis) all refer to internal inflammation or wound. Because the community uses antibiotics for external wounds, injuries and inflammation the family will seek antibiotics to heal all 'internal' pain or illnesses they perceive to be caused by inflammation or internal 'wound'.

"I usually take one para [paracetamol] and one ampi [ampicillin]. Then I don't feel any more pain in my stomach." Family Member #3-NPH

"Phsas (healing) in case we have inflammation, intestinal inflammation, gastric inflammation, other wound we can take ampi [ampicillin]." Family Member #4-KCH

After having taken a cocktail of drugs and when family members perceived that symptoms were unrelenting and severe such unendurable pain, colic or fever they would attend a community primary healthcare centre or hospital. If their finances permitted they would visit a private healthcare provider.

"In case of minor sickness, I go to buy medicines but I go to a healthcare centre if it is a severe illness." Family Member # 2-KRV

"I go to hospital when I have a sharp pain in my stomach and/or bowel....like when there is an inside pain, which we cannot know what it is. I cannot go to a pharmacy." Family Member # 7-BT

"We always go to a [private] clinic if we have a severe sickness." Family Member # 10-MBR

These patients will also consult several healthcare providers when they perceive their treatment has been ineffective including unofficial healthcare providers known in the community as village *Petts.* The community 'prescriber-shopper' would request after-hours private care from physicians, nurses or village Petts.

Interviewer: Did you go to physician H; how many consultations? 5 consultations?
Participant: We visited physician H 3 times. He gave medicines and my husband got better. After he was better, he relapsed.
Interviewer: Then you went to another healthcare provider?
Participant: Yes, after thinking that the hospital was [too] far we went to Pett K.
Interviewer: How many times did you consult Pett K?
Participant: Two times. He injected [my husband] and he gave medicines. When we came the third time he told us that he couldn't treat [him]; couldn't continue any more. He told us to come to this hospital.

Healthcare providers are often referred to as Pett and this term includes unofficial "village Pett". The unofficial village Petts were healthcare providers during the Khmer Rouge genocide period (between 1975 and 1979) or unofficially trained in the Cambodia-Thai border camps during civil unrest after the Khmer Rouge period, and those who have unknown medical training history. These unofficial suppliers have remained practitioners in the community making house calls where they provide their patients with a diagnosis and treatment that includes antibiotics.

Interview of Family Member # 001_A_002 KP
Interviewer: Who is that private Pett? Is he a doctor? Where does he work?
Participant: I heard that he is a military Pett coming from the camp [Cambodian-Thai camp during civil unrest].
Interview of Family Member #4-KCH
Participant: I fetched a Pett to give treatment at my home, the Pett in the village.

Interviewer: Village Pett ... is he a staff from a health centre?
Participant: He is not a staff in a health centre. He just gives treatment to villagers; but he is not a health centre staff.

Despite perceptions of the severity of an illness that influences healthcare-seeking behaviour, family members described other factors that include:

a) Convenience

"I generally go to the healthcare centre near my house. I only pay 1000 riels and I'm given medicines for three days." Family Member # 3-KTL

b) Burden of balancing demands of earning an income, taking care of children, the elderly and their properties at home, with providing basic care in the hospital to their family member during their admission;

"I have small grandchildren, their parents go to work. I said to the hospital staff 'if my husband has typhoid fever please give him IV injections at home'. I don't want to go to hospital because there's no one to take care of him in hospital as I'm at home with the grandchildren." Family Member # 1-KRV

c) Ability to pay healthcare providers and purchase of medicine.

"If I have money I buy medicines, to take two doses. But if I don't have money I can only buy medicines to take once only." Family Member # 4-KTL

d) Trust in the safety of the healthcare provider and effectiveness of the treatment;

"It is safer to come to this hospital than to buy medicines outside. We meet the doctor and he advised us to take this or that [medicine] which is effective." Family Member # 8-MBR

Nurses from primary healthcare centres and a trained pharmacist at a provincial pharmacy explained how the financial constraints of the patients prevented them from initially consulting a physician and how this drives poor medication behaviour:

"In real practice as I have experienced the patients just let us inject for one or two days. If they are better, they stop because they don't have the money [to continue treatment]." Nurse #1-SLL5
"For minor cases mostly patients come to buy one or two doses of medicines at the pharmacy because they don't have much money. They do this because they don't have money to see a physician." Pharmacist # 2-SRP

Unrestricted access to antibiotics

Access to antibiotics is unrestricted and facilitated by various community enablers who include trained private pharmacists and untrained pharmacy attendants, drug outlet suppliers, unofficial village Pett suppliers, nurses and trained physicians. The community is so familiar with the antibiotics that are freely available that they know the name of many such as pen [penicillin], amox [amoxicillin], ampi [ampicillin], tetra [tetracycline] and cotrim [co-trimoxazole]. These antibiotics are even freely available in small village grocery shops in remote regions.

"When I have a high temperature or a cold, amox [amoxicillin] and ampi [ampicillin] are given to me mixed together. If I have a runny nose the drug sellers give me ampi, and if this isn't available it's replaced with amox." Family Member #2-NPH

"After I realize that cotrim [cotrimoxazole] can cure diarrhoea I always buy it. I buy only one tablet and I crush and grind it with water for my children to drink." Family Member #1-SRP

Most drug sellers in pharmacies or drugs outlets were untrained. But training does not always guarantee appropriate antibiotic use. When asked when antibiotics were indicated both trained pharmacists and untrained suppliers believed that antibiotics were indicated when their patients had diarrhoea and respiratory symptoms such as sore throat, fever and cough. Both trained and untrained suppliers drive the antibiotic-seeking behavior by providing a cocktail of drugs based on symptoms and this cocktail includes non-prescription medications plus an antibiotic such as amoxicillin, ampicillin, cephalexin, cefixime or co-amoxyclavulanic acid for upper respiratory infections and co-trimoxazole for diarrhoea.

"For normal colds without high temperature, patients can take amoxicillin. If they cough or have a high temperature, they take augmentin or cefixime. It depends on the seriousness of the sickness." Untrained pharmacy attendant #1-PP

"It is like what I told you earlier. Antibiotics are mostly used in case of diarrhoea, high temperature, cold and cough." Untrained pharmacy attendant # 1-NL
"Antibiotics should be prescribed for sicknesses such as respiratory inflammation." Untrained pharmacy attendant #1-KCH

"As my routine, I listen to their [patient's] sickness first. If they have a headache, then I give Alaxan [ibuprofen and paracetamol] or Para [paracetamol]; if they have a cold, I give them Decolgen [anti allergic, decongestant and paracetamol] and vitamin. I can use amox or ampi in the case that they have a sore throat or have a fever for many days ago." Trained pharmacist #2-SRP

Nurses from public hospitals and community primary healthcare centres commonly provide private after-hours services that offer a diagnosis and treatment. When asked "Have you ever invited nurses to your house for treatment?" family members indicated they provide injections and antibiotics:

"Yes. It [occurs] in the case [when] we are very busy at home and don't have enough time to get treatment at [a] clinic, then we can call the nurse to treat us at our house." Family Member #9-MBR

"He (nurse) told me that I had gastric inflammation and then he wrote ceftri [ceftriaxone] injection on a piece of paper. He asked me 'do you want drugs at the healthcare centre or want me to give the injection at home.' I thought I wanted him to give the injection [at home] because I don't have time to go to the healthcare centre to take drugs." Family Member #6-KCH

Nurses who are employed in primary healthcare centres also have a private practice and prescribe fluoroquinolones and 3rd generation cephalosporin and often provide injections.

"If it's typhoid fever we prescribe oflocet [fluoroquinolones] for 5 days. If they [patients] don't recover we prescribe ceftri [cetriaxone]." Nurse #3-NL

"If the sickness becomes more severe, we have to use IV injection and ceftri [cetriaxone]. If the sickness is just a simple fever, which is not serious, we continue using oflocet [fluoroquinolone] for 3-5 days." Nurse #2-NL

Unofficial village Petts are unregistered or have undefined training and supply medications and antibiotics including broad-spectrum antibiotics in the community.

"Village Pett are Pett from Pol Pot regime [Khmer Rouge] who have experience (providing health care during that time). They sell medicines and if we need ampi [ampicillin] or amox [amoxicillin], they will sell them to us. They provide injections too." Family Member #3-BT

"It is the same for both treatment at the healthcare centre and treatment from door to door. Some people use Amox as Thnam Psas (antibiotic). Village Petts providing treatment from door to door mostly prescribe Ceftri [ceftriaxone]. They prescribe the high ones. Ceftri is generally used." Nurse #2-NL

Official healthcare providers were concerned about these village Petts providing care and antibiotics but did not recognise their own professions' role in misusing antibiotics.

"Yes, there are [unofficial Petts] but far from here in the remote rural area. There are also some Petts who just learn from each other and never went to school. Now we still cannot stop this problem." Nurse # 1-SLL5

Poor knowledge about antibiotics

Family members were asked about the benefit of antibiotics with the interviewer who used the local term *Thnam Phsas* or the antibiotics by name such as amoxicillin, ampicillin or penicillin. They described how *Thnam Phsas* could heal minor wounds ('dambao'), injuries ('robuos') or cuts ('mout') and inflammation ('roleak') such as throat inflammation ('roleak bampongkor').

"If there is a wound [dambao], mostly people take Thnam Phsas. It can heal both inside and outside of the body." Family Member #8-MBR

"We take ampi [ampicillin] when we have cuts [mout] on arms or legs or when we have a motorbike accident or other small accident. When we take it [ampicillin], it helps to heal the injury [robuos]." Family Member # 2-NMCH

"If we have cough and we're afraid that it will cause throat inflammation we take Thnam Phsas. When I tell drug sellers that I have a cough, cold or sore throat, then they will cocktail it [Thnam Phsas] for me." Family Member #13-SRP

"Based on my understanding, Thnam Phsas [antibiotic] is for throat inflammation." Family Member #4-NL

Trained pharmacists, untrained pharmacy attendants and nurses from community primary healthcare centers upheld the community's belief about the benefits of antibiotics that they use to treat inflammation.

"Generally drug cocktail is for common cold, cough or mild sore throat. For common cold and cough I don't give antibiotic in the cocktail. I only give antibiotics for throat inflammation." Trained pharmacist #001_A_007 PP

> *"Antibiotics should be prescribed for sicknesses such as respiratory inflammation." Untrained pharmacy Attendant #3-KCH*
>
> *"For those who have minor sicknesses, sometimes I do not prescribe antibiotics for them, never. Mostly I prescribe them as long as they have throat inflammation. It is like this." Untrained pharmacy attendant #3-NL*
>
> *"If we see that they have upper breathing inflammation or bronchitis, we prescribe antibiotics for them [patients]." Nurse #5-KRV*
>
> *"We think that the disease could be something related to inflammation, and then we use antibiotics." Nurse #3-SLL5*

Besides a belief that antibiotics were beneficial for injuries, wounds and inflammation, family members described further misconceptions that antibiotics could be beneficial for the common cold, high temperature, pain and even malaria.

> *"Ampi [ampicillin] and amox [amoxicillin] help us, for example, when I have a stuffy nose, it helps to reduce the clogging and I can breathe more easily, feel better, reduces the temperature and so on." Family Member #2-NPH*
>
> *"When I have pain, we take it [amoxicillin]. It helps to reduce pain." Family Member #2-KRV*
>
> *"Yes. Ampi [ampicillin] for less severe disease has less phsas (healing) substance but it has cooling substance inside. For malaria, we can take it [ampicillin] in a mixture as well. For ampi [ampicillin], if there is amox [amoxicillin], we still use ampi [ampicillin] because it has cooling substance. I use [it] like this." Family Member #4-KCH*

Discussion

Misuse of antibiotics was widespread in the community that was driven by a determined antibiotic-seeking behaviour facilitated by both trained and untrained healthcare providers who supplied and enabled the community's antibiotic use. All actors held poor knowledge about the indications and uses of antibiotics: the community, trained pharmacists and unofficial suppliers who include untrained pharmacy attendants, drug outlets, nurses and village Petts. The source of the unrestricted access to antibiotics was pharmacies and drug outlets. Through these sources self-medication with antibiotics and drug-cocktails has become a community norm that may expedite antibiotic resistance [7]. These sources also provided nurses and village Petts with easy access to antibiotics that they would supply the community during house-calls.

The services provided by village Petts are unsafe because most would have received training without examinations to ensure that they had reached a minimum acceptable level of medical knowledge. In 2014, an unofficial village Pett was responsible for an outbreak of HIV infections among Cambodian villagers from unsafe injecting practices [35]. In November 2016 a new law was passed requiring all healthcare professionals to register with their relevant professional body for licensing. At the same time new penalties of up to 2 years jail were legislated that outlawed unregistered providers of diagnoses and treatments but it is too early to determine whether the legislation will be success. To date, the current implementation of laws and regulations pertaining to the registration of trained pharmacists is not working [36, 37] to stem the flow of non-prescription antibiotics. Methods of improving the effective enforcement of existing pharmaceutical law and regulation need to be developed that would prevent antibiotics from being sold outside registered pharmacies. Improved regulations should carry fines for pharmacies that do not have a trained pharmacist on the premises during trading hours and fines where antibiotic usage does not match prescription numbers.

Limited household finances impede safe healthcare-seeking behaviour in developing countries [8, 12, 13] and this was an important barrier for our community. Poor understanding about the importance of the correct indication for and dosage of antibiotics in our community has aided supplier-shopping and in other communities [8, 38]. Although poor knowledge facilitated the practice of purchasing one or two doses of antibiotics neither the pharmacists nor the home-visiting nurses corrected this practice. There are an estimated 13,000 village drug outlets across Cambodia [23] that provide antibiotics over-the-counter without a prescription. During our fieldwork we sent in a mystery shopper who easily purchased a cocktail of drugs for his common cold symptoms. Our mystery shopper was given two doses of 500 mg amoxicillin and several unknown medications for his symptoms (Fig. 1). Apart from the misuse of antibiotic for the common cold [39] one or two doses of amoxicillin may cause resistance in commensal bacteria [40, 41]. One or two doses of antibiotics is insufficient treatment for the majority of bacterial infections. As an example the treatment of amoxicillin sensitive group A β-hemolytic streptococcal pharyngitis is 1000 mg of amoxicillin once-daily for 10 days [42]. In addition to the contribution by drug outlets to inappropriate dispensing of antibiotics the drug outlets also flood the community with counterfeit and substandard antibiotics [43]. Counterfeit antibiotics place pathogens under pressure to develop antibiotic resistance and if antibiotics are eventually prescribed appropriately for patients who

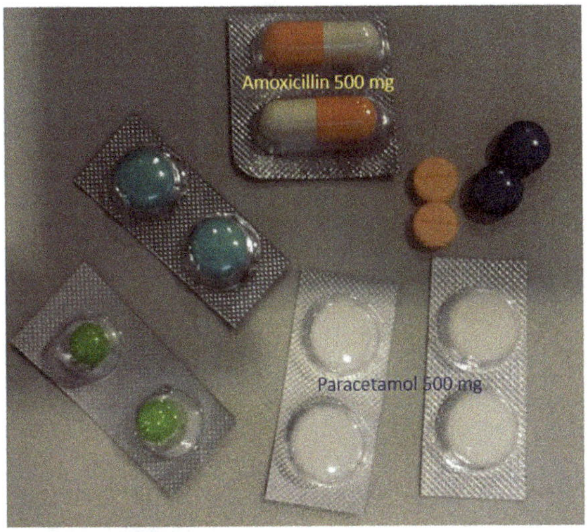

Fig. 1 Drug cocktails for common cold purchased from a village drug outlet

has recently used counterfeit antibiotics the treatment may be ineffective [44]. The Cambodian Ministry of Health enforced the closure in 2010 of nearly 65% of illegal pharmacies across the country [37] but the implementation of these laws and regulation remains weak [45]. The community's expressed appreciation of trained healthcare providers for a serious illness may help the success of the 2016 legislation of only registered physicians to provide treatment, but only if there was an unrelenting public education campaign that runs in conjunction with fines for unlawful antibiotic supply.

Conclusions

The magnitude of antibiotic misuse in the Cambodian community was driven by antibiotic-seeking behaviour that would not be rewarded without unrestricted access to antibiotics. The misconceptions of the indications for antibiotics would have less impact on antibiotic-seeking behaviour if unfettered access to antibiotics were prevented. The control of antibiotic access requires the immediate outlawing of antibiotic access from source other than a registered pharmacist and a prescription. This would also prevent the direct access to antibiotics by nurses and village Petts who supply antibiotics during home visits. Educational programs about the serious consequences of antibiotic misuse could be dealt with by providing appropriate and affordable healthcare-seeking pathways to become the first point-of-care for strictly regulated antibiotic prescribing.

Abbreviations

DALY: Disability-adjusted life year; FGD: Focus group discussion; UNSW: University of New South Wales; WHO: World Health Organization

Acknowledgements

We are grateful for the financial support provided by Fondation Mérieux, Cambodia, and Institute of Tropical Medicine, Belgium. We thank the Department of Hospital Services, Ministry of Health, for collaboration and coordination of our fieldwork. We are grateful for the invaluable contributions from family members, pharmacy attendants, and community healthcare centre nurses who were open and forthright during our discussions.

Funding

Dr Chhorvoin Om is supported by a four-year Australia Awards scholarship for his PhD under the supervision of Prof McLaws and the scholarship providers had no role in this study. The Institute of Tropical Medicine, Belgium and the Fondation Mérieux, Cambodia financially supported the fieldwork.

Authors' contributions

CO and MM designed the study and the interview guides, conduct data coding and analysis, and wrote the manuscript. CO conducts FGDs and interviews, FD, JM and EV provided guidance during the fieldwork and critical feedback of the manuscript. All authors gave approval for publishing this manuscript.

Competing interests

"The authors declare that they have no competing interests."

Consent for publication

Not applicable.

Author details

[1]School of Public Health and Community Medicine, UNSW Medicine, UNSW, Level 3 Samuels Building, Sydney 2052, NSW, Australia. [2]Diagnostic Microbiology Development Program, # 23 (First Floor), Street 310, BKK 1, Khan Chamcar Morn, Phnom Penh, Cambodia. [3]Department of Clinical Sciences, Institute of Tropical Medicine, Nationalestraat 155, 2000 Antwerp, Belgium.

References

1. WHO. Worldwide country situation analysis: response to antimicrobial resistance. Geneva, 2015. http://www.ac2bmr.fr/images/WHO_Response.pdf. Accessed 20 Aug 2016
2. Ventola CL. The antibiotic resistance crisis: part 1: causes and threats. P T. 2015;40(4):277–83.
3. Bhutta ZA, Sommerfeld J, Lassi ZS, Salam RA, Das JK. Global burden, distribution, and interventions for infectious diseases of poverty. Infect Dis Poverty. 2014;3:21.
4. WHO. The Global Burden of Disease: 2004 Update. Geneva, 2008. http://www.who.int/healthinfo/global_burden_disease/GBD_report_2004update_full.pdf?ua=1. Accessed 07 Oct 2016.
5. WHO. Interventions and Strategies to Improve the use of antimicrobials in developing countries: a review. Geneva, 2001. http://www.who.int/drugresistance/Interventions_and_strategies_to_improve_the_use_of_antim.pdf. Accessed 15 Aug 2016.
6. Okeke IN, Laxminarayan R, Bhutta ZA, Duse AG, Jenkins P, O'Brien TF, et al. Antimicrobial resistance in developing countries. Part I: recent trends and current status. Lancet Infect Dis. 2005;5(8):481–93.
7. Morgan DJ, Okeke IN, Laxminarayan R, Perencevich EN, Weisenberg S. Non-prescription antimicrobial use worldwide: a systematic review. Lancet Infect Dis. 2011;11(9):692–701.
8. Isturiz RE, Carbon C. Antibiotic use in developing countries. Infect Control Hosp Epidemiol. 2000;21(6):394–7.
9. Gwatkin DR, Guillot M. The Burden of Disease Among the Global Poor. Current Situation, Future Trends, and Implications for Strategy. Washington, DC, The World Bank. 2000. http://siteresources.worldbank.org/INTPAH/Resources/Publications/Seminars/burden.pdf. Accessed 07 Oct 2016

10. Hogerzeil HV, Bimo, Ross-Degnan D, Laing RO, Ofori-Adjei D, Santoso B et al. Field tests for rational drug use in twelve developing countries. Lancet. 1993;342:1408-10.
11. Planta MB. The role of poverty in antimicrobial resistance. J Am Board Fam Med. 2007;20(6):533–9.
12. Okeke IN, Lamikanra A, Edelman R. Socioeconomic and behavioral factors leading to acquired bacterial resistance to antibiotics in developing countries. Emerg Infect Dis. 1999;5(1):18–27.
13. Radyowijati A, Haak H, Radyowijati A, Haak H. Improving antibiotic use in low-income countries: an overview of evidence on determinants. Soc Sci Med. 2003;57(4):733–44.
14. Radyowijati A, Haak H. Determinants of antimicrobial use in the developing world: child health research project special report. USAID Bureau of Global Health: Washington D.C.; 2002. http://www.childhealthresearch.org/doc/AMR_vol4.pdf. Accessed 03 Oct 2016.
15. Okumura J, Wakai S, Umenai T, Okumura J, Wakai S, Umenai T. Drug utilisation and self-medication in rural communities in Vietnam. Soc Sci Med. 2002;54(12):1875–86.
16. Stoesser N, Moore CE, Pocock JM, An KP, Emary K, Carter M, et al. Pediatric bloodstream infections in Cambodia, 2007 to 2011. Pediatr Infect Dis J. 2013;32(7):E272–E6.
17. Emary K, Moore CE, Chanpheaktra N, An KP, Chheng K, Sona S, et al. Enteric fever in Cambodian children is dominated by multidrug-resistant H58 Salmonella enterica serovar Typhi with intermediate susceptibility to ciprofloxacin. Trans Roy Soc Trop Med Hyg. 2012; 106(12):718–24.
18. Kasper MR, Sokhal B, Blair PJ, Wierzba TF, Putnam SD, Kasper MR, et al. Emergence of multidrug-resistant Salmonella enterica serovar Typhi with reduced susceptibility to fluoroquinolones in Cambodia. Diagn Microbiol Infect Dis. 2010;66(2):207–9.
19. Vlieghe ER, Phe T, De Smet B, Veng HC, Kham C, Lim K, et al. Bloodstream infection among adults in Phnom Penh, Cambodia: Key pathogens and resistance patterns. PLoS One. 2013;8(3):e59775.
20. Chareonkul C, Khun VL, Boonshuyar C. Rational drug use in Cambodia: study of three pilot health centers in Kampong Thom Province. Southeast Asian J Trop Med Public Health. 2002;33(2):418–24.
21. WHO. Annual Report 2002 Essential Drugs and Medicines Policy: Supporting countries to close the access gap. Geneva, 2002. http://apps.who.int/medicinedocs/pdf/s4863e/s4863e.pdf. Accessed 10 Oct 2016.
22. Emary KRW, Carter MJ, Pol S, Sona S, Kumar V, Day NPJ, et al. Urinary antibiotic activity in paediatric patients attending an outpatient department in north-western Cambodia. Trop Med Int Health. 2015;20(1):24–8.
23. Ramage I. Assessment of official private providers and delivery of health care services to children under five. Phnom Penh, Cambodia: WHO; 2011. http://citeseerx.ist.psu.edu/viewdoc/download?doi=10.1.1.548.3332&rep=rep1&type=pdf. Accessed 12 Oct 2016.
24. The World Bank. Cambodia Country Overview. 2016. http://www.worldbank.org/en/country/cambodia/overview. Accessed 21 Oct 2016.
25. Asian Development Bank. Cambodia: Country poverty analysis 2014. Mandaluyong City, Philippines, 2014. https://www.adb.org/sites/default/files/institutional-document/151706/cambodia-country-poverty-analysis-2014.pdf. Accessed 10 Oct 2016.
26. Department of Planning and Health Information. Annual health statistics report 2012. Phnom Penh, Cambodia: Ministry of Health; 2012.
27. National Institute of Statistics. Cambodia Demographic and Health Survey 2010. Ministry of Planning, Phnom Penh, Cambodia, 2010. https://dhsprogram.com/pubs/pdf/FR249/FR249.pdf. Accessed 12 Oct 2016.
28. Giacomini MK, Cook DJ. Users' guides to the medical literature: XXIII. Qualitative research in health care A. Are the results of the study valid? evidence-based medicine working group. JAMA. 2000;284(3):357–62.
29. Om C, Vlieghe E, McLaughlin JC, Daily F, McLaws ML. Antibiotic prescribing practices: A national survey of Cambodian physicians. Am J Infect Control. 2016;44(10):1144–8.
30. Morse JM. The significance of saturation. Qual Health Res. 1995;5(2):147–9.
31. Francis JJ, Johnston M, Robertson C, Glidewell L, Entwistle V, Eccles MP, et al. What is an adequate sample size? Operationalising data saturation for theory-based interview studies. Psychol Health. 2010;25(10):1229–45.
32. Braun V, Clarke V. Using thematic analysis in psychology. Qual Res Psychol. 2006;3(2):77–101.
33. Sandelowski M, Leeman J. Writing usable qualitative health research findings. Qual Health Res. 2012;22(10):1404–13.
34. Joffe H, Yardley L. Research methods for clinical and health psychology. London: SAGE Publications Ltd; 2004. p. 56–68. Content and Thematic Analysis.
35. Vun MC, Galang RR, Fujita M, Killam W, Gokhale R, Pitman J, et al. Cluster of HIV infections attributed to unsafe injection practices–Cambodia, December 1, 2014-February 28, 2015. MMWR Morb Mortal Wkly Rep. 2016;65(6):142–5.
36. Ministry of Health. Medicines Policy of the Kingdom of Cambodia. Phnom Penh, Cambodia, 2010. http://apps.who.int/medicinedocs/documents/s22477en/s22477en.pdf. Accessed 15 Feb 2017.
37. Burki T. The real cost of counterfeit medicines. Lancet Infect Dis. 2010;10(9):585–6.
38. Byarugaba DK. A view on antimicrobial resistance in developing countries and responsible risk factors. Int J Antimicrob Agents. 2004;24(2):105–10.
39. Nair H, Nokes DJ, Gessner BD, Dherani M, Madhi SA, Singleton RJ, et al. Global burden of acute lower respiratory infections due to respiratory syncytial virus in young children: a systematic review and meta-analysis. Lancet. 2010;375(9725):1545–55.
40. Arroll B, Kenealy T. Antibiotics for the common cold. Cochrane Database Syst Rev. 2002;(3):Cd000247.
41. Robinson J. Antibiotics for the common cold—do they work? Evidence-Based Child Health. 2013;8(5):1512–3.
42. Andrews M, Condren M. Once-daily amoxicillin for pharyngitis. J Pediatr Pharmacol Ther. 2010;15(4):244–8.
43. Almuzaini T, Choonara I, Sammons H. Substandard and counterfeit medicines: a systematic review of the literature. BMJ Open. 2013;3(8):e002923.
44. Kelesidis T, Kelesidis I, Rafailidis PI, Falagas ME. Counterfeit or substandard antimicrobial drugs: a review of the scientific evidence. J Antimicrob Chemother. 2007;60(2):214–36.
45. Lon CT, Tsuyuoka R, Phanouvong S, Nivanna N, Socheat D, Sokhan C, et al. Counterfeit and substandard antimalarial drugs in Cambodia. Trans R Soc Trop Med Hyg. 2006;100(11):1019–24.

15

Key features of *mcr-1*-bearing plasmids from *Escherichia coli* isolated from humans and food

Katrin Zurfluh[1*], Magdalena Nüesch-Inderbinen[1], Jochen Klumpp[2], Laurent Poirel[3,4], Patrice Nordmann[3,4] and Roger Stephan[1]

Abstract

Background: *Mcr-1*-harboring Enterobacteriaceae are reported worldwide since their first discovery in 2015. However, a limited number of studies are available that compared full-length plasmid sequences of human and animal origins.

Methods: In this study, *mcr-1*-bearing plasmids from seven *Escherichia coli* isolates recovered from patients (n = 3), poultry meat (n = 2) and turkey meat (n = 2) in Switzerland were further analyzed and compared. Isolates were characterized by multilocus sequence typing (MLST). The *mcr-1*-bearing plasmids were transferred by transformation into reference strain *E. coli* DH5α and MCR-1-producing transformants were selected on LB-agar supplemented with 2 mg/L colistin. Purified plasmids were then sequenced and compared.

Results: MLST revealed six distinct STs, illustrating the high clonal diversity among *mcr-1*-positive *E. coli* isolates of different origins. Two different *mcr-1*-positive plasmids were identified from a single *E. coli* ST48 human isolate. All other isolates possessed a single *mcr-1* harboring plasmid. Transferable IncI2 (size ca. 60–61 kb) and IncX4 (size ca. 33–35 kb) type plasmids each bearing *mcr-1* were found associated with human and food isolates. None of the *mcr-1*-positive IncI2 and IncX4 plasmids possessed any additional resistance determinants. Surprisingly, all but one of the sequenced *mcr-1*-positive plasmids lacked the IS*Apl1* element, which is a key element mediating acquisition of *mcr-1* into various plasmid backbones.

Conclusions: There is strong evidence that the food chain may be an important transmission route for *mcr-1*-bearing plasmids. Our data suggest that some "epidemic" plasmids rather than specific *E. coli* clones might be responsible for the spread of the *mcr-1* gene along the food chain.

Keywords: Colistin, *Mcr-1*, Plasmid, IS*Apl1*

Background

The increasing number of multidrug-resistant Gram-negative bacteria and the lack of novel antimicrobials has led to the reintroduction of polymyxins as last-resort antimicrobials in human medicine, although once avoided because of its nephro- and neurotoxicity [1, 2]. By contrast, in veterinary medicine, colistin is still widely used for the treatment of diarrhea in food-producing animals such as calves and pigs in most countries [3]. Until late 2015, only chromosomally-encoded mechanisms of resistance to polymyxins were known [4]. The mobile colistin resistance gene, *mcr-1,* was first described on a conjugative IncI2 plasmid from Chinese isolates. It encodes a phosphoethanolamine transferase that adds phosphoethanolamine to the lipid A [5]. Retrospective studies performed worldwide revealed that the gene had been circulating undetected for at least twenty years and animals have been suggested to be its main reservoir [6]. The dissemination of *mcr-1* is associated with a large variety of plasmids including incompatibility groups IncI2, IncX4, IncF, IncHI1, IncHI2, IncP and IncY [7–10]. Most of these groups are well

* Correspondence: katrin.zurfluh@uzh.ch
[1]Institute for Food Safety and Hygiene, Vetsuisse Faculty University of Zurich, Winterthurerstrasse 272, 8057 Zurich, Switzerland
Full list of author information is available at the end of the article

known to be involved in the spread of a diversity of antibiotic resistance genes in Enterobacteriaceae.

The aim of this study was to characterize *mcr-1*-bearing plasmids from *E. coli* originating from humans and food isolated at the same location (Switzerland) in order to improve the understanding of the epidemiology and spreading potential of the *mcr-1* gene.

Methods

In total, seven *E. coli* isolates harboring *mcr-1* plasmids were used in the present study, including one uropathogenic *E. coli* (UPEC) isolate recovered from human urinary tract infection (CDF8), two isolates from humans with diarrhea and history of travel to Asia (ColR598 and ColR644SK1), and two isolates respectively from retail poultry meat (PC11 and PF11) and retail turkey meat (PF52 and PF91). UPEC strain CDF8 was obtained from a patient hospitalized in Switzerland in 2016 (unpublished) and food isolates PC11, PF11, PF52 and PF91 had been isolated in 2016 from food imported from Germany and sold in retail stores in Switzerland [11] ColR598 and ColR644SK1 were obtained from a stool sample screening from patients with diarrhea during the June to December 2016 period. Briefly, a total of 320 non-duplicate samples were screened for the presence of colistin-resistant Enterobacteriaceae by enriching one loopful of stool in 5 ml *Enterobacteriaceae* enrichment (EE) broth (BD, Franklin Lakes, NJ, USA) for 24 h at 37 °C, followed by streaking one loopful onto LB agar plates containing 4 mg/L colistin, 10 mg/L vancomycin and 5 mg/L amphotericin B for selection of colistin-resistant Gram-negative bacteria. The isolates were identified using API ID 32 E (bioMérieux, Marcy l'Etoile, France) and analyzed for the presence of *mcr-1* by PCR as described previously [5]. Minimal inhibitory concentration of colistin was determined for *mcr-1*-positive isolates using broth dilution tests as recommended by EUCAST. Moreover, isolates were subjected to susceptibility testing against 13 antimicrobial agents by the disc diffusion method according to CLSI protocols and evaluated according to CLSI criteria [12].

Multilocus sequence typing (MLST) was performed as described previously [13], and isolates were assigned to sequence types (ST) and clonal complexes (CC) according to the Achtman scheme (http://mlst.ucc.ie/mlst/dbs/Ecoli).

The *mcr-1*-positive plasmids were extracted using the Qiagen Midi kit (Qiagen, Hombrechtikon, Switzerland) and transferred by transformation using electroporation into *E. coli* DH5α. Colistin-resistant transformants were selected on LB-agar supplemented with 2 mg/L colistin (Sigma-Aldrich, Buchs SG, Switzerland). The *mcr-1* plasmids were extracted using the Large-Construct Kit (Qiagen, Hombrechtikon, Switzerland) according the manufacturer's protocol and sequenced on a PacBio RS2 device (Pacific Biosciences, Menlo Park, USA) with a 10 kb size-selected insert library and P6/C4 chemistry. De novo assembly (using the HGAP3 algorithm) was performed using SMRTanalysis version 2.3.0 (Pacific Biosciences). The HGAP3 settings were kept at the defaults, except for the expected genome size, which was set between 50 kb and 100 kb. The plasmid sequence was automatically annotated using the online Rapid Annotation Subsequencing Technology (RAST) [14] and CLC Main Workbench Version 7.8.1 (CLC bio, Aarhus, Denmark). Automated annotation was manually refined using the BLASTn and BLASTp programs (http://blast.ncbi.nlm.nih.gov/Blast.cgi).

Results and discussion

The results of this study analyzing seven distinct *mcr-1*-harbouring isolates of different sources are summarized in Table 1. Noticeably, all *mcr-1*-harbouring isolates were *E. coli* that correspond to the most important reservoir of MCR-1 producers identified so far. MLST analysis did not show any close clonal relationship between the seven *mcr-1*-positive *E. coli* isolates, suggesting that the dissemination of the *mcr-1* gene is so far not primarily associated with any specific clonal lineage.

From the seven *E. coli* isolates, a total of eight *mcr-1*-bearing plasmids was recovered, with the human isolate ColR598 yielding two distinct *mcr-1*-positive plasmids. Li and colleagues showed in a recent study that coexistence of two *mcr-1* bearing plasmids seems to be common [15]. Nevertheless, the MIC's for colistin were not affected by the number of *mcr-1* bearing plasmids present in one isolate [15]. The eight plasmids belonged to two plasmid types that have been often shown to be involved in the spread of *mcr-1* [16]. Three IncI2 plasmids (pPC11, pCoR598_2 and pColR644SK1) were ca. 60 kb in-size, and were similar to pHNSHP45 (Fig. 1), the original sequenced *mcr-1* plasmid published in 2015 [5]. The three IncI2 plasmids shared a common plasmid backbone, however, in the case of pPC11 the *mcr-1* cassette [17] was located in an inverted orientation compared to the others (data not shown). Additionally, the IncI2 plasmids from human isolates (pColR598_2 and pColR644SK1) varied greatly compared to the plasmid pPC11 (poultry isolate) in the shufflon region, which is a clustered inversion region encoding components of the pilV protein involved in plasmid transmission [18]. The components are rearranged by Rci, a recombinase encoded by the *rci* gene (Fig. 1). This observation is in accordance with recently sequenced IncI2 plasmids carrying *mcr-1* detected in *E. coli* from swine and cattle in Japan [19].

The other five plasmids (pPF11, pPF52, pPF91, pCDF8 and pColR598_1) all belonged to the plasmid incompatibility group IncX4 and were ca. 33 kb in-size. Their

Table 1 Features of the eight *mcr-1*-harboring plasmids from seven *E. coli* isolated from humans and from food

Host strain ID	Origin	Source	ST (CC)	MIC colistin [mg/L]	Resistance profile	*mcr-1* harbouring plasmid	Plasmid size (bp)	Inc group	*Mcr-1* gene cassette	Additional resistance genes on the *mcr-1* harbouring plasmid	Reference
PC11	Chicken	Meat	ST1251	8	AM, CF	pPC11	59.830	IncI2	IS*Apl1*-*mcr-1*-orf	none	[11]
PF11	Chicken	Meat	ST156 (CC156)	8	AM, CF, NA, CIP, TE	pPF11	33.308	IncX4	*mcr-1*-orf	none	[11]
PF52	Turkey	Meat	ST58 (CC155)	4	AM, CF, SMZ	pPF52	33.300	IncX4	*mcr-1*-orf	none	[11]
PF91	Turkey	Meat	ST1431	8	AM, CF, TE, C, SMZ	pPF91	33.310	IncX4	*mcr-1*-orf	none	[11]
CDF8	Human	UTI	nd	4	AM, CZ, CTX, FEP, NA, CIP, S, K	pCDF8	33.660	IncX4	*mcr-1*-orf	none	this study
ColR598	Human	Diarrhea	ST48 (CC10)	4	NA, CIP, TE	pColR598_1	33.299	IncX4	*mcr-1*-orf	none	this study
ColR598	Human	Diarrhea	ST48 (CC10)	4	NA, CIP, TE	pColR598_2	60.939	IncI2	*mcr-1*-orf	none	this study
ColR644SK1	Human	Diarrhea	ST117	4	AM, CF, TE, C, SMZ, TMP	pColR644SK1	60.952	IncI2	*mcr-1*-orf	none	this study

Abbreviations: *CC* clonal complex; *Inc.* plasmid incompatibility group; *ST* sequence type; *UTI* urinary tract infection, not determined; *MIC* minimal inhibitory concentration; *AM* ampicillin; *CF* cephalothin; *CZ* cefazolin; *CIP* ciprofloxacin; *NA* nalidixic acid; *K* kanamycin; *S* streptomycin; *SMZ* sulfamethoxazole; *TMP* trimethoprim; *TE* tetracycline; *C* chloramphenicol

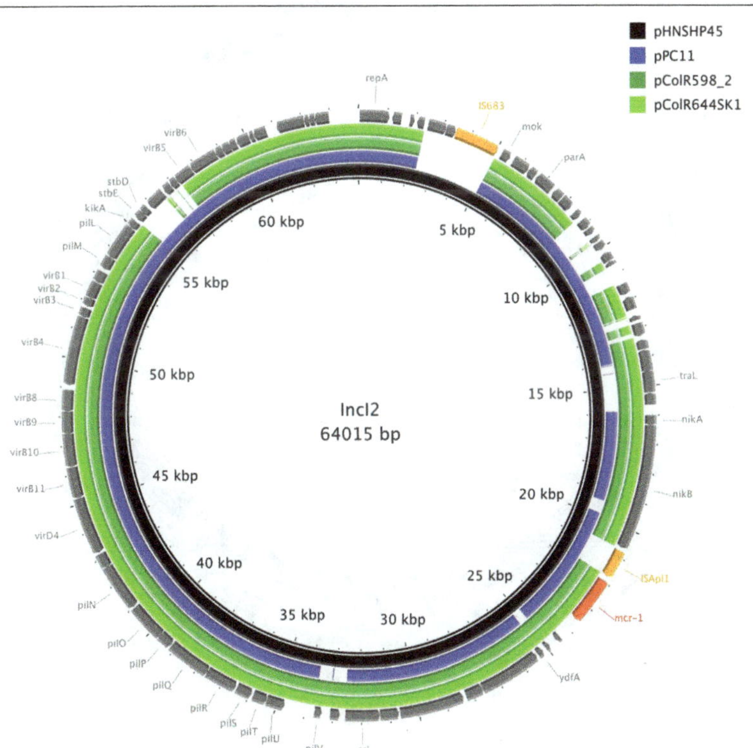

Fig. 1 Sequencing alignment of IncI2-type *mcr-1*-harboring plasmids. The first *mcr-1*-harboring plasmid, pHNSHP45 (Accession-Nr. KP347127), which was isolated in China, was used as reference plasmid (black circle). The outmost circle in grey arrows shows the annotations of the reference plasmid. The insertions element and the *mcr-1* gene were highlighted in orange and red arrows, respectively. Gaps indicate regions that were missing in the respective plasmid compared to the reference plasmid

sequences varied only by very few nucleotides (≥99% homology), mostly located in non-coding regions (Fig. 2). In the case of pDCF8 the *mcr-1* cassette was located in an inverted orientation compared to the others (data not shown). Of note, those almost identical IncX4 plasmids originate from humans, poultry and turkey meat, illustrating their wide dissemination throughout multiple sources, and providing further evidence of the likely association of *mcr-1*-mediated colistin resistance through food-producing animals.

An open reading frame (*orf*) encoding an hypothetical protein with similarities to a PAP2 superfamily protein was detected immediately downstream of the *mcr-1* gene (both together hereafter referred to as *mcr-1* cassette) was identified on all eight plasmids.

The insertion sequence IS*Apl1*, has been shown to play a key role in the mobilization of *mcr-1* [20], but was absent upstream of *mcr-1* in most of our isolates. Further evidence for the importance of IS*Apl1* in the mobilization of *mcr-1* was the presence of IS*Apl1* next to the *mcr-1* gene on the chromosome of an *E. coli* veal calf isolate from Netherland [21]. Moreover, transposition of the *mcr-1* gene by an IS*Apl1*-made composite transposon was recently demonstrated [17]. Highly similar inverted repeat (IRR) and direct repeat (DR) sequences were identified on IncX4, IncHI1 and IncHI2 backbones immediately downstream of the *mcr-1* cassette, resembling the target insertion site resulting from the IS*Apl1*-mediated transposition [16], although the IS element itself was not always present. In a recent study, no putative inverted repeat sequences were identified at the extremities of the *mcr-1* cassette [22]. Furthermore, Snesrud and colleagues [20] proposed the loss of one or both IS*Apl1* elements as an explanation for the minor variations (mismatches and deletions) at the 3'end of the *mcr-1* element. Accordingly, in this study, IS*Apl1* was present only on a single IncI2 plasmid (pPC11) and was located upstream of the *mcr-1* gene.

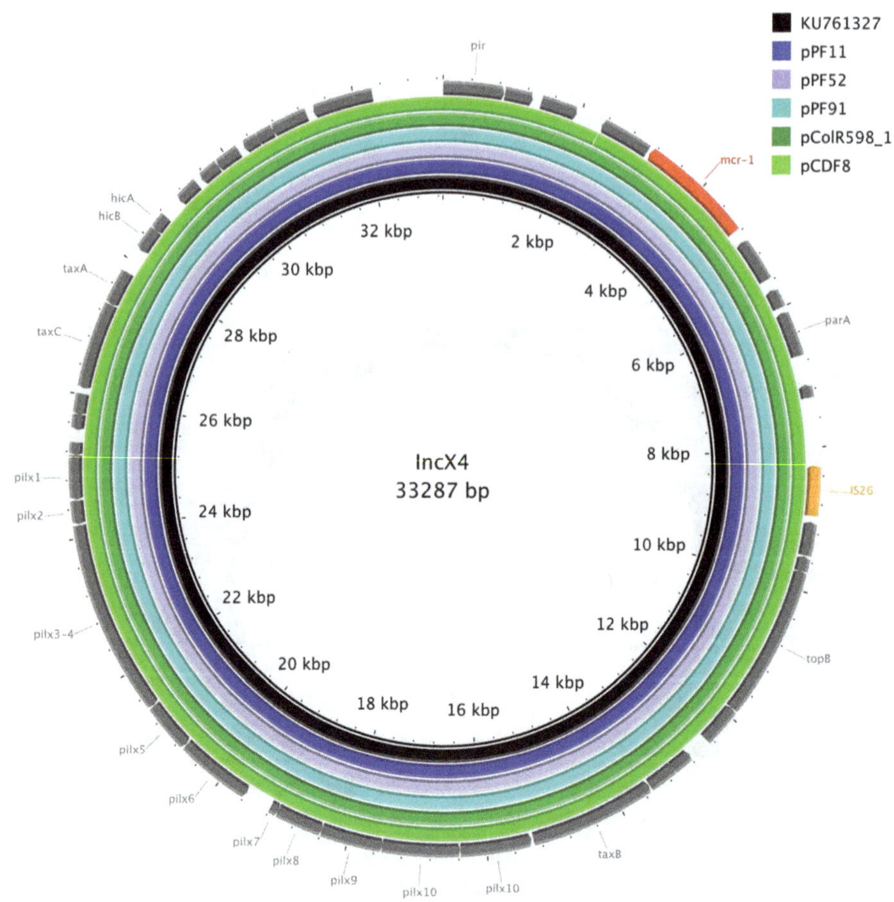

Fig. 2 Sequencing alignment of IncX4-type *mcr-1*-harboring plasmids. The *mcr-1* harboring plasmid, pmcr-1_X4 (Accession-Nr. KU761327), which was obtained from two *Klebisiella pneumonia* isolates and one *Escherichia coli* isolate from patients in eastern China and which was one of the first sequenced IncX4 *mcr-1* positive plasmids, was used as reference plasmid (black circle). The outmost circle in grey arrows shows the annotations of the reference plasmid. The insertions element and the *mcr-1* gene were highlighted in orange and red arrows, respectively. The figure indicates the high degree of homology of the *mcr-1* harboring IncX4 plasmids independently of their isolation source and geographical origin

Noticeably, none of the sequenced plasmids carried additional antibiotic resistance determinants. This is in agreement with other observations [5, 9, 22] and appears to be quite a specificity to the *mcr-1* gene, considering that most antibiotic resistance plasmids often carry multiple resistance genes. It is therefore tempting to speculate that this specificity is related to selection of those MCR-1 determinants by treatment containing polymyxins in animals. Moreover, the food samples described in this study originated from Germany, a country with high use of colistin in animal husbandry, and both humans with diarrhea had visited countries in Asia, where colistin is applied widely to treat animals [3]. However, the extended-spectrum ß-lactamase gene $bla_{CTX\text{-}M\text{-}64}$ has recently been detected on an *mcr-1*-harboring IncI2 plasmid [23]. There are some further data were the *mcr*-1 gene was located on large multidrug resistance plasmids for example in combination with extended-spectrum beta-lactamase genes [9, 15, 24]. In these studies *mcr-1* was mainly harboured on IncHI2 or IncF plasmids. It is to be expected that *mcr-1* harboring plasmids co-harboring resistances to antimicrobials crucial to human treatment become more frequent in future.

Conclusion

Transferable IncI2 and IncX4 type plasmids harbouring *mcr-1* were found in *E. coli* of different clonal backgrounds isolated from humans and from food. The high similarity between the plasmids belonging to the same incompatibility groups shows that these "epidemic" plasmids may be responsible for the spread of the *mcr-1* gene along the food chain and humans, rather than single specific *E. coli* clones. A single strain may even contain more than one *mcr-1*-harboring plasmid. Further studies are needed in order to determine the mechanisms that lead to the acquisition or even accumulation of *mcr-1*-harboring plasmids within Enterobacteriaceae.

Abbreviations

bla: ß-lactamase gene; CC: Clonal complex; EE: *Enterobacteriaceae* enrichment; Inc: Plasmid incompatibility group; MLST: Multilocus sequence type; NENT: National Centre for Enteropathogenic Bacteria and *Listeria*; ST: Sequence type; UPEC: Uropathogenic *E. coli*; UTI: Urinary tract infection

Acknowledgements

We are grateful to the staff of the Functional Genomics Center Zurich, particularly Simon Grüter and Andrea Patrignani for excellent technical support and bioinformatics support.

Funding

This work was funded by the Swiss Federal Office of Public Health, Division Communicable Diseases.

Authors' contributions

RS, LP and PN designed the study. KZ carried out the microbiological and molecular biological tests. KZ and JK did the bioinformatic analysis. KZ, MNI and RS analyzed and interpreted the data. KZ and MNI drafted the manuscript. All authors read and approved the final manuscript.

Consent for publication

Not applicable.

Competing interests

The authors declare that they have no competing interest.

Author details

[1]Institute for Food Safety and Hygiene, Vetsuisse Faculty University of Zurich, Winterthurerstrasse 272, 8057 Zurich, Switzerland. [2]Institute of Food, Nutrition and Health, ETH Zurich, Schmelzbergstr. 7, 8092 Zurich, Switzerland. [3]Emerging Antibiotic Resistance, Medical and Molecular Microbiology Unit, Department of Medicine, University of Fribourg, Fribourg, Switzerland. [4]National Reference Center for Emerging Antibiotic Resistance, University of Fribourg, Fribourg, Switzerland.

References

1. Paterson DL, Harris PNA. Colistin resistance: a major breach in our last line of defense. Lancet Infect Dis. 2016;16:132–3.
2. Poirel L, Jayol A, Nordmann P. Polymyxins: antibacterial activity, susceptibility testing and resistance mechanisms encoded by plasmids or chromosomes. Clin Microbiol Rev. 2017;30:557–96.
3. Irrgang A, Roschanski N, Tenhagen B-A, Grobbel M, Skladnikiewicz-Ziemer T, Thomas K, et al. Prevalence of *mcr-1* in *E. coli* from livestock and food in Germany, 2010–2015. PLoS One. doi: 10.1371/journal.pone.0159863.
4. Olaitan AO, Morand S, Rolain JM. Mechanisms of polymyxin resistance: acquired and intrinsic resistance in bacteria. Front Microbiol. 2014;5:1–18.
5. Liu YY, Wang Y, Walsh TR, Yi LX, Zhang R, Spencer J, et al. Emergence of plasmid-mediated colistin resistance mechanism MCR-1 in animals and human beings in China: a microbiological and molecular biological study. Lancet Infect Dis. 2015;16:161–8.
6. Schwarz S, Johnson AP. Transferable resistance to colistin: a new but old threat. J Antimicrob Chemother. 2016;71:2066–70.
7. Zhi C, Lv L, Yu LF, Doi Y, Liu JH. Dissemination of the *mcr-1* colistin resistance gene. Lancet Infect Dis. 2016;16:292–3.
8. McGann P, Snesrud E, Maybank R, Corey B, Ong AC, Clifford R, et al. *Escherichia coli* harboring *mcr-1* and $bla_{CTX\text{-}M}$ on a novel IncF plasmid: first report of *mcr-1* in the USA. Antimicrob Agents Chemother. 2016;60:4420–1.
9. Zurfluh K, Klumpp J, Nüesch-Inderbinen M, Stephan R. Full-length nucleotide sequences of *mcr-1*-harboring plasmids isolated from extended-spectrum-β-lactamase-producing *Escherichia coli* isolates of different origins. Antimicrob Agents Chemother. 2016;60:5589–91.
10. Zhang C, Feng Y, Liu F, Jiang H, Qu Z, Lei M, et al. Phage-like IncY plasmid carrying the *mcr-1* gene in *Escherichia coli* from a pig farm in China. Antimicrob Agents Chemother. 2016; doi: 10.1128/AAC.02035-16.
11. Zurfluh K, Buess S, Stephan R, Nüesch-Inderbinen M. Assessment of the occurrence of MCR producing Enterobacteriaceae in Swiss and imported poultry meat. J Food Sci Tech. 2016; doi: 10.15436/JFST.1.4.5.
12. Clinical and Laboratory Standards Institute. 2016. M100S. Performance standards for antimicrobial susceptibility testing, 26st informational supplement. Clinical and Laboratory Standards Institute, Wayne, PA.
13. Wirth T, Falush D, Lan R, Colles F, Mensa P, Wieler LH, et al. Sex and virulence in *Escherichia coli:* an evolutionary perspective. Mol Microbiol. 2006;60:1136–51. doi: 10.1111/j.1365-2958.2006.05172.x.
14. Aziz RK, Bartels D, Best AA, DeJongh M, Disz T, Edwards RA, et al. The RAST server: rapid annotations using subsystems technology. BMC Genomics. 2008; doi: 10.1186/1471-2164-9-75.

15. Li R, Xie M, Zhang J, Yang Z, Liu L, Liu X, et al. Genetic characterization of *mcr-1*-bearing plasmids to depict molecular mechanisms underlying deissemination of the colistin resistance determinant. J Antimicrob Chemother. 2017;72:393–401.
16. Sun J, Fang L-X, Zuowei W, Deng H, Yang R-S, Li X-P, et al. Genetic analysis of the IncX4 plasmids: implications for a unique pattern in the *mcr-1* acquisition. Sci Rep. 2017;7:424.
17. Poirel L, Kieffer N., Nordmann P. In vitro study of ISApa1 mobilization of the colistin resistance gene *mcr-1*. Antimicrob Agents Chemother. 2017 pii: AAC. 00127–17. doi: 10.1128/AAC.00127-17.
18. Gyohda A, Furuya N, Kogure N, Komano T. Sequence-specific and non-specific binding of the Rci protein to the asymmetric recombination sites of the R64 shuffflon. J Mol Biol. 2002;318:975–83.
19. Sekizuka T, Kawanishi M, Ohnishi M, Shima A, Kato K, Yamashita A, et al. Elucidation of quantitative structural diversity of remarkable rearrangement regions, shufflons, in IncI2 plasmids. Sci Rep. 2017;7:928.
20. Snesrud E, He S, Chandler M, Dekker JP, Hickmann AB, McGann P, Dyda F. A model for transposition of the colistin resistance gene *mcr-1* by IS*Apl1*. Antimicrob Agents Chemother. 2016;60:6973–6.
21. Veldman K, van Essen-Zandbergen A, Rapallini M, Wit B, Heymans R, van Pelt W, et al. Location of colistin resistance gene *mcr-1* in Enterobacteriaceae from livestock and meat. J Antimicrob Chemother. 2017;71:2340–2.
22. Poirel L, Kieffer N, Brink A, Coetze J, Jayol A, Nordmann P. Genetic features of MCR-1-producing colistin-resistant *Escherichia coli* isolates in South Africa. Antimicrob Agents Chemother. 2016;60:4394–7. doi: 10.1128/AAC.00444-16.
23. Sonnevend Á, Ghazawi A, Alqahtani M, Shibl A, Jamal W, Hashmey R, Pal T. Plasmid-mediated colistin resistance in *Escherichia coli* from the Arabian peninsula. Int J Infect Dis. 2016;50:85–90. doi: 10.1016/j.ijid.2016.07.007.
24. McGann P, Snesrud E, Maybank R, Corey B, Ong AC, Clifford R, et al. *Escherichia coli* harboring *mcr-1* and $bla_{CTX\text{-}M}$ on a novel IncF plasmid: first report of *mcr-1* in the United States. Antimicrob Agents Chemother. 2016; 60:4420–1. doi: 10.1128/AAC.01103-16.

16

Risk factors and outcomes of organ-space surgical site infections after elective colon and rectal surgery

Aina Gomila[1,2], Jordi Carratalà[1,2,3], Daniel Camprubí[1,2], Evelyn Shaw[1,2], Josep Mª Badia[2,4], Antoni Cruz[2,5], Francesc Aguilar[2,6], Carmen Nicolás[2,7], Anna Marrón[2,8], Laura Mora[2,9], Rafel Perez[2,10], Lydia Martin[2,11], Rosa Vázquez[2,4], Ana Felisa Lopez[2,12], Enric Limón[2,3], Francesc Gudiol[2,3], Miquel Pujol[1,2,13*] and on behalf of VINCat colon surgery group

Abstract

Background: Organ-space surgical site infections (SSI) are the most serious and costly infections after colorectal surgery. Most previous studies of risk factors for SSI have analysed colon and rectal procedures together. The aim of the study was to determine whether colon and rectal procedures have different risk factors and outcomes for organ-space SSI.

Methods: A multicentre observational prospective cohort study of adults undergoing elective colon and rectal procedures at 10 Spanish hospitals from 2011 to 2014. Patients were followed up until 30 days post-surgery. Surgical site infection was defined according to the Centers for Disease Control and Prevention criteria. Oral antibiotic prophylaxis (OAP) was considered as the administration of oral antibiotics the day before surgery combined with systemic intravenous antibiotic prophylaxis.

Results: Of 3,701 patients, 2,518 (68%) underwent colon surgery and 1,183 (32%) rectal surgery. In colon surgery, the overall SSI rate was 16.4% and the organ-space SSI rate was 7.9%, while in rectal surgery the rates were 21.6% and 11.5% respectively ($p < 0.001$). Independent risk factors for organ-space SSI in colon surgery were male sex (Odds ratio -OR-: 1.57, 95% CI: 1.14–2.15) and ostomy creation (OR: 2.65, 95% CI: 1.8–3.92) while laparoscopy (OR: 0.5, 95% CI: 0.38–0.69) and OAP combined with intravenous antibiotic prophylaxis (OR: 0.7, 95% CI: 0.51–0.97) were protective factors. In rectal surgery, independent risk factors for organ-space SSI were male sex (OR: 2.11, 95% CI: 1.34–3.31) and longer surgery (OR: 1.49, 95% CI: 1.03–2.15), whereas OAP with intravenous antibiotic prophylaxis (OR: 0.49, 95% CI: 0.32–0.73) was a protective factor. Among patients with organ-space SSI, we found a significant difference in the overall 30-day mortality, being higher in colon surgery than in rectal surgery (11.5% *vs* 5.1%, $p = 0.04$).

Conclusions: Organ-space SSI in colon and rectal surgery has some differences in terms of incidence, risk factors and outcomes. These differences could be considered for surveillance purposes and for the implementation of preventive strategies. Administration of OAP would be an important measure to reduce the OS-SSI rate in both colon and rectal surgeries.

Keywords: Surgical site infections, Organ-space surgical site infections, Colorectal surgery, Surveillance

* Correspondence: mpujol@bellvitgehospital.cat
[1]Hospital Universitari de Bellvitge-IDIBELL, Barcelona, Spain
[2]VINCat program, Catalonia, Spain
Full list of author information is available at the end of the article

Background

Due to the clean-contaminated nature of the wound, rates of surgical site infections (SSI) after colorectal surgery are the highest among elective procedures, exceeding 20% in some institutions [1–3]. It has been suggested that the rates and risk factors for developing an SSI after colon and rectal surgery may be different [4, 5], due to the differences found in the surgical approach and the degree of bacterial contamination between both surgeries. Nevertheless, most studies carried out to date have analysed colon and rectal surgeries together [6, 7]. Separate assessments of patients undergoing colon and rectal surgery are scarce [4, 8].

It has been proposed that incisional SSI (I-SSI) and organ-space SSI (OS-SSI) may have distinct pathogenesis and risk factors. Incisional SSI has been associated with increased body mass index or the presence of an ostomy [6, 9]. On the other hand, OS-SSI has been more frequently related to blood transfusion, previous abdominal surgery or poor nutritional status [6, 7, 10]. Interestingly, the development of an OS-SSI has more severe consequences than the development of an I-SSI; in many cases OS-SSI requires reoperation and increases morbidity and length of stay (LOS) [11, 12]. Moreover, while many of the most significant advances in colon and rectal surgery such as laparoscopy and other minimally invasive techniques have decreased I-SSI rates, they have had a lesser impact on OS-SSI [13, 14].

Remarkably, the administration of mechanical bowel preparation (MBP) was discontinued in the last decades in most Spanish hospitals due to the lack of effectiveness [15]. In this scenario, and for reasons not well established, the administration of oral antibiotic prophylaxis (OAP) was discontinued too. Currently, only some hospitals use it in the elective surgery of the colon and rectum in Spain. This situation contrasts with that of other European and American countries, where the OAP is part of the daily practice.

The aim of this study was to compare the incidence, risk factors and outcomes of OS-SSI in patients undergoing elective surgery of the colon or rectum in a large, representative cohort of Spanish hospitals.

Methods

Patients, design and setting

We performed a multicentre observational study of a prospective cohort of adult patients (≥18 years old) undergoing elective colon and rectal surgery from January 2011 to December 2014 at 10 hospitals participating in the VINCat program. All consecutive patients hospitalized in any surgical department at the different hospitals were included and followed up until 30 days after surgery. Patients with a pre-existing SSI at the time of surgery were excluded. Post-discharge surveillance of SSI was mandatory and consisted of a review of electronic clinical records (primary and secondary care), checking readmissions and emergency visits, and reviewing microbiological and radiological data. For the purposes of the present study, patients were differentiated according to whether colon or rectal surgery was performed.

VINCat surveillance program

The VINCat program [16] is a healthcare-associated infection surveillance program in Spain, based on the National Healthcare Safety Network (NHSN) model [17]. It recruits hospitals on a voluntary basis and currently receives surveillance data from trained infection control staff at 66 hospitals, who submit information on preoperative demographics, comorbidities, operative characteristics, microbiology and treatment data, and 30-day postoperative outcomes for eligible surgical procedures [18].

Definitions

SSIs were defined according to the Centers for Disease Control and Prevention (CDC) criteria [19] and divided into superficial incisional, deep incisional and OS. Surgical procedure categories were stratified according to the risk of surgical infection (–1 to 3) as defined by the NHSN.

Independent variables

Predictor variables considered for the development of an OS-SSI were: age, sex, American Society of Anesthesiologists (ASA) physical status classification, MBP, OAP, adequacy of intravenous antibiotic prophylaxis, surgical risk index category according to the National Nosocomial Infections Surveillance (NNIS) modified system criteria [20], date and prolonged operation time (≥75th percentile of the procedure), laparoscopy, wound classification, date of SSI, site of SSI (I-SSI or OS-SSI), microbiology and underlying disease (neoplasia, inflammatory bowel disease –IBD- or others). Age (<65 and ≥ 65 years), ASA (I-II and III-IV) score and NNIS modified risk index (–1-0 and 1–2) were dichotomized for the analysis.

Adequacy of intravenous antibiotic prophylaxis was established when all the following three factors were met: antibiotics administered according to local protocol at each hospital, completion of the infusion within 60 min before the surgical incision, and perioperative antibiotic redosing if indicated.

The OAP was always considered as the administration of oral antibiotic prophylaxis the day before surgery in combination with systemic intravenous antibiotic prophylaxis perioperatively. The administration was not mandatory and was done according to local protocols at each hospital. It was applied in 4 of the 10 participating hospitals.

Dependent variables

The development of overall SSI and OS-SSI in both colon and rectal populations, readmission, LOS and mortality within 30 days of initial surgery were recorded. Readmission for any cause within 30 days of initial surgery was documented. LOS included readmission if there was. Overall mortality was defined as death due to any cause within 30 days of initial surgery.

Statistical analysis

Categorical variables were described as totals and frequencies; continuous variables were described as medians and interquartile ranges (IQR) and mean and standard deviation (SD) in some cases. Univariate analysis comparing the two populations was carried out using the chi-square test or Fisher exact test for categorical variables and the *t*-test or Mann-Whitney test for continuous variables. Comparisons between patients who developed an OS-SSI and those who did not (no OS-SSI) were performed separately for colon and rectal populations. Finally, multivariate analysis with all statistically significant variables ($p \leq 0.05$) associated with OS-SSI in colon and rectal populations were performed separately to determine independent predictive factors for the development of OS-SSI. In these cases, results were given as odds ratios (OR) and 95% confidence intervals (95% CI). The final model's goodness-of-fit was assessed by the Hosmer-Lemeshow test. Data were analysed with IBM SPSS 20.0 (Chicago, Ill.).

Results

Characteristics of patients and incidence of SSI in colon and rectal surgery

During the study period, a total of 3,701 patients undergoing elective colorectal surgery were prospectively followed-up, 68% after colon surgery and 32% after rectal surgery.

Characteristics of patients undergoing colon or rectal surgery are shown in Table 1. Patients who underwent colon surgery were older (median age 70.6 years, interquartile range [IQR] 62–79 *vs* 68 years [IQR 60–76], $p < 0.001$) and had higher proportions of ASA score III-IV (42.2% *vs* 36.7%, $p = 0.002$) than patients undergoing rectal surgery. In contrast, patients undergoing rectal procedures were more likely to be male (67.2% *vs* 59.3%, $p = 0.001$), to have neoplasia (97% *vs* 93.5%, $p < 0.001$), to have a longer duration of surgery (42.7% *vs* 37.6%, $p = 0.003$), and to have an ostomy (64% *vs* 8.3%, $p < 0.001$). The administration of correct intravenous antibiotic prophylaxis was 84% in colon surgery and 81.6% in rectal surgery, $p = 0.4$. In colon surgery, the overall SSI rate was 16.4% and the OS-SSI rate 7.9%, while in rectal surgery, the overall SSI was 21.6% and the OS-SSI 11.5% ($p < 0.001$), as shown in Fig. 1. When patients who received OAP combined with correct intravenous antibiotic prophylaxis ($n = 1.345$) were analysed, significant differences in

Table 1 Characteristics of patients in colon and rectal surgery

Variable	Colon ($n = 2518$)	Rectum ($n = 1183$)	*p*-value
Age, median (IQR) years	70.6 (62–79)	68 (60–76)	<0.001
Age ≥65, *n* (%)	1711 (67.95%)	724 (61.20%)	0.001
Males, *n* (%)	1494 (59.33%)	795 (67.20%)	0.001
ASA III-IV, *n* (%)	1062 (42.18%)	434 (36.69%)	0.002
Neoplasia, *n* (%)	2355 (93.5%)	1147 (97%)	<0.001
Inflammatory bowel disease, *n* (%)	75 (3%)	16 (1.4%)	0.003
Other, *n* (%)	86 (3.4%)	17 (1.4%)	0.001
Duration of surgery ≥75th-percentile[a], *n* (%)	947 (37.61%)	505 (42.69%)	0.003
NNIS Risk index 1–2, *n* (%)	909 (36.10%)	398 (33.64%)	0.15
Laparoscopy, *n* (%)	1515 (60.17%)	782 (66.10%)	0.001
Correct IV antibiotic prophylaxis, *n* (%)	2117 (84.07%)	966 (81.66%)	0.41
Previous radiotherapy, *n* (%)	33 (1.31%)	545 (46.07%)	<0.001
Previous chemotherapy, *n* (%)	78 (3.10%)	533 (45.05%)	<0.001
Oral antibiotic prophylaxis, *n* (%)	1078 (42.81%)	489 (41.34%)	0.41
Mechanical bowel preparation, *n* (%)	1749 (69.46%)	1038 (87.74%)	<0.001
- Missing	58 (2.30%)	20 (1.69%)	
Ostomy, *n* (%)	208 (8.26%)	754 (63.74%)	<0.001

IQR interquartile range, *ASA* American Society of Anesthesiologists physical status classification, *NNIS* National Nosocomial Infections Surveillance, *IV* intravenous
[a]Greater than 75th percentile for the duration of surgery (180 min, 3 h)

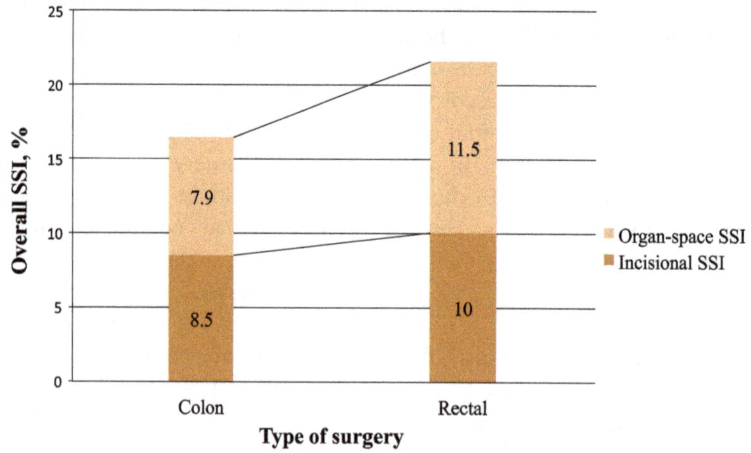

Fig. 1 Incidence of surgical site infection in colon and rectal surgery. Shows the incidence of overall surgical site infection, incisional surgical site infection and organ-space surgical site infection in colon and rectal surgery separately. SSI: surgical site infection

overall SSI rate between colon and rectal surgery (12.3% *vs* 19.9%, $p < 0.001$) were found, while there were no differences in the OS-SSI rate (6.2% vs 8.4%, $p = 0.1$).

Risk factors for OS-SSI in colon and rectal surgery

Univariate analyses of risk factors for OS-SSI in colon and rectal surgery are shown separately in Table 2. In colon surgery, male sex, NNIS ≥1 and ostomy creation were significantly associated with OS-SSI, while laparoscopic surgery and OAP had lower associations with OS-SSI. In rectal surgery, male sex, longer duration of surgery and NNIS ≥1 were associated with OS-SSI, whereas OAP had a lower association with OS-SSI.

A logistic regression multivariate analysis using significant predictive factors found in the univariate analysis is shown in Table 3. Independent risk factors for OS-SSI after colon surgery were male sex (OR 1.57, 95% CI 1.14–2.15) and ostomy creation (OR 2.65, 95% CI 1.8–3.9), while laparoscopy (OR 0.5, 95% CI 0.38–0.69) and the administration of OAP (OR 0.7, 95% CI 0.51–0.97) were independent protective factors. Independent risk factors for OS-SSI in rectal surgery were male sex (OR 2.11, 95% CI 1.34–3.31) and longer duration of surgery

Table 2 Univariate analysis of risk factors for organ-space surgical site infection in colon and rectal surgery

	Colon			Rectum		
Risk factor	No OS-SSI (*n* = 2318)	OS-SSI (*n* = 200)	*p*- value	No OS-SSI (*n* = 1043)	OS-SSI (*n* = 136)	*p*- value
Age, median (IQR) years	70 (61–79)	73 (63–79)	0.3	68 (60–76)	66.5 (58–74)	0.07
Age ≥ 65 years, (%)	67.6	72	0.2	61.5	58.8	0.5
Male sex, (%)	58.4	70	0.001	65.4	80.9	<0.001
ASA ≥ III, (%)	41.9	45.5	0.3	36.1	41.2	0.25
Correct IV antibiotic prophylaxis, (%)	84.3	81.5	0.3	81.4	83.8	0.5
Duration of operation ≥ p75th[a], (%)	37.5	39	0.7	41.2	54.4	0.003
Laparoscopy, (%)	61.6	44	<0.001	66.3	64.7	0.7
NNIS ≥ 1, (%)	35.5	43	0.03	32.7	41.2	0.05
Neoplasia, (%)	93.6	93	0.7	97.2	94.9	0.13
Inflammatory bowel disease, (%)	2.9	4	0.38	1.1	2.9	0.1
Chemotherapy, (%)	3.1	3.5	0.7	45.1	45.2	1
Radiotherapy, (%)	1.2	2.5	0.18	46	47.4	0.7
Oral antibiotic prophylaxis, (%)	43.7	33	0.004	43.3	26.5	<0.001
Mechanical bowel preparation, (%)	71.4	67.2	0.2	89.1	90.4	0.6
Ostomy, (%)	7.3	20	<0.001	63.8	65.2	0.7

No OS-SSI no organ-space surgical site infections (include patients with incisional SSI and patients without SSI), *OS-SSI* organ-space SSI, *IQR* interquartile range, *ASA* American Society of Anesthesiologists physical status classification, *IV* intravenous, *NNIS* National Nosocomial Infections Surveillance Risk Index.
[a]Greater than 75th percentile for the duration of surgery (180 min, 3 h)

Table 3 Multivariate analysis of risk factors for organ-space surgical site infection in colon and rectal surgery

	Colon				Rectum		
Risk factor	OR	95% CI	*p*-value	Risk factor	OR	95% CI	*p*-value
Male sex	**1.57**	**1.14–2.15**	**0.004**	Male sex	**2.11**	**1.34–3.31**	**0.001**
Laparoscopy	**0.5**	**0.38–0.69**	**<0.001**	Duration of operation ≥ p75th[a]	**1.49**	**1.03–2.15**	**0.07**
NNIS ≥ 1	1.17	0.83–1.64	0.36	NNIS ≥ 1	1.1	0.74–1.66	0.6
Oral antibiotic prophylaxis	**0.7**	**0.51–0.97**	**0.03**	Oral antibiotic prophylaxis	**0.49**	**0.32–0.73**	**0.001**
Ostomy	**2.65**	**1.8–3.92**	**<0.001**				

Signifficant OR and 95% CI appear in bold text
OR Odds ratio, *95%CI* 95% confidence interval, *NNIS* National Nosocomial Infections Surveillance Risk Index.
[a]Greater than 75th percentile for the duration of surgery (180 min, 3 h)

(OR 1.49, 95% CI 1–2.15), whereas the administration of OAP (OR 0.49, 95% CI 0.32–0.73) was the only independent protective factor.

Outcomes of patients with OS-SSI in colon and rectal surgery

Table 4 shows the outcomes of patients who developed an OS-SSI in colon and rectal surgery. There were no significant differences between colon and rectal procedures regarding median LOS (25 days [IQR 18–31] *vs* 23 days [IQR 16–33], $p = 0.1$), mean LOS (30.2 days ± SD 25 *vs* 32 days ± SD 28, $p = 0.19$) and readmission rate (19.5% *vs* 24.3%, $p = 0.3$). Overall 30-day mortality was significantly higher after colon surgery than after rectal surgery (11.5% [23/200] *vs* 5.1% [7/136], $p = 0.04$).

Discussion

This large multicentre cohort study found significant differences in the incidence, predictive factors and outcomes of OS-SSI after elective colon and rectal surgery. This suggests that the two procedures should be considered as different surgical interventions.

The separation of procedures according to patients' characteristics may allow more accurate assessment of their specific risk factors. Comparing colon and rectal populations, we found that they had different characteristics in terms of risk factors for SSI. Patients undergoing colon surgery were older, had more IBD and less laparoscopy, factors related to SSI. On the other hand, patients undergoing rectal surgery were younger but had more rate of malignancy; more frequently received chemoradiotherapy and had longer surgery duration. The surgical techniques were also different, something inherent to the anatomical location of the disease, in special with more ostomies performed in rectal resections. These factors, associated with the fact that the rectum has higher bacterial contamination load, conferred it greater risk of SSI. Accordingly, overall SSI and OS-SSI rates were higher in rectal surgery than in colon surgery. Although these rates were high, they were similar to these reported in previous studies [8, 21]. Data from surveillance systems in Europe an US vary widely [22, 23], being in most cases lower than ours, though post-discharge surveillance is not always performed.

We found significant differences in the predictive factors for developing an OS-SSI in colon and rectal surgeries. In colon surgery, independent risk factors predisposing to OS-SSI were male sex and ostomy creation, while laparoscopic surgery and OAP were protective factors. In rectal surgery, independent risk factors for OS-SSI were male sex and longer duration of surgery, whereas OAP was the only protective factor. Male sex was a common risk factor for developing OS-SSI in both colon and rectal surgeries; this association is well established [5, 7, 24], although the reasons are not known.

Ostomy creation was a strong risk factor for the development of OS-SSI in colon surgery but not in rectal surgery, as previously reported elsewhere [8]. Ostomies are normally used to divert the faecal stream from a newly created immature anastomosis, or to definitively disconnect the gastrointestinal tract in some extensive colorectal

Table 4 Outcomes of patients with organ-space surgical site infection in colon and rectal surgery

Variable	Colon ($n = 200$)	Rectum ($n = 136$)	Overall ($n = 336$)	*p*-value
Readmission, *n* (%)	39 (19.5)	33 (24.3)	72 (21.4)	0.3
Readmission due to SSI, *n* (%)	34 (17)	30 (22.1)	64 (19)	0.2
Length of stay, median (IQR) days	25 (18–31)	23 (16–33)	24 (17–36)	0.1
Length of stay, mean (SD) days	30.2 (25)	32 (28)	27.6 (19.7)	0.1
Mortality, *n* (%)	23 (11.5)	7 (5.1)	30 (8.9)	0.04
Mortality attributed to SSI, *n* (%)	21 (10.5)	6 (4.4)	27 (8)	0.04

SSI surgical site infection, *IQR* interquartile range, *SD* standard deviation

surgeries. Nevertheless, ostomies have been associated with increased rates of SSI in previous studies [4–6, 9] because they allow organisms from the air, contaminated hands, or skin flora to reach the subcutaneous fat and the wound, and eventually the intraabdominal cavity [25]. In our study, patients with colon surgery who received an ostomy more frequently underwent laparotomy due to complex pathology like IBD or diverticulitis. These diseases have been associated with OS-SSI [26], and ostomy creation may act, in part, as a marker of this complex pathology.

The laparoscopic approach significantly reduced SSI rates in several large-database studies and also offered other benefits such as faster recovery of pulmonary function, less pain and shorter postoperative stay [13, 14]. In our study it served as an independent protective factor for the development of OS-SSI in colon surgery, but not in rectal surgery. Probably, the beneficial effect of laparoscopy was exceeded by the higher frequency of risk factors for SSI inherent in rectal surgery.

Importantly, we found that OAP was a protective factor for the development of OS-SSI in both colon and rectal surgeries, although the impact was higher in rectal surgery, probably because the rectum has a higher level of bacterial contamination. During the study period there was not a national or regional recommendation for the application of OAP, and for this reason the use of the measure was decided by each participating hospital (it was only applied in 4 of the 10 hospitals). The findings of the present study lead to a change in the clinical practice of hospitals participating in the VINCat program and in 2016 the use of OAP was institutionally recommended. The OAP combined with intravenous prophylaxis and MBP significantly reduces SSI rates after colon and rectal surgery by decreasing the intraluminal bacterial load [27–30]; in a previous meta-analysis of randomized controlled trials comparing the effectiveness of OAP plus intravenous antibiotic prophylaxis *vs* intravenous antibiotic prophylaxis alone, the association of OAP was estimated to reduce the incidence of SSI by 43% [31]. Nevertheless, the use of MBP has been widely questioned, due to its unpleasant gastrointestinal effects, and in many studies it has failed to reduce SSI rates [15]. Currently, since almost all studies that demonstrate the effectiveness of OAP have been performed in combination with MBP, the use of MBP will have to be raised again. Last World Health Organization (WHO) recommendations on preoperative measures for surgical site infection prevention suggest using OAP with MBP in all adults undergoing elective colorectal surgery [32, 33].

Longer duration of surgery was an independent risk factor for the development of an OS-SSI in rectal surgery. This association has often been described in the colorectal surgery population [21, 34, 35], and it also favours other risk factors for SSI like the hyperglycaemia or hypothermia [33]. Given the capacity of this parameter to predict SSI, it was included as one of the components of the NNIS risk index. Rectal tumours close to the anal verge usually require extensive surgery with additional organ resection, requiring longer operative time and causing greater bleeding, factors that have been associated with an increased risk of SSI [24, 36]. Moreover, in these prolonged surgeries, antibiotic redosing is not always administered correctly.

Significantly, mortality of patients with OS-SSI after colon surgery was higher than after rectal surgery. The fact that patients in the colon group were older and more frequently had complicated diseases other than neoplasia could explain this result.

Among the strengths of the study is its multicentre nature, the large number of patients included and the fact that all data were collected by trained infection control staff. However, the study has a number of limitations that should be acknowledged. Firstly, the retrospective analysis of prospectively collected data may lead to bias and is unable to control for confounding factors. Secondly, certain risk factors that have been linked to SSI such as perioperative hyperglycaemia, hypothermia and blood transfusion were not recorded here.

Conclusions

We found differences in the incidence, risk factors and outcomes of overall SSI and OS-SSI between colon and rectal surgery, suggesting that they could be considered as different surgical procedures. These differences should be borne in mind for the purpose of surveillance and for the implementation of preventive strategies. Administration of OAP would be an important measure to reduce the OS-SSI rate in both colon and rectal surgeries.

Abbreviations

95% CI: 95% confidence interval; ASA: American Society of Anesthesiologists; CDC: Centers for disease control and prevention; IBD: Inflammatory bowel disease; IBM SPSS: International business machines Corp. Statistical package for the social sciences; IQR: Interquartile range; I-SSI: Incisional SSI; LOS: Length of stay; MBP: Mechanical bowel preparation; NHSN: National Healthcare Safety Network; NNIS: National Nosocomial Infection Surveillance; OAP: Oral antibiotic prophylaxis; OR: Odds ratio; OS-SSI: Organ-space surgical site infection; SD: Standard deviation; SSI: Surgical site infection; WHO: World Health Organization

Acknowledgments

We want to thanks the other collaborators at *Hospital Universitari de Bellvitge*, Doménico Fraccavieri, Rosa Escofet, at *Corporació Sanitària Parc Taulí*, Xavier Serra-Aracil, Marta Piriz, at *Parc Sanitari Sant Joan de Déu de Sant Boi*, Vicens Diaz-Brito, Encarna Moreno, at *Hospital Universitari Sant Joan de Reus*, Antoni Castro, Simona Iftimie, at *Consorci Sanitari de Terrassa*, Elena Espejo, Lurdes Pagespetit, at *Consorci Sanitari de l'Anoia*, Montse Brugués, at *Fundació Althaia*, Fina Obradors, at *Hospital de Viladecans*, Ana Lérida, Camilo Sanz, at *Fundació Privada Hospital Asil de Granollers*, Jordi Cuquet, Nares Arroyo and at *Hospital Universitari Mútua de Terrassa*, Albert Navarro, Núria Freixas.
Writing assistance was provided by the Department of Languages in the Faculty of Medicine of Barcelona University.

Funding

No specific grant was received for this research from funding agencies in the public, commercial, or not-for-profit sectors.

Authors' contributions

AG and MP conceived and designed the study, AG analyzed and interpreted the patient data regarding surgical site infections after colon and rectal surgery. AG, JC and MP were major contributors in writing the manuscript. All authors read and approved the final manuscript.

Competing interests

The authors declare that they have no competing interests.

Consent for publication

Not applicable.

Author details

[1]Hospital Universitari de Bellvitge-IDIBELL, Barcelona, Spain. [2]VINCat program, Catalonia, Spain. [3]University of Barcelona, Barcelona, Spain. [4]Hospital General de Granollers, Universitat Internacional de Catalunya, Barcelona, Spain. [5]Parc Sanitari Sant Joan de Déu de Sant Boi, Barcelona, Spain. [6]Consorci Sanitari de Terrassa, Barcelona, Spain. [7]Hospital Universitari Mútua de Terrassa, Barcelona, Spain. [8]Consorci Sanitari de l'Anoia, Barcelona, Spain. [9]Corporació Sanitària Parc Taulí, Barcelona, Spain. [10]Fundació Althaia, Barcelona, Spain. [11]Hospital de Viladecans, Barcelona, Spain. [12]Hospital Universitari Sant Joan de Reus, Tarragona, Spain. [13]Infectious Diseases Department, Hospital Universitari de Bellvitge, Feixa Llarga s/n, 08907 L'Hospitalet de Llobregat, Barcelona, Spain.

References

1. Kirby A, Burnside G, Bretsztajn L, Burke D. Postoperative infections following colorectal surgery in an english teaching hospital. Infect Dis (Lond). 2015;47:825–9.
2. Limón E, Shaw E, Badia JM, Piriz M, Escofet R, Gudiol F, et al. Post-discharge surgical site infections after uncomplicated elective colorectal surgery: impact and risk factors. The experience of the VINCat Program. J Hosp Infect. 2014;86:127–32.
3. Petrosillo N, Drapeau CMJ, Nicastri E, Martini L, Ippolito G, Moro ML, et al. Surgical site infections in Italian Hospitals: a prospective multicenter study. BMC Infect Dis. 2008;8:34.
4. Konishi T, Watanabe T, Kishimoto J, Nagawa H. Elective colon and rectal surgery differ in risk factors for wound infection: results of prospective surveillance. Ann Surg. 2006;244:758–63.
5. Morikane K, Honda H, Yamagishi T, Suzuki S, Aminaka M. Factors associated with surgical site infection in colorectal surgery: the Japan nosocomial infections surveillance. Infect Control Hosp Epidemiol. 2014;35:660–6.
6. Blumetti J, Luu M, Sarosi G, Hartless K, Mcfarlin J, Parker B, et al. Surgical site infections after colorectal surgery: do risk factors vary depending on the type of infection considered? Surgery. 2007;142:704–11.
7. Tang R, Chen HH, Wang YL, Changchien CR, Chen J-S. Risk factors for surgical site infection after elective resection of the colon and rectum : a single-center prospective study of 2, 809 consecutive patients. Ann Surg. 2001;234:181–9.
8. Serra-Aracil X, Espin-Basany E, Biondo S, Guirao X, Orrego C, Sitges-Serra A, et al. Surgical site infection in elective operations for colorectal cancer after the application of preventive measures. Arch Surg. 2011;146:606.
9. Ho VP, Stein SL, Trencheva K, Barie PS, Milsom JW, Lee SW, et al. Differing risk factors for incisional and organ/space surgical site infections following abdominal colorectal surgery. Dis Colon Rectum. 2011;54:818–25.
10. Frasson M, Granero-Castro P, Ramos Rodriguez JL, Flor-Lorente B, Braithwaite M, Martí Martínez E, et al. Risk factors for anastomotic leak and postoperative morbidity and mortality after elective right colectomy for cancer: results from a prospective, multicentric study of 1102 patients. Int J Colorectal Dis. 2016;31:105–14.
11. de Lissovoy G, Fraeman K, Hutchins V, Murphy D, Song D, Vaughn BB. Surgical site infection: incidence and impact on hospital utilization and treatment costs. Am J Infect Control. 2009;37:387–97.
12. Eagye KJ, Nicolau DP. Deep and organ/space infections in patients undergoing elective colorectal surgery: incidence and impact on hospital length of stay and costs. Am J Surg. 2009;198:359–67.
13. Aimaq R, Akopian G, Kaufman HS. Surgical site infection rates in laparoscopic versus open colorectal surgery. Am Surg. 2011;77:1290–4.
14. Kiran RP, El-Gazzaz H, Vogel JD, Remzi FH. Laparoscopic approach significantly reduces surgical site infections after colorectal surgery: data from national surgical quality improvement program. J Am Coll Surg. 2010;211:232–8.
15. Dahabreh IJ, Steele DW, Shah N, Trikalinos TA. Oral mechanical bowel preparation for colorectal surgery: systematic review and meta-analysis. Dis Colon Rectum. 2015;58:698–707.
16. VINCat Program. Generalitat de Catalunya. http://vincat.gencat.cat/ca/. Accessed 8 May 2016.
17. National Healthcare Safety Network | Centers for Disease Control and Prevention. http://www.cdc.gov/nhsn/. Accessed 8 May 2016.
18. Pujol M, Limón E, López-Contreras J, Sallés M, Bella F, Gudiol F. Surveillance of surgical site infections in elective colorectal surgery. Results of the VINCat program (2007–2010). Enferm Infecc Microbiol Clin. 2012;30 Suppl 3:20–5.
19. CDC Surgical Site Infection (SSI) Event definition. http://www.cdc.gov/nhsn/pdfs/pscmanual/9pscssicurrent.pdf. Accessed 8 May 2016.
20. Horan TC, Emori G, Atlanta M. Definitions of key terms used in the NNIS system. Am J Infect Control. 1997;25:112–6.
21. Hennessey DB, Burke JP, Ni-Dhonochu T, Shields C, Winter DC, Mealy K. Risk factors for surgical site infection following colorectal resection: a multi-institutional study. Int J Colorectal Dis. 2016;31:267–71.
22. Surveillance of surgical site infections in NHS hospitals in England 2015/16. https://www.gov.uk/government/uploads/system/uploads/attachment_data/file/577418/Surgical_site_infections_NHS_hospitals_2015_to_2016.pdf.. Accessed Mar 2017.
23. Young H, Knepper B, Moore EE, Johnson JL, Mehler P, Price CS. Surgical site infection after colon surgery: national healthcare safety network risk factors and modeled rates compared with published risk factors and rates. J Am Coll Surg. 2012;214:852–9.
24. Bakker IS, Grossmann I, Henneman D, Havenga K, Wiggers T. Risk factors for anastomotic leakage and leak-related mortality after colonic cancer surgery in a nationwide audit. Br J Surg. 2014;101:424–32. discussion 432.
25. Fraccalvieri D, Biondo S, Saez J, Millan M, Kreisler E, Golda T, et al. Management of colorectal anastomotic leakage: differences between salvage and anastomotic takedown. Am J Surg. 2012;204:671–6.
26. Eskicioglu C, Nelson J, Roberts PL, Marcello PW, Read TE, Hall JF, et al. Is patient diagnosis a risk factor for organ space infection after colorectal resections? Dis Colon Rectum. 2014;57:733–9.
27. Morris MS, Graham LA, Chu DI, Cannon JA, Hawn MT. Oral antibiotic bowel preparation significantly reduces surgical site infection rates and readmission rates in elective colorectal surgery. Ann Surg. 2015;261:1034–40.
28. Englesbe MJ, Brooks L, Kubus J, Luchtefeld M, Lynch J, Senagore A, et al. A statewide assessment of surgical site infection following colectomy: the role of oral antibiotics. Ann Surg. 2010;252(3):514–9. discussion 519–20.
29. Scarborough JE, Mantyh CR, Sun Z, Migaly J. Combined mechanical and oral antibiotic bowel preparation reduces incisional surgical site infection and anastomotic leak rates after elective colorectal resection: an analysis of colectomy-targeted ACS NSQIP. Ann Surg. 2015;262:331–7.
30. Machuca I, Gutiérrez-Gutiérrez B, Pérez Cortés S, Gracia-Ahufinger I, Serrano J, Madrigal MD, et al. Oral decontamination with aminoglycosides is associated with lower risk of mortality and infections in high-risk patients colonized with colistin-resistant, KPC-producing Klebsiella pneumoniae. J Antimicrob Chemother. 2016;71:3242–9.
31. Bellows CF, Mills KT, Kelly TN, Gagliardi G. Combination of oral non-absorbable and intravenous antibiotics versus intravenous antibiotics alone

in the prevention of surgical site infections after colorectal surgery: a meta-analysis of randomized controlled trials. Tech Coloproctol. 2011;15:385–95.

32. De Jonge S, Atema JJ, Gans S, Boermeester MA, Gomes SM, Solomkin JS, et al. New WHO recommendations on preoperative measures for surgical site infection prevention: an evidence-based global perspective. Lancet Infect Dis. 2016;16: e276–87.
33. Allegranzi B, Zayed B, Bischoff P, Kubilay NZ, de Jonge S, de Vries F, et al. New WHO recommendations on intraoperative and postoperative measures for surgical site infection prevention: an evidence-based global perspective. Lancet Infect Dis. 2016;16:e288–303.
34. Gervaz P, Bandiera-Clerc C, Buchs NC, Eisenring M-C, Troillet N, Perneger T, et al. Scoring system to predict the risk of surgical-site infection after colorectal resection. Br J Surg. 2012;99:589–95.
35. Watanabe M, Suzuki H, Nomura S, Hanawa H, Chihara N, Mizutani S, et al. Performance assessment of the risk index category for surgical site infection after colorectal surgery. Surg Infect (Larchmt). 2015;16:84–9.
36. Kwaan MR, Melton GB, Madoff RD, Chipman JG. Abdominoperineal resection, pelvic exenteration, and additional organ resection increase the risk of surgical site infection after elective colorectal surgery: An American College of Surgeons National Surgical Quality Improvement Program Analysis. Surg Infect (Larchmt). 2015;16:675–83.

17

Reducing unnecessary culturing: a systems approach to evaluating urine culture ordering and collection practices among nurses in two acute care settings

Robert Redwood[1], Mary Jo Knobloch[1,2], Daniela C. Pellegrini[3], Matthew J. Ziegler[4], Michael Pulia[5] and Nasia Safdar[1,2*]

Abstract

Background: Inappropriate ordering and acquisition of urine cultures leads to unnecessary treatment of asymptomatic bacteriuria (ASB). Treatment of ASB contributes to antimicrobial resistance particularly among hospital-acquired organisms. Our objective was to investigate urine culture ordering and collection practices among nurses to identify key system-level and human factor barriers and facilitators that affect optimal ordering and collection practices.

Methods: We conducted two focus groups, one with ED nurses and the other with ICU nurses. Questions were developed using the Systems Engineering Initiative for Patient Safety (SEIPS) framework. We used iterative categorization (directed content analysis followed by summative content analysis) to code and analyze the data both deductively (using SEIPS domains) and inductively (emerging themes).

Results: Factors affecting optimal urine ordering and collection included barriers at the person, process, and task levels. For ED nurses, barriers included patient factors, physician communication, reflex culture protocols, the electronic health record, urinary symptoms, and ED throughput. For ICU nurses, barriers included physician notification of urinalysis results, personal protective equipment, collection technique, patient body habitus, and Foley catheter issues.

Conclusions: We identified multiple potential process barriers to nurse adherence with evidence-based recommendations for ordering and collecting urine cultures in the ICU and ED. A systems approach to identifying barriers and facilitators can be useful to design interventions for improving urine ordering and collection practices.

Keywords: Acute care, Antibacterial agents, Asymptomatic bacteriuria, Inappropriate prescribing, Prevention & Control, Emergency department, Intensive care unit, Nursing, SEIPS, Urinalysis, Urine culture

Background

Asymptomatic bacteriuria (ASB), also known as an asymptomatic urinary tract infection, is defined as isolation of bacteria in an appropriately collected urine sample from an individual without signs or symptoms referable to the urinary tract [1]. While the prevalence of ASB varies by population, it is a common phenomenon and occurs in 1–5% of healthy adult women and 2–10% of pregnant women. It is highly prevalent in diabetic women (9–27%), nursing home residents (25–50%), and spinal-cord injury patients (23–89%) [1].

The Infectious Disease Society of America (IDSA) recommends against routine screening for ASB (except in pregnant women and patients undergoing urological surgery), rejection of all samples with greater than five squamous epithelial cells per low-power field, and consideration of an alternate diagnosis to UTI in patients without urinary symptoms [2]. Treatment of ASB in most clinical settings is not recommended [3]. In addition, the American Geriatrics Society and the American Board of Internal Medicine

* Correspondence: ns2@medicine.wisc.edu
[1]Division of Infectious Disease, Department of Medicine, University of Wisconsin-Madison School of Medicine and Public Health, 750 Highland Ave, Madison, Wisconsin 53705, USA
[2]William S. Middleton Memorial Veterans Hospital, 2500 Overlook Terrace, Madison, Wisconsin 53705, USA
Full list of author information is available at the end of the article

recently identified treatment of ASB as an overused intervention in their "Choosing Wisely" campaign [4]. Even with these guidelines, however, recent studies have shown a 20–80% gap between what is recommended and what is practiced [5–7].

Previous studies have identified barriers to appropriate management of ASB with an emphasis on knowledge gaps. Trautner et al. surveyed 169 providers at a tertiary care center and found that decreased knowledge regarding the recognition and management of ASB was associated with poor familiarity with guidelines and cognitive biases (i.e. organism type, patient age, and presence of pyuria influenced the inappropriate use of antibiotics) [7]. Drekonja et al. identified a similar knowledge gap among 100 surveyed resident physicians with 14% reporting that they had read the IDSA guideline on management of ASB and a mean of 37% correct answers when provided with five clinical vignette questions regarding the management of ASB in nonsurgical scenarios [8].

Additional studies have investigated non-sterile urine collection techniques and the unnecessary ordering of urine cultures as upstream factors that contribute to the unnecessary treatment of ASB [9, 10]. However, there is little known regarding the barriers and facilitators that affect nurse initiated ordering and collection practices in the emergency department (ED) and intensive care unit (ICU) where time constraints may increase the risk of over testing or improper collection techniques [11].

We undertook a qualitative study to investigate urine culture ordering and collecting practices among ED and ICU nurses at an academic medical center. Our aim was to identify key systems and human factors that affect concordance with recommended urine ordering and collection practices among nurses. At the time the study was conducted, reflex urine culture testing was in place-urinalyses with pyuria were automatically processed for urine cultures.

Methods

Conceptual framework and focus group design

We conducted focus groups to investigate both the systems and human factors elements that affect urine sample collection and urine collection techniques. ED and ICU nurses were chosen as our subjects of interest because acute care nurses face unique challenges (uncertainty of diagnosis in hemodynamically unstable patients, resuscitation/stabilization concerns, time constraints, and incomplete clinical information). Additionally, antibiotic decisions made in these challenging settings heavily influence subsequent outpatient and inpatient care plans. We used the Systems Engineering Initiative for Patient Safety (SEIPS) model, a framework for understanding structures, processes and outcomes in healthcare to model our focus group questions [12]. The work system elements included in the SEIPS model are person, process, task, organization, tools/technology, physical environment. These elements can affect patient and employee/organizational outcomes, and can be used to improve patient safety. Systems engineering principles are becoming increasingly common for care redesign in acute care settings where teamwork and multi-step care is common [13]. The strengths of this model include its focus on work system design while taking a broad view of care processes and outcomes. Fig. 1 shows the SEIPS model adapted to this study [12].

Two 45-min focus groups were held at our 592-bed tertiary care medical center, between the months of

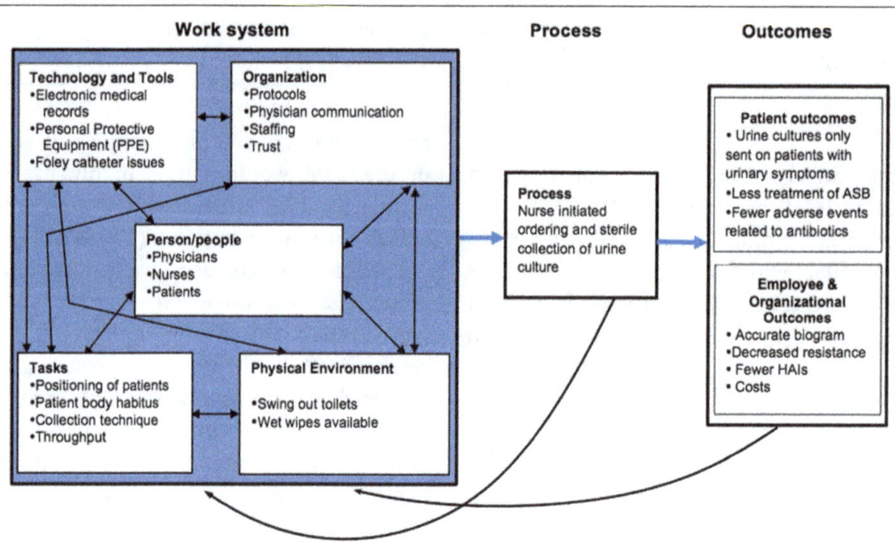

Fig. 1 The Systems Engineering Initiative for Patient Safety (SEIPS) model, adapted from Carayon et al. 2006

October 2014 and February 2015. Participants were selected by convenience sampling: all nurses in each unit were invited to participate and all who responded were included. We asked a series of open-ended questions regarding system elements impacting urine ordering and collection practices. The distinction between asymptomatic bacteriuria and UTIs was not addressed. Focus groups were audio-recorded and transcribed by authors MZ and DP. Specific questions are listed in Tables 1 and 2. This was a QI project which was deemed exempt and IRB review was not required.

Data analysis

We used iterative categorization for our data analysis, a systematic technique for analyzing qualitative data that is designed to incorporate the pre-selected framework that researchers deem important (in this case the SEIPS framework) and also inductively include emerging themes from the data [14].

We divided analysis into two stages: descriptive and interpretative. In the descriptive stage, we performed line-by-line coding of the interview transcripts using deductive as well as inductive processes. We constrained our deductive coding to the aforementioned SEIPS domains and then counted the number of appearances for each domain and tabulated the results as a frequency plot. During the inductive coding process, we did not constrain the coding by a framework and instead assigned a free-text theme to each statement or segment of the transcript. We then tabulated this more expansive set of inductive coding themes as a unique frequency plot. Two researchers (RR and MJK) performed the coding and we compared agreement between the researchers using Cohen's kappa statistic for inter-rater reliability. We combined coding results from RR and MJK and averaged the results to yield a set of four preliminary frequency plots. For both the inductive and deductive frequency plots, we considered the top 50% of themes to be dominant themes and selected those for further analysis. Having thus completed the descriptive stage of the analysis, we were left with four final frequency plots, each narrowed to the top 50% of themes: (1) ED Nurses-Deductive, (2) ICU Nurses-Deductive, (3) ED Nurses-Inductive, and (4) ICU Nurses-Inductive.

In the interpretation stage of the analysis, we combined the two inductive frequency plots to identify shared themes that acute care nurses face regarding ordering urine cultures and sterile collection techniques and then did the same for the deductive frequency plots. We present the results both quantitatively as the percentage of the interview content dedicated to each theme and qualitatively as central concepts with representative quotations.

Table 1 ED RN focus group questions (SEIPS framework domain in parentheses)

How often do you look at a patient's urine sample? (Task)
Walk us through the steps of what you would do if you have concerns about a patient's urine when you are first evaluating them in the ED? (Process)
What challenges are there for collecting an adequate urine sample and how do they effect whether or not you order a urine culture? (Physical environment)
Which guidelines are you aware of for the ordering of urine cultures? (Organization)
What do you think about the communication between nursing and physicians regarding urine culture ordering? (Person)
What clinical presentations other than dysuria would prompt you to think about ordering a urine culture or a urinalysis with reflex culture? (Task)
Do you feel that there is a role for the electronic health record for decision support in terms of when to order a urine culture? (Technology and tools)
How do you feel this issue affects patient safety or quality of care? (Patient outcome)
How do your job demands influence the ordering of urine cultures? (Organization)
How does this topic affect your job satisfaction or stress? (Employee and organizational outcome)

Table 2 ICU RN focus group questions (SEIPS framework domain in parentheses)

What is the longest, oldest catheter that has been in one of your patients? (Person)
Could you walk us through the steps of what you would do if you were concerned about a patient's urine? What prompts you to order a urine culture? (Organization)
How do you collect a urine sample from both a patient who is with and without a catheter or nephrostomy tube? (Task)
Would you say that there are challenges or difficult processes about collecting a clean catch sample compared to doing it with a Foley or nephrostomy tube? (Task)
When do you assess patients for urinary symptoms or changes in urine appearance/output? How does that fit into your work day? (Process)
Suppose you have collected a urine sample or you are concerned about urinary symptoms, what kinds of barriers or challenges have you noticed when communicating these concerns to the provider? (Technology and tools)
Is there anything about the work environment that makes it challenging or affects your ability to get a urine sample? (Physical environment)
Do you feel that there is any difference between experienced nurses vs. younger nurses in terms of how to approach ordering urine cultures? (Person)
How do you feel this issue affects patient safety or quality of care? (Patient outcome)
How does this topic affect your job satisfaction or stress? (Employee or organizational outcome)

Results

Participants included five ED nurses and six ICU nurses. All participants were white females with a bachelor degree in nursing, ages ranged from 24 to 54 years old and practice experience ranged from 2 to 25 years. The average weighted Cohen's kappa statistic for inter-rater reliability was 0.70 for the deductive coding, 0.91 for the inductive coding, and 0.81 overall. This indicates fair agreement between the two researchers for deductive coding, excellent agreement for inductive coding, and good agreement overall (Table 3).

Deductive results (combined ED and ICU nurses)

Systems-based coding results (structured, deductive) were similar for both ED and ICU nurses with person (25% ED, 30% ICU), process (24% ED, 26% ICU), and task (17% ED, 17% ICU) comprising the dominant themes. For example, one ICU nurse expressed that rarely do physicians not trust her judgment: "If I say, 'boy that [urine] really smells and you should check that out', the provider will say 'ok' and they will write the [urinalysis with urine culture] order." This quotation is a representative ICU nurse comment that was coded under "person" [nurse-physician dyad] in the deductive analysis. Similarly, the quotation, "Nurses will have a patient void in a hat and then will collect that as a UA when that really isn't the best sample because that really isn't sterile," was an ED nurse comment that was coded under "process" [collection process] and "I feel that the urine [in Foley catheters] looks suspicious for infection" was an ED nurse comment that was coded under "task" [interpretation of urine appearance]. Table 4 contains a list of dominant themes paired with illustrative quotations.

Inductive results

In terms of human factors (inductive process), dominant themes for ED nurses included patient factors (13%), physician communication/availability (12%), reflex culture protocols (9%), the electronic health record (7%), urinary symptoms (6%), and ED throughput (5%). For example, the quotation "basically every geriatric patient should get a urinalysis. I'm actually being kind of serious" is a representative ED nurse comment that was coded under "patient factors" [geriatric patients] in the inductive analysis.

Dominant human factor themes for ICU nurses included physician notification of urinalysis results (24%), personal protective equipment (13%), collection technique (13%), patient body habitus (12%), and Foley catheter issues (12%). For example, the quotation "if I were straight cathing [sic] a large person I probably would gown up to protect my arms since you are going to be in there" is a representative ICU nurse comment that was coded under "personal protective equipment" [protective gown facilitating proper collection technique] in the inductive analysis.

Tables 5 and 6 contain a full list of dominant themes paired with illustrative quotations for ED and ICU focus groups, respectively.

Table 3 Inter-rater reliability results for each focus group transcript

	κ Statistic	95% CI	*p*-value
ED RN Inductive	0.890	0.7612–0.9180	0.02
ICU RN Inductive	0.931	0.8650–0.9967	0.04
ED RN Deductive (SEIPS framework)	0.641	0.4421–0.8399	<0.05
ICU RN Deductive (SEIPS framework)	0.772	0.5774–0.8999	0.04

Table 4 Deductive Results: Dominant Themes and Illustrative Quotations

Dominant Theme	Illustrative Quotation
(Percent of focus group content pertaining to SEIPS framework domain)	
Person (25% ED, 30% ICU)	"Finding the physician [is a challenge to obtaining a urinalysis order]" –ED RN A "Rarely do [the physicians] not trust me. If I say boy that [urine] really smells and you should check that out, the provider will say ok and they will write the [urinalysis with urine culture] order." –ICU RN A
Process (24% ED, 26% ICU)	"Nurses will have a patient void in a hat and then will collect that as a UA when that really isn't the best sample because that really isn't sterile." –ED RN D "[Nurses] who are new will ask someone who is more senior, if they would ask the doctor for an order if a urine [sample] looked weird." –ICU RN F
Task (17% ED, 17% ICU)	"I feel that the urine [in Foley catheters] looks suspicious for infection." "It always does." –ED RNs D & E "If it's a change in the [Foley catheter urine appearance] and [the patient] is communicative and they haven't complained of anything, I probably would just get the sample before I would think to ask if they were having any urinary symptoms." –ICU RN F

Discussion

We identified multiple potential process barriers to nurse compliance with evidence-based recommendations for ordering and collecting urine cultures in the ICU and ED. Process facilitators (i.e. technology, materials, work systems, people that help the process) were rarely mentioned and questions designed to extract information about facilitators were typically answered with comments about barriers.

Within the work system, barriers related to the acute care environment at the person, process, and task level tended to dominate the conversation. The emphasis on nurses' difficulty in locating physicians to discuss results (person) and nurse-initiated ordering protocols that

Table 5 ED Nurse Inductive Results: Dominant Themes and Illustrative Quotations

Dominant Theme	Illustrative Quotation
(Percent of focus group content pertaining to theme)	
Patient Traits (13%)	"Basically every geriatric patient should get a urinalysis. I'm actually being kind of serious." –ED RN E "[Patients need to have] the supplies to clean themselves adequately because that little piece of paper…really? The people that come down sometimes definitely have some issues that they need to deal with before they give us a sample." –ED RN C
Physician Communication and Availability (12%)	"If we think the urine looks really nasty and then I'll go ahead and add the [urine culture] order." –ED RN D "There wasn't communication [between nurses and physicians]; the order would just go in and the physician would see it." –ED RN B
Reflex Culture Protocol (9%)	"We did not order [isolated] urine cultures; it was always reflex urinalysis with culture" –ED RN C
Electronic Health Record (7%)	"That's annoying when [a clinical care reminder] pops up; it's already being addressed." –ED RN E "I think that in my head I say, 'that's the protocol,' but I don't actually go into the computer to review it" –ED RN B
Symptoms (6%)	"I always thought that it was lab that looked at the results; said that there the white blood cells were up and then setup the culture. It wasn't my decision or the physician's decision, or patient presentation that drove that, rather objective data." –ED RN D
Throughput (5%)	"People call back the next day and say that the urine was clean while they were in the ER but then their culture grew bacteria, so what about those people? They say that '[my] primary care doctor called me and told me that I need to be put on antibiotics.'" –ED RN A

Table 6 ICU Nurse Inductive Results: Dominant Themes and Illustrative Quotations

Dominant Theme	Illustrative Quotation
(Percent of focus group content pertaining to theme)	
Physician Notification of Urinalysis Results (24%)	"If you have a new patient and [the physicians] are questioning what kind of sepsis they were having, then I would be more cognizant of if there was bacteria or white blood cells in the patient's urine. But otherwise, not really." –ICU RN E
Personal Protective Equipment (13%)	"If I were straight cathing a large person I probably would gown up to protect my arms since you are going to be in there. If you are going to be doing something that's fluidy, I would still wear them because they are outside of the rooms, whether they are ordered or not." –ICU RN F (on PPE being a facilitator of proper straight catheterization technique)
Collection Technique/ Clean Catch (13%)	"If you are going to get a straight cath [sample] sterilely for a female, at least, you need two nurses, regardless of their size." "Right, and then if it's a bigger person, then it can take five to six potentially." –ICU RNs E & C
Patient Body Habitus (12%)	"Trying to get a clean catch on patients who don't mobilize and can't stand over a toilet, that is [an environmental barrier] too because we don't really have bathrooms, we have swing out toilets that are too low for most of our patients anyways." –ICU RN F
Foley Catheter (12%)	"If you are super swamped in another room and a nurse helps you by dumping your Foley bag, [they may help you out by saying], 'hey, did you notice that your urine looks terrible?'" –ICU RN D

default to a urinalysis with reflex culture (process) demonstrates how communication breakdown can lead to work-arounds or sub-optimal practice. Similarly, the emphasis on patient body habitus compromising sterile collection technique or expectations of rapid collection (tasks) underscores how the pace of work can lead to skipping key steps in favor of work-flow efficiency. It is not surprising that ED and ICU nurses identified similar system-level barriers since both environments are fast-paced and rely heavily on both nurse autonomy and teamwork between nurses and physicians. In healthcare, teamwork can create checks and balances that contribute to patient safety, but autonomy can promote efficiency. For example, ideal care may be for a nurse and physician to take a moment and discuss together whether a patient requires a urine culture, which may be challenging to achieve with high fidelity [15]. Similarly, obtaining a truly sterile straight catheter urine sample on an obese patient may require more resources in personnel time than are readily available. In such situations, there may be a trade-off between autonomy over teamwork essentially compromising one care process (sterile technique) in favor of another (efficiency). Increasing our understanding of the competing priorities that health care providers may face in the complex system of healthcare organizations is an essential step in optimizing high reliability systems that promote best practices.

The following findings from the inductive analysis merit attention: First, nurses in both settings displayed either a misinterpretation or a desire for more knowledge in terms of when it is recommended to order a urine culture. Common misconceptions were that—in the absence of symptoms—dark or foul-smelling urine, change in Foley catheter urine appearance, or presence of bacteruria/pyuria justified sending a urine culture. One ED nurse also identified a system design flaw in which unnecessary urine cultures were sent from the ED and primary care physicians would recommend antibiotics for their patients a few days later at follow up based on positive culture results [16]. This nurse observation mirrors a larger trend that has been identified in the inpatient literature; namely that 61% of admitted patients with positive urine cultures may have ASB [17, 18]. System interventions like requiring a guideline-concordant indication for ordering of urine cultures (as protocol) may enhance adherence to national guidelines. Person/environment-level interventions such as targeted education campaigns or guideline pocket cards in the department can complement system level interventions [19].

Second, the ED nurse cohort called attention to physician communication as a barrier. This attributed to increased time constraints in the ED (rapid patient turnover and throughput) and lack of standardized electronic communication tools (as opposed to the ICU nurses who had a universally-used pager system in place to communicate with the physicians). ED nurses also had urinalysis ordering protocols in place that provided more autonomy in terms of nurse-initiated ordering than the ICU protocols. Rapid ED throughput is essential to patient safety, since ED crowding is a known risk factor for medical error and delays of care [20]. Nevertheless, communication issues are often solvable without drastic compromises in throughput. Examples of system interventions include a team huddle (as protocol) at various times throughout an ED shift or the inclusion of an antibiotic stewardship item on the departmental rounds checklist. Person/tools-level interventions could include staff cell phones or "post-it" messages in the electronic health record to facilitate rapid communication of changes in patient status or urinalysis results, even when providers are not in close proximity [21].

Third, we found that a trusting relationship between physicians and nurses may paradoxically pose a barrier to appropriate urine culture ordering. While trust between providers is certainly a positive part of effective teamwork, trust without shared understanding can result in miscommunication and medical error. In our focus groups, some nurses were not familiar with the IDSA guidelines that urine cultures should typically only be ordered in the presence of urinary symptoms, but then went on to voice that physicians trust them to order cultures using their judgement, including when patients are asymptomatic but the urine appears cloudy or had a foul smell. These knowledge gaps may often go unnoticed and interventions that address these gaps are needed.

Fourth, we found that challenges with following proper urine culture collection techniques existed in both clinical settings, but varied based on patient factors. In the ED, the primary concern was that patients did not use pre-collection cleansing kits in the proper manner, thus providing contaminated samples. Rather than slow down patient movement through the ED by re-sending a clean catheter sample, providers sometimes sent cultures on contaminated samples. In the ICU, sedated patients or obese patients were often a barrier to collecting a proper sample, although nurses did note that PPE was a facilitator of proper collection techniques; primarily, because they felt more comfortable cleansing the patient's perineum when they were protected from skin and body fluid contact. This was particularly true in the most obese patients, where straight catheter collection required close physical contact. Our understanding of interventions to improve sterile urine collection continues to evolve and interventions that emphasize patient education or standardized cleansing techniques have produced equivocal results [22]. Further research in this area is needed.

Fifth, ED nurses found it was inconvenient to look up urine culture protocols and guidelines in the electronic health record and, in one instance, commented that the alerts associated with sending inappropriate cultures were a nuisance. These observations underscore a larger systems issue; namely, alert fatigue and its ability to compromise the utility of clinical decision support systems [23]. One illustrative example of a solution for alert fatigue was proposed by Rush et al. who found that having a multidisciplinary committee audit the electronic health record to minimize low-yield alerts helped to ensure that the clinical decision support system enhances, rather than hinders patient care [24].

Sixth, both groups stated that older patients and patients with an indwelling Foley catheter were more likely to have urine cultures sent. Since these two groups often suffer from cognitive impairment and deficits in sensation, they are high-risk for diagnostic uncertainty and inappropriate treatment of ASB and may represent a high-yield starting point for targeted interventions. One low-cost intervention that is supported in the long-term care literature is the use of an ASB algorithm for older patients and patients with an indwelling catheter. Loeb et al. (2005) provide an effective algorithm for long term care environments that has not been validated in acute care settings [25].

Our literature search revealed two studies that addressed this issue. Jones et al. (2016) surveyed 394 RNs from five hospitals regarding appropriate reasons and methods to obtain urine culture specimens on patients with indwelling Foley catheters [11]. They found that 58% of RNs reported that their colleagues follow recommended collection techniques when collecting urine samples in patients with an indwelling catheter. In March 2017, Fakih and Khatib emphasized in a letter to the editor that "improving the culture of culturing should be viewed as an integral component of antimicrobial stewardship [and] is likely to encourage clinicians to use their clinical judgment in their patient evaluations and to move from a reflexive process to a more reflective one, leading to better care" [26]. They recommended a two-pronged approach to eliminating CAUTIs that includes optimizing care pathways and educating frontline providers on best practices.

We found two studies that specifically investigated nurse initiated ordering and collection practices in a general patient population. Richards et al. (2012) found that replacing a routine urinalysis and culture protocol for all patients in a urology clinic with a nurse practitioner-initiated protocol resulted in a 10% drop in the number of urinalyses and cultures ordered with no change in clinical management [27]. Frazee et al. (2012) found that 61% of 129 surveyed female ED patients received proper midstream parted-labia urinalysis catch instructions from their nurses and 82% of the cohort that received instructions actually understood them [28].

Limitations of this study include small sample size and results derived from a single institution. Convenience sampling of participants also creates a risk of selection bias. Potential disadvantages of using focus groups rather than interviews in this study included disagreements among participants, irrelevant side discussions, and participants feeling under pressure to agree with the dominant view. While we found several misperceptions among nurses related to ordering of the urine cultures, it may be such misperceptions occur among other members of the treating team. We did not conduct focus groups for other members of the treating team in this study as our main focus was on the collection and ordering of urine specimens-a task performed most often by nurses at our institution.

Our findings have implications for infection preventionists and clinicians in the ICU and the ED. When analyzing the complexity of ordering urine culture and urine collection, those working in EDs and ICUs should consider a system level approach that identifies the work system barriers and facilitators to compliance with guidelines. Our study findings can assist in guiding targeted interventions within these acute care settings.

Conclusions

In this study, we found barriers to appropriate ordering and collection of urine cultures, using a human factors framework. These included common knowledge misconceptions, communication barriers, unfamiliarity with IDSA guidelines/hospital protocols, and a perception that urine cultures were more likely needed in those with a foley catheter or of older age. Our findings may be used to identify interventions to address these barriers and improve quality of care.

Abbreviations

ASB: Asymptomatic bacteriuria; ED: Emergency department; ICU: Intensive care unit; IDSA: The Infectious Disease Society of America; SEIPS: Systems engineering initiative for patient safety

Acknowledgements

Not applicable.

Funding

Nasia Safdar is supported by a VA funded patient safety center of inquiry.

Authors' contributions

Authors MZ, DP, RR, and MJK participated in data collection and analysis. Authors RR, MP, and MJK participated in manuscript preparation. Author NS provided oversight to the project and edited the manuscript. All authors read and approved the final manuscript.

Consent for publication

Not applicable.

Competing interests

The authors declare that they have no competing interests.

Author details

[1]Division of Infectious Disease, Department of Medicine, University of Wisconsin-Madison School of Medicine and Public Health, 750 Highland Ave, Madison, Wisconsin 53705, USA. [2]William S. Middleton Memorial Veterans Hospital, 2500 Overlook Terrace, Madison, Wisconsin 53705, USA. [3]Department of Infectious Disease, University of Chicago Medical Center, 5841 S Maryland Ave, Chicago, Illinois 60637, USA. [4]Division of Infectious Disease, Perelman School of Medicine, University of Pennsylvania, 3400 Civic Center Blvd, Philadelphia, Pennsylvania 19104, USA. [5]BerbeeWalsh Department of Emergency Medicine, University of Wisconsin-Madison School of Medicine and Public Health, 800 University Bay Drive, Madison, Wisconsin 53705, USA.

References

1. Nicolle LE, et al. Infectious Diseases Society of America guidelines for the diagnosis and treatment of asymptomatic bacteriuria in adults. Clin Infect Dis. 2005;40(5):643–54.
2. Gupta K, et al. International clinical practice guidelines for the treatment of acute uncomplicated cystitis and pyelonephritis in women: a 2010 update by the Infectious Diseases Society of America and the European Society for Microbiology and Infectious Diseases. Clin Infect Dis. 2011;52(5):e103–20.
3. Nicolle LE. Asymptomatic bacteriuria: review and discussion of the IDSA guidelines. Int J Antimicrob Agents. 2006;28(Suppl 1):S42–8.
4. Foundation, A. Choosing Wisely [cited 2017 February 20]; Available from: www.choosingwisely.org/doctor-patient-lists/american-geriatrics-society.
5. Cope M, et al. Inappropriate treatment of catheter-associated asymptomatic bacteriuria in a tertiary care hospital. Clin Infect Dis. 2009;48(9):1182–8.
6. Trautner BW. Asymptomatic bacteriuria: when the treatment is worse than the disease. Nat Rev Urol. 2011;9(2):85–93.
7. Trautner BW, et al. Overtreatment of asymptomatic bacteriuria: identifying provider barriers to evidence-based care. Am J Infect Control. 2014;42(6):653–8.
8. Drekonja DM, et al. A survey of resident physicians' knowledge regarding urine testing and subsequent antimicrobial treatment. Am J Infect Control. 2013;41(10):892–6.

9. Fridkin S, et al. Vital signs: improving antibiotic use among hospitalized patients. MMWR Morb Mortal Wkly Rep. 2014;63(9):194–200.
10. Schulz L, et al. Top ten myths regarding the diagnosis and treatment of urinary tract infections. J Emerg Med. 2016;51(1):25–30.
11. Jones K, et al. How and when nurses collect urine cultures on catheterized patients: a survey of 5 hospitals. Am J Infect Control. 2016;44(2):173–6.
12. Carayon P, et al. Work system design for patient safety: the SEIPS model. Qual Saf Health Care. 2006;15(Suppl 1):i50–8.
13. Xie A, Carayon P. A systematic review of human factors and ergonomics (HFE)-based healthcare system redesign for quality of care and patient safety. Ergonomics. 2015;58(1):33–49.
14. Neale J. Iterative categorization (IC): a systematic technique for analysing qualitative data. Addiction. 2016;111(6):1096–106.
15. Walker S, et al. Why are antibiotics prescribed for asymptomatic bacteriuria in institutionalized elderly people? A qualitative study of physicians' and nurses' perceptions. CMAJ. 2000;163(3):273–7.
16. Humphries RM, Dien Bard J. Point-counterpoint: reflex cultures reduce laboratory workload and improve antimicrobial stewardship in patients suspected of having urinary tract infections. J Clin Microbiol. 2016;54(2):254–8.
17. Hartley S, et al. Overtreatment of asymptomatic bacteriuria: identifying targets for improvement. Infect Control Hosp Epidemiol. 2015;36(4):470–3.
18. Hartley S, et al. Inappropriate testing for urinary tract infection in hospitalized patients: an opportunity for improvement. Infect Control Hosp Epidemiol. 2013;34(11):1204–7.
19. Hartley SE, et al. Evaluating a hospitalist-based intervention to decrease unnecessary antimicrobial use in patients with asymptomatic Bacteriuria. Infect Control Hosp Epidemiol. 2016;37(9):1044–51.
20. Carter EJ, Pouch SM, Larson EL. The relationship between emergency department crowding and patient outcomes: a systematic review. J Nurs Scholarsh. 2014;46(2):106–15.
21. Breslin S, Greskovich W, Turisco F. Wireless technology improves nursing workflow and communications. Comput Inform Nurs. 2004;22(5):275–81.
22. Teo S, Cheek JA, Craig S. Improving clean-catch contamination rates: a prospective interventional cohort study. Emerg Med Australas. 2016;28(6):698–703.
23. Farley HL, et al. Quality and safety implications of emergency department information systems. Ann Emerg Med. 2013;62(4):399–407.
24. Rush JL, et al. Improving patient safety by combating alert fatigue. J Grad Med Educ. 2016;8(4):620–1.
25. Loeb M, et al. Effect of a multifaceted intervention on number of antimicrobial prescriptions for suspected urinary tract infections in residents of nursing homes: cluster randomised controlled trial. BMJ. 2005;331(7518):669.
26. Fakih MG, Khatib R. Improving the culture of culturing: critical asset to antimicrobial stewardship. Infect Control Hosp Epidemiol. 2017;38(3):377–9.
27. Richards KA, et al. Utility of routine urinalysis and urine culture testing in an ambulatory urology clinic: a quality improvement initiative in a veterans healthcare facility. Can J Urol. 2017;24(1):8627–33.
28. Frazee BW, et al. Urine collection in the emergency department: what really happens in there? West J Emerg Med. 2012;13(5):401–5.

18

One-year molecular surveillance of carbapenem-susceptible *A. baumannii* on a German intensive care unit: diversity or clonality

Andreas F. Wendel[1*], Monika Malecki[1], Robin Otchwemah[1], Carlos J. Tellez-Castillo[2], Samir G. Sakka[3] and Frauke Mattner[1]

Abstract

Background: *A. baumannii* is a common nosocomial pathogen known for its high transmission potential. A high rate of carbapenem-susceptible *Acinetobacter calcoaceticus-Acinetobacter baumannii* (ACB)-complex in clinical specimens led to the implementation of a pathogen-based surveillance on a 32-bed surgical intensive care unit (SICU) in a German tertiary care centre.

Methods: Between April 2017 and March 2018, ACB-complex isolates with an epidemiological link to the SICU were further assessed. Identification to the species level was carried out using a multiplex PCR targeting the *gyrB* gene, followed by RAPD, PFGE (ApaI) and whole genome sequencing (WGS, core genome MLST, SeqSphere+ software, Ridom). Additional infection prevention and control (IPC) measures were introduced as follows: epidemiological investigations, hand hygiene training, additional terminal cleaning and disinfection incl. UV-light, screening for carbapenem-susceptible *A. baumannii* and environmental sampling. Hospital-acquired infections were classified according to the CDC definitions.

Results: Fourty four patients were colonized/infected with one or two (different) carbapenem-susceptible ACB-complex isolates. Fourty three out of 48 isolates were classified as hospital-acquired (detection on or after 3rd day of admission). Nearly all isolates were identified as *A. baumannii*, only four as *A. pittii*. Twelve patients developed *A. baumannii* infections. Genotyping revealed two pulsotype clusters, which were confirmed to be cgMLST clonal cluster type 1770 ($n = 8$ patients) and type 1769 ($n = 12$ patients) by WGS. All other isolates were distinct from each other. Nearly all transmission events of the two clonal clusters were confirmed by conventional epidemiology. Transmissions stopped after a period of several months. Environmental sampling revealed a relevant dissemination of *A. baumannii*, but only a few isolates corresponded to clinical strains. Introduction of the additional screening revealed a significantly earlier detection of carbapenem-susceptible *A. baumannii* during hospitalization.

Conclusions: A molecular and infection surveillance of ACB-complex based on identification to the species level, classic epidemiology and genotyping revealed simultaneously occurring independent transmission events and clusters of hospital-acquired *A. baumannii*. This underlines the importance of such an extensive surveillance methodology in IPC programmes also for carbapenem-susceptible *A. baumannii*.

Keywords: Infection control, Surveillance, Bacterial typing, *Acinetobacter baumannii*

* Correspondence: wendela@kliniken-koeln.de
[1]Institute of Hygiene, University Hospital I of Witten/Herdecke, Cologne Merheim Medical Centre, Cologne, Germany
Full list of author information is available at the end of the article

Background

Acinetobacter baumannii is a pathogen of emerging clinical significance causing a broad range of hospital-acquired infections [1]. Its excellent capacity to survive in the hospital environment results in a high transmission propensity [2]. Additionally, rapid antibiotic resistance development makes effective therapy challenging [1]. *Acinetobacter baumannii* cannot be reliably differentiated by phenotypic or biochemical methods from other *Acinetobacter* species like *Acinetobacter pittii* (formerly genomic species 3) or *Acinetobacter nosocomialis* (formerly genomic species 13TU). These species are grouped together amongst others into the *Acinetobacter calcoaceticus-Acinetobacter baumannii* (ACB)-complex [3, 4]. However, these species differ in virulence, antibiotic resistance rates and natural habitat [1, 5]. Recent methods like MALDI-TOF/MS promise to identify the species just as accurately as molecular methods [1, 3].

Compared to other *Acinetobacter* species, *A. baumannii* is not a ubiquitous organism. It is mostly found in the hospital setting (human and environment); a natural reservoir still needs to be assessed. Healthy humans do not appear to be colonized by *A. baumannii* [1]. The population of *A. baumannii* is genetically more homogenous compared to those of *A. pittii* or *A. nosocomialis* [3, 6].

Numerous nosocomial outbreaks have been described so far, mostly with multidrug-resistant (MDR) *A. baumannii* [7]. Recent infection control and prevention (IPC) recommendations focus on multidrug-resistant *Acinetobacter* spp., taking the environment-to-patient and patient-to-patient transmission into consideration [8].

At the beginning of 2017, we retrospectively observed a high (apparently endemic) rate of carbapenem-susceptible *A. baumannii* in clinical specimens on the surgical intensive care unit in comparison to other intensive care units. Therefore, we decided to install a pathogen-based surveillance. In the present study we report on a complex increase of clonal and non-clonal *A. baumannii*, describe the local epidemiology and the IPC measures applied in a German tertiary care centre.

Methods

Setting

The study was conducted at a 724-bed tertiary care hospital. The surgical intensive care unit (SICU) has 32 beds (14 single rooms and 9 double rooms). Only four single patient rooms are equipped with washbasins. Adult patients from various surgical specialties are treated on the unit: general surgery, visceral surgery, vascular surgery, neurosurgery, orthopaedics, trauma, and solid organ transplantations such as kidney. The average ICU length of stay was 5.2 days in 2017. The IPC service is provided by the Institute of Hygiene. The protocol of the German healthcare-associated infection surveillance on intensive care units (ITS-KISS) was implemented on the SICU in 2012 [9].

Microbiological sampling and analysis

A rectal and nose/throat screening for multidrug-resistant Gram-negative organisms was performed on every patient at admission and once weekly. Swabs were subsequently inoculated on chromogenic chromID® ESBL (bioMérieux) media. Additionally, tracheal secretions were sampled from intubated patients once weekly (inoculation on standard media). Identification and antimicrobial susceptibility testing (imipenem, meropenem, gentamicin, tobramycin, amikacin, ciprofloxacin, sulfamethoxazole/trimethoprim) were performed with the VITEK 2 system (VITEK 2 GN-ID and AST-N248, bioMérieux). Uncertain identification results were further investigated by MALDI-TOF (Brucker Diagnostic). Identification of *Acinetobacter* species was done to the complex level. EUCAST standards were used for interpretation. Only ACB-complex isolates being at least non-susceptible to one carbapenem and/or ciprofloxacin (in accordance with the German classification for multidrug-resistant Gram-negative organisms [10]) were reported in screening specimens at the beginning of the study in April 2017. Screening for carbapenem-susceptible ACB-complex was included in September 2017 until the end of the study because of the increasing number of isolates detected in clinical specimens. Therefore, all ACB-complex isolates growing on the cefpodoxime-containing media were reported.

Pathogen-based epidemiology

From April 2017 onwards, microbiological data was retrieved from the laboratory surveillance information system (Hybase v.6, epiNET AG, Germany) and searched for ACB-complex isolates once daily. Only patients with an epidemiological link to the SICU were further assessed (stay on the SICU within the last month). Epidemiological data of the colonized or infected patients was collected by the infection control nurse from the patients' clinical records and from the attending physicians or nurses.

Bacterial isolates and infections were considered as community-acquired if the collection of the specimen or the start of infection occurred on or before the 2nd day of admission. Afterwards, bacterial isolates and infections were defined as hospital-acquired. Transmission analysis was based on epidemiological data (direct room or ward contact and/or documented care by the same staff) and genetic data. Definite transmission events were defined as isolation of genetically-related isolates from two patients who were on the same ward at the same time (at least 24 h, patient-to-patient transmission) or in the same single/double room with a maximum gap of 7 days (room-to-patient transmission). Hospital-acquired infections were classified according to the Centers for Disease Control and Prevention (CDC) definitions [11]. Patients without related signs of infection were considered to be colonized.

Molecular surveillance and genotyping

Further identification to the species level was carried out using a multiplex PCR targeting the *gyrB* gene [3]. First strain relatedness was assessed using random amplification of polymorphic DNA (RAPD) with the three primers (ERIC-1, ERIC-2 and ST272 [12, 13]) and including at least the preceding five isolates in each run. Isolates with the same banding patterns were considered to be related. Later on, pulsed-field gel electrophoresis (PFGE) was performed by using ApaI (New England Biolabs, USA). DNA separation was performed in 1% agarose in 0.5× Trisborate-EDTA (TBE) buffer in a CHEF-DR III System (Bio-Rad, LaJolla, CA, USA) using 6 V/cm for 19 h with pulse times of 5 s to 20 s. The strain relatedness was calculated with GelCompar II version 5.1 software (Applied Maths NV, Belgium) and in accordance to the criteria of Tenover et al. [14, 15].

Representative isolates of clinical and environmental samples with the same pulsotype were further assessed by whole genome sequencing (five out of eight isolates of pulsotype A and seven out of 15 isolates of pulsotype B). In short, genomic DNA was extracted with the DNeasy UltraClean Microbial Kit (Qiagen, Germany) following the manufacturer's instructions. The library preparation using proprietary methods und subsequent sequencing using Illumina HiSeq instruments in 150 bp paired-end read mode was performed by GATC Biotech (Konstanz, Germany). Before assembly, quality control of the reads was carried out with FastQC version 0.11.5 [16]. De novo assembly was performed using Velvet (version 1.1.04) software integrated into the SeqSphere+ software version 5.0 (Ridom, Münster, Germany) using default parameters [17]. An average N50 of 582,568 bp across isolates was achieved. Afterwards, WGS-based species identification with the assembled genomes was performed using JSpeciesWS (version 3.0.18) [18]. Acquired resistance genes on assembled sequences were identified by ResFinder (version 2.1; threshold of 98% identity and minimum length of 60%) [19]. Subsequently, we applied a core genome multilocus sequence type (cgMLST) genotyping approach using the publicly available core genome MLST scheme for *A. baumannii* (2390 targets) published by Higgins et al. (SeqSphere+ software) [20]. During comparison of the allelic profile the "pairwise ignoring missing values" option was turned on. Genomes containing at least 95% of the defined cgMLST targets were included. Isolates with less than 10 different alleles in the cgMLST target gene set were considered as highly related (clonal cluster) [20].

Infection control management and interventions

Contact (and standard) precautions were applied for every patient colonized or infected with ciprofloxacin-non-susceptible ACB-complex and/or carbapenem-non-susceptible ACB -complex (barrier nursing in two-bed room or single room, use of gowns and gloves), whereas standard precautions were applied for carbapenem- and ciprofloxacin-susceptible ACB-complex isolates. Standard or contact precautions did not change during the study period. Infection control nurses visited the SICU at least twice weekly during the whole study period.

During the surveillance of ACB-complex isolates, possible transmissions were suspected. Therefore, additional infection control measures were introduced. Hand hygiene compliance and correct use of gloves was intensified with additional standard hygiene training sessions for the health care workers (including the radiology and cleaning staff) from June to November 2017. Hand hygiene compliance observations ($n = 200$) were carried out in July and August 2017. Standard terminal cleaning and disinfection was performed once with Glucoprotamin 0.5% (Incidin plus, Ecolab Healthcare, Germany). In August and September 2017, an intensified terminal cleaning and disinfection was performed in all 23 patient's rooms at least once as follows: disinfection two times with Glucoprotamin 0.5% and subsequently disinfection with a portable UV-light (Verilux CleanWave Sanitizing Wand, Verilux, USA) targeting complex surfaces [21]. The use of disposable patient medical equipment was encouraged. Local health authorities were informed about the clonal spread in September 2017. Environmental sampling was performed several times between June and November 2017. Sampling was conducted using moistened rayon swabs with amies transport medium (Copan, Italy). Samples were inoculated on MacConkey agar, blood agar (Oxoid, Germany) and tryptic soy broth (Merck Millipore, Germany) and incubated for a maximum of 48 h at 37 °C. Identification and susceptibility testing were performed as stated above. Sampled inanimate surfaces were as follows: patient rooms (bedside table, reusable medical equipment, washbasins, touchscreens, hand -touch sites of the endotracheal suction system), storage rooms (cupboards, shelves), electrocardiography machines, mobile x-ray systems (incl. cassettes) and disinfectant dosing systems.

Statistical analysis

Statistical analysis was performed with PSPP 1.0.1. The Student *t* test was used for continuous normally distributed variables, the Mann-Whitney *U* test for variables that did not follow a normal distribution and the χ^2 test or Fisher's exact test for categorical variables.

Nucleotide sequence accession number

Sequence reads of the strains have been deposited as a project at the European Nucleotid Archive under the accession number PRJEB27660.

Results

Isolate and patient characteristics

Between April 2017 and March 2018, 44 patients who had at least one epidemiological link to the SICU were found to be colonized or infected with a carbapenem-susceptible ACB-complex. Overall, 37 patients carried a fully susceptible (susceptible to all antimicrobial agents tested) ACB-complex isolate, three patients a ciprofloxacin- and sulfamethoxazole/trimethoprim-resistant ACB-complex isolate and four patients ACB-complex isolates with both phenotypes. Nearly all isolates (43 out of 48) were classified as hospital-acquired. The five community-acquired isolates (three *A. pittii*, two *A. baumannii*) were detected within 24 h; the four affected patients were not hospitalized in the preceding 30 days. The patient colonized with the two different community-acquired *A. baumannii* isolates was from a nursing home. During the same time period two patients were detected with a carbapenem -resistant ACB-complex.

All ACB-complex isolates, except four, were available for further identification and genotyping. Of those, two hospital-acquired and three community-acquired isolates were identified as *A. pittii*; all other isolates were identified as *A. baumannii.*

Relevant clinical and epidemiologic data of the subgroup of 36 patients with hospital-acquired colonisation/ infection with carbapenem-susceptible *A. baumannii* (excluding patients with *A. pittii* or non-available ACB-complex) are displayed in Table 1. Twelve patients developed hospital-acquired infections. Seven patients died during their hospital stay. None of the patients died from an infection with ACB-complex. The anatomic site of first detection was sampled and *A. baumannii*-negative in 30 out of 36 patients during the week preceding the first detection.

Table 1 Epidemiologic characteristics of 36 patients with hospital-acquired *A. baumannii*

Characteristics	Value
Age (years)	
median (range)	62 (21; 80)
Gender	
female	13 (36%)
Hospital stay at first isolation (days)	
median (range)	19 (5; 62)
Source of first positive specimen[a]	
respiratory tract	14 (38.8%)
nose/throat (screening)	12 (33.3%)
rectum (screening)	7 (19.4%)
wound	4 (11,1%)
urine	2 (5.6%)
blood culture	1 (2.8%)
Infection	
pneumonia	7 (19.4%)
wound infection	2 (5.6%)
urinary tract infection	1 (2.8%)
CLABSI	2 (5.6%)
Antibiotic treatment[b]	30 (83.3%)
Surgery[b]	20 (55.5%)
Non-surgical intervention[b]	24 (66.7%)
Mechanical ventilation[b]	14 (38.8%)
Dialysis[b]	5 (13.8%)

[a]exceeds 100% as first identification was done in two different specimens in four patients; [b]Within a maximal interval of seven days before first isolation; *CLABSI* central line associated blood stream infections

Genotyping and transmission analysis

Based on conventional genotyping by PFGE, we were able to show two genetically highly-related clonal clusters of fully susceptible *A. baumannii* isolates: clonal cluster 1 containing eight patients and clonal cluster 2 containing 12 patients and three environmental isolates. All other clinical and environmental isolates were distinct. Both clusters were confirmed by whole genome sequencing. The maximum distance of targets within clonal cluster 1 (cgMLST cluster type 1770, ST Oxford 753, ST Pasteur 494) were two targets, within clonal cluster 2 (cgMLST cluster type 1769, ST with Oxford or Pasteur scheme unknown) four targets and in between the clusters 2227 targets (Fig. 1).

Genetic in silico search for *bla* genes displayed the cephalosporinase-encoding bla_{ADC-25}-like gene in both clusters, the $bla_{OXA-106}$-like gene in cluster 1-isolates and the bla_{OXA-51} gene in cluster 2-isolates. The $bla_{OXA-106}$ gene belongs to the bla_{OXA-51} gene subgroup [22]. Both clonal clusters emerged over a period of nearly 6 months. The epidemiologic and genetic data of the *A. baumannii*-surveillance are displayed in Fig. 2.

Analysing spatiotemporal links based on room occupancy, we were not able to identify index patients admitted with the clones. By conventional epidemiology, nearly all transmission events were confirmed as "definite" except for one patient in each cluster where an epidemiological link to other patients or rooms could not be established. Although most definite transmissions occurred within the SICU, two patients in clonal cluster 1 and two patients in cluster 2 must have acquired the respective clone on other wards than the SICU (Fig. 3).

The two carbapenem-resistant *A. baumannii* isolates detected during the study period were neither

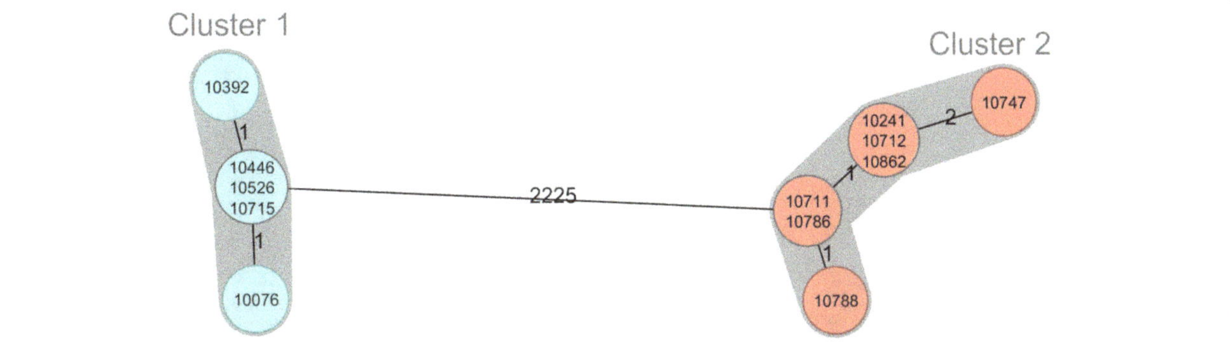

Fig. 1 Minimum-spanning tree of the representative 12 *A. baumannii* isolates showing the genetic relationship based on the cgMLST scheme (Ridom SeqSphere+, 2359 targets). Each circle displays a single genotype and numbers on the connecting lines in between the allele difference. Clonally related genetic clusters (< 10 alleles difference) containing more than one patient are encircled in grey

epidemiologically nor genetically linked to each other or the other carbapenem-susceptible isolates.

Infection control management

Observations carried out by infection control nurses revealed actions resulting in patient contamination from washbasins and vice versa. The hand hygiene compliance before patient contact, before aseptic tasks, after body fluid exposure risk, after patient contact and after contact with patient surroundings was at 75, 67, 54, 70 and 69% respectively (national reference data from the German national hand hygiene campaign AKTION Saubere Hände (ASH) from 2017: 53, 49, 74, 70 and 69% resp. [23]).

Environmental sampling revealed six ACB-complex -positive specimens out of a total of 206 specimens collected. *A. pittii*, not related to any clinical isolates, was found on one mobile x-ray system cassette. *A. baumannii* was found in a washbasin, on a fixation tape and on the pressure regulator of the endotracheal suction system at three beds. The latter isolates were genetically related to the clinical isolates of the *A. baumannii*-colonized/infected patients cared for at the time of sampling (clonal cluster 2). All mentioned positive surfaces and the pressure regulators of all endotracheal suction systems on the SICU were properly disinfected and resampled afterwards (negative). We were not able to link the acquisition of the clonal cluster strains to (non-) invasive procedures or contact to radiology.

As mentioned above, screening for susceptible *A. baumannii* was introduced in September 2017. This led to a significantly earlier detection (median: 19 days before vs. 12 days after; $p = 0.04$) of fully susceptible ACB-complex. Also, first detection of fully susceptible ACB-complex was performed significantly more from screening specimens than from clinical specimens (83.3% after vs. 22.2% before; $p < 0.0001$). All five community-acquired ACB-complex isolates were detected after the introduction of the additional screening procedures. Interestingly, no ACB-complex isolates were detected in August 2017, in February 2018 and in March 2018 (Fig. 2). However, we did not observe any change in patient numbers or screenings compliance during these months.

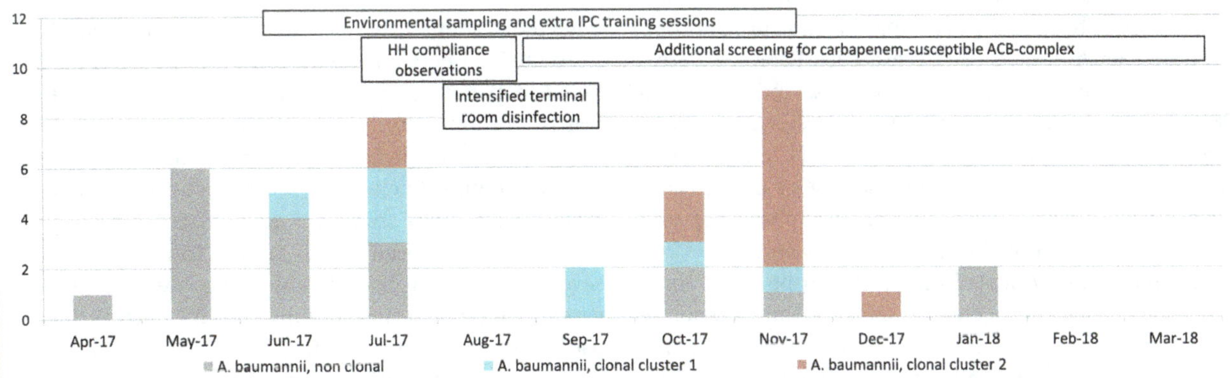

Fig. 2 Overview of new cases with a hospital-acquired carbapenem-susceptible *A. baumannii* with an epidemiological link to the SICU (39 isolates from 36 patients). Boxes indicate additional infections control measures and their duration; HH, hand hygiene

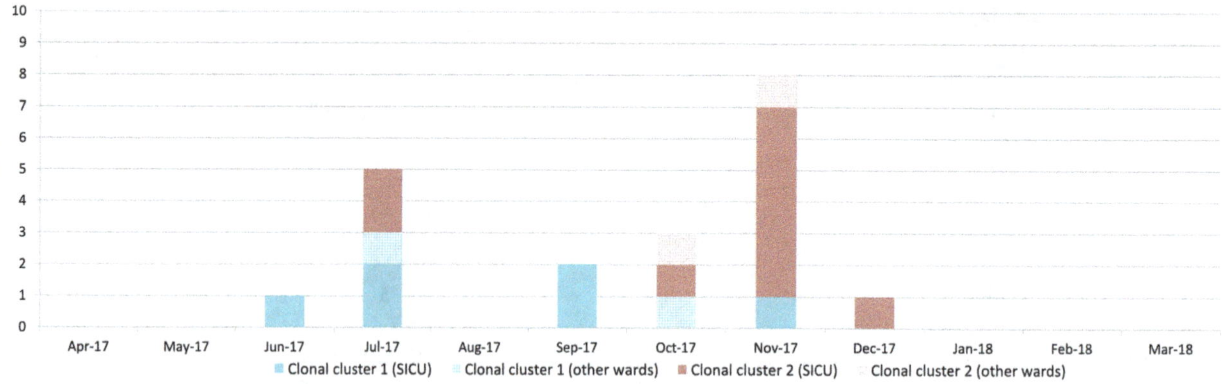

Fig. 3 Overview of the most likely ward of acquisition of the two carbapenem-susceptible *A. baumannii* clones

Discussion

In this study, we report on a molecular and infection surveillance of carbapenem-susceptible *A. baumannii* on a surgical intensive care unit in a tertiary care centre. During the one-year study period, an initial polyclonal increase of *A. baumannii* was observed, followed by the emergence of two dominant clones.

A pathogen-based surveillance is part of the vertical approach in infection control [24]; it is mostly conducted for MDR bacteria, e.g. carbapenem-resistant *A. baumannii*, in German hospitals [9]. Hence, there is no detailed surveillance data about the occurrence and epidemiology of carbapenem-susceptible *A. baumannii*. Furthermore, we found only a few descriptions of outbreaks of carbapenem -susceptible *A. baumannii* in the literature, e.g. [25]. A recent meta-analysis reported that three quarter of *Acinetobacter* outbreaks in the literature were attributed to MDR bacteria. However, the definition of MDR is used inconsistently, and is not always in line with international recommendations [7]. The underreporting of outbreaks of non-MDR *A. baumannii* might be due to a surveillance bias, as IPC programmes put the main focus on MDR bacteria. Another reason might be a publication bias, as MDR infections are more difficult to treat and as MDR *A. baumannii* has high transmission rates [1, 7]. Moreover, MDR *A. baumannii* has become endemic in a lot of countries. The carbapenem-resistance rate exceeded 75% in invasive isolates in some south-eastern European countries in 2016 [26]. On German intensive care units, 43% of clinical isolates were resistant to imipenem in 2015 [27]. This study was conducted in a low endemic setting of carbapenem -resistant *A. baumannii* (only sporadic appearance and almost exclusively related to a hospital stay abroad).

The epidemiology of *A. baumannii* can be quite complex. Simultaneously occurring endemic and epidemic MDR *A. baumannii* clones are described in the literature, making detection and control difficult [1, 28]. The worldwide emergence of carbapenem-resistant *A. baumannii* is caused by a few successful clonal lineages [29]. The molecular epidemiology of non-MDR *A. baumannii* is less clear, but the population of non-MDR isolates is described as less homogenous [6]. Based on our results, the dynamics of transmission cannot simply be explained by an "endemic setting" of *A. baumannii*. Noteworthy, nearly all acquisitions were hospital-acquired. Moreover, the general reservoir of *A. baumannii* is unknown, as it is found almost exclusively in the hospital environment [1, 5]. Appearance and transmission of *A. baumannii* is quite common on intensive care units [7, 28] and occurs via contaminated hands after contact with the inanimate environment or colonized/infected patients. A recent review showed a positive association between infection/colonization with *A. baumannii* and exposure to rooms previously occupied by patients with *A. baumannii* [30]. In our study, we found direct and indirect evidence for both modes of transmission (patient-to-patient or environment-to-patient). The variety of environmental *A. baumannii* isolates, clonally and non-clonally related to clinical isolates, found on frequently touched surfaces, demonstrates the widespread environmental contamination and supports the importance of hand hygiene. We were not able to find definitive epidemiological links for all patients. Of course, colonized health-care workers or colonized (undetected) patients cannot be completely ruled out. It can be quite cumbersome to establish spatiotemporal links between patients, who are often transferred to several wards and units during their hospital stay. Interestingly, we also found evidence for transmissions from the SICU to and within other wards. Some electronic surveillance systems can help to detect patient contacts, e.g. the Hybase software used in this study. However, they fail if several patients from different wards are affected or in cases of indirect transmissions (room contact). Easy to use software solutions are lacking to analyse and visualize complex patient transfers.

The transmissions of the clonal strains were stopped with a combination of standard hygiene measures, intensified environmental cleaning and disinfection and rectal screening for carbapenem-susceptible ACB-complex. Contact precautions were only applied to a minority of patients as stated above. The expanded screening was introduced in the middle of the study period and resulted in a significantly earlier detection of ACB-complex. Before the introduction, community-acquired isolates might have been misclassified as hospital-acquired due to the late detection. Neither the sensitivity of patient screening for (MDR) *A. baumannii* colonization nor the ideal screening loci are well known. Recent studies showed a low sensitivity of detection in colonized patients [31] or demonstrated that perirectal screening might be more appropriate than rectal screening for *A. baumannii* [32]. Nevertheless, in our opinion the combination of three screening loci (rectal and nose/throat) and subsequent inoculation on a cefpodoxime -containing media, as performed in our study, reach a sufficient sensitivity.

We also applied UV light to disinfect complex surfaces [21] in combination with two times standard cleaning and disinfection over a period of 2 months. As rooms were blocked for hours during this procedure, these additional measures were stopped. Therefore, the impact of additional environmental cleaning and disinfection remains unclear in our study. However, intensified room cleaning and disinfection was described as an effective IPC measure during outbreak periods [33]. We also observed a relevant environmental contamination, especially on difficult-to-clean regulators of the endotracheal suction system. As nearly all of them were contaminated with skin flora and other pathogens (e.g. *Klebsiella pneumoniae, Enterococcus faecium*), they might have been a reservoir of transmission. As there is no dedicated cleaning staff for terminal cleaning and disinfection of medical products in our hospital during the late and night shifts, this task is assigned to the nurse at times of patient-to-nurse ratios of sometimes 3:1 or worse. This ratio is not unusual on German intensive care units [34].

The *A. baumannii* infection rate of approx. 50% was described during outbreaks, with no difference between MDR- and non-MDR infected patients [7]. In our cohort, we observed a hospital-acquired *A. baumannii* infection rate of 33.3% (12 out of 36 patients). The majority of our patients showed the relevant risk factors for colonization/infection with *A. baumannii,* already well described for MDR *Acinetobacter,* such as prolonged hospital stays at an ICU, mechanical ventilation or prior antimicrobial therapy [7, 28]. Selective pressure of broad-spectrum penicillins or third-generation cephalosporins, both favoured in our hospital, might have played a decisive role.

We encountered some pitfalls of such surveillance. A proper and reliable (molecular) identification of the isolates to the species level is needed, as the different ACB-complex species differ in their hospital epidemiology. Especially *A. baumannii* and to a certain extent *A. nosocomialis* are known to cause outbreaks in hospital settings [1, 5]. In our opinion, it is important to consider microbiological results after the patients' transfer to other wards. We would have missed seven patients if we had only included specimens collected on the SICU. Hence, a hospital-wide surveillance appears more appropriate to identify possible transmission pathways, but requires extended IPC resources. Furthermore, a typing method with high discriminatory power is crucial. In our opinion, RAPD and PFGE are suitable methods for typing of *A. baumannii.* However, in times of next generation sequencing (NGS), a "random access" database may be more appropriate. For example, a gene-by-gene approach with an accepted allele scheme (cgMLST) can be used over longer periods [35]. The application of a cgMLST scheme was recently demonstrated by Willems et al. in an outbreak of *A. baumannii* [36].

There are a few limitations to this study. First, we only analysed one isolate per resistance pattern per patient. Patients colonized/infected with more than one strain might have remained undetected. Secondly, a formal case–control study to determine risk factors for carriage of carbapenem-susceptible *A. baumannii* was not performed. However, our aim was to describe the surveillance results and the molecular epidemiology. Thirdly, we only applied NGS for isolates that were highly related using PFGE and RAPD for economic reasons. Related isolates showing different PFGE/RAPD patterns, though unlikely, might have gone unnoticed.

Conclusions

A molecular and infection surveillance of ACB-complex based on identification to the species level, classic epidemiology and genotyping revealed simultaneously occurring independent transmission events and clusters of hospital-acquired *A. baumannii.* This underlines the importance of such an extensive surveillance methodology in IPC programmes also for carbapenem-susceptible *A. baumannii.*

Abbreviations

ACB: *Acinetobacter calcoaceticus-Acinetobacter baumannii*; cgMLST: Core genome multilocus sequence type; CLABSI: Central line associated blood stream infections; HH: Hand hygiene; IPC: Infection prevention and control; ITS-KISS: Intensivstation-Krankenhaus-Infektions-Surveillance-System = German national nosocomial infections surveillance on intensive care units; MDR: Multidrug-resistant; NGS: Next generation sequencing; PFGE: Pulsed-field gel electrophoresis; RAPD: Random amplification of polymorphic DNA; SICU: Surgical ICU; WGS: Whole genome sequencing

Acknowledgements

We thank Ingo Winterfeld for technical help and the infection control nurses Regine Galante, Andreas Kirchler, Gudrun Gaksch and Michael Loeper, who took part in the infection control surveillance at the surgical intensive care unit (all from the Institute of Hygiene, Cologne). We also thank Dr. Paul Higgins (Institute for Medical Microbiology, Immunology and Hygiene,

University of Cologne, Germany) for help with interpretation of the molecular epidemiology. We also thank the team of the Department of Clinical Microbiology (MVZ synlab Leverkusen GmbH) for collection of the isolates during the study period.

Funding
None.

Authors' contributions
AFW and FM: Conception and design of the study, acquisition, analysis and interpretation of the data. MM and RO: Acquisition, analysis and interpretation of data, revising article critically. SGS and CTC: Acquisition of the data. AFW: writing and original draft. All authors read and approved the final manuscript.

Consent for publication
Not applicable.

Competing interests
The authors declare that they have no competing interests.

Author details
[1]Institute of Hygiene, University Hospital I of Witten/Herdecke, Cologne Merheim Medical Centre, Cologne, Germany. [2]Department of Clinical Microbiology, MVZ synlab Leverkusen GmbH, Köln-Merheim, Germany. [3]Department of Anesthesiology and Operative Intensive Care Medicine, University of Witten/Herdecke, Cologne Merheim Medical Centre, Cologne, Germany.

References
1. Antunes LC, Visca P, Towner KJ. Acinetobacter baumannii: evolution of a global pathogen. Pathog Dis. 2014;71:292–301.
2. Wendt C, Dietze B, Dietz E, Ruden H. Survival of Acinetobacter baumannii on dry surfaces. J Clin Microbiol. 1997;35:1394–7.
3. Higgins PG, Lehmann M, Wisplinghoff H, Seifert H. gyrB multiplex PCR to differentiate between Acinetobacter calcoaceticus and Acinetobacter genomic species 3. J Clin Microbiol. 2010;48:4592–4.
4. Mari-Almirall M, Cosgaya C, Higgins PG, Van Assche A, Telli M, Huys G, et al. MALDI-TOF/MS identification of species from the Acinetobacter baumannii (Ab) group revisited: inclusion of the novel A. seifertii and A. dijkshoorniae species. Clin Microbiol Infect. 2017;23:210 e1- e9.
5. Al Atrouni A, Joly-Guillou ML, Hamze M, Kempf M. Reservoirs of non-baumannii Acinetobacter species. Front Microbiol. 2016;7:49.
6. Schleicher X, Higgins PG, Wisplinghoff H, Korber-Irrgang B, Kresken M, Seifert H. Molecular epidemiology of Acinetobacter baumannii and Acinetobacter nosocomialis in Germany over a 5-year period (2005-2009). Clin Microbiol Infect. 2013;19:737–42.
7. Wieland K, Chhatwal P, Vonberg RP. Nosocomial outbreaks caused by Acinetobacter baumannii and Pseudomonas aeruginosa: results of a systematic review. Am J Infect Control. 2018;46:643–8.
8. Tacconelli E, Cataldo MA, Dancer SJ, De Angelis G, Falcone M, Frank U, et al. ESCMID guidelines for the management of the infection control measures to reduce transmission of multidrug-resistant gram-negative bacteria in hospitalized patients. Clin Microbiol Infect. 2014;20(Suppl 1):1–55.
9. Schroder C, Schwab F, Behnke M, Breier AC, Maechler F, Piening B, et al. Epidemiology of healthcare associated infections in Germany: nearly 20 years of surveillance. Int J Med Microbiol. 2015;305:799–806.
10. Muller J, Voss A, Kock R, Sinha B, Rossen JW, Kaase M, et al. Cross-border comparison of the Dutch and German guidelines on multidrug-resistant gram-negative microorganisms. Antimicrob Resist Infect Control. 2015;4:7.
11. Horan TC, Andrus M, Dudeck MA. CDC/NHSN surveillance definition of health care-associated infection and criteria for specific types of infections in the acute care setting. Am J Infect Control. 2008;36:309–32.
12. Mahenthiralingam E, Campbell ME, Foster J, Lam JS, Speert DP. Random amplified polymorphic DNA typing of Pseudomonas aeruginosa isolates recovered from patients with cystic fibrosis. J Clin Microbiol. 1996;34:1129–35.
13. Versalovic J, Koeuth T, Lupski JR. Distribution of repetitive DNA sequences in eubacteria and application to fingerprinting of bacterial genomes. Nucleic Acids Res. 1991;19:6823–31.
14. Tenover FC, Arbeit RD, Goering RV, Mickelsen PA, Murray BE, Persing DH, et al. Interpreting chromosomal DNA restriction patterns produced by pulsed-field gel electrophoresis: criteria for bacterial strain typing. J Clin Microbiol. 1995;33:2233–9.
15. Wendel AF, Kaase M, Autenrieth IB, Peter S, Oberhettinger P, Rieber H, et al. Protracted regional dissemination of GIM-1-producing Serratia marcescens in Western Germany. Antimicrob Agents Chemother. 2017;61(3). https://doi.org/10.1128/AAC.01880-16.
16. FastQC. http://www.bioinformatics.babraham.ac.uk/projects/fastqc/. Accessed 22 Oct 2018.
17. Junemann S, Sedlazeck FJ, Prior K, Albersmeier A, John U, Kalinowski J, et al. Updating benchtop sequencing performance comparison. Nat Biotechnol. 2013;31:294–6.
18. Richter M, Rossello-Mora R, Oliver Glockner F, Peplies J. JSpeciesWS: a web server for prokaryotic species circumscription based on pairwise genome comparison. Bioinformatics. 2016;32:929–31.
19. Zankari E, Hasman H, Cosentino S, Vestergaard M, Rasmussen S, Lund O, et al. Identification of acquired antimicrobial resistance genes. J Antimicrob Chemother. 2012;67:2640–4.
20. Higgins PG, Prior K, Harmsen D, Seifert H. Development and evaluation of a core genome multilocus typing scheme for whole-genome sequence-based typing of Acinetobacter baumannii. PLoS One. 2017;12:e0179228.
21. Petersson LP, Albrecht UV, Sedlacek L, Gemein S, Gebel J, Vonberg RP. Portable UV light as an alternative for decontamination. Am J Infect Control. 2014;42:1334–6.
22. Evans BA, Brown S, Hamouda A, Findlay J, Amyes SG. Eleven novel OXA-51-like enzymes from clinical isolates of Acinetobacter baumannii. Clin Microbiol Infect. 2007;13:1137–8.
23. Database ASH. https://www.aktion-sauberehaende.de/fileadmin/ash/downloads/pdf/Compliance/Compliance__Funktionsbereiche_201701_201712_ComplianceReference_Alle_Funktionsbereiche.pdf. Accessed 22 Oct 2018.
24. Wenzel RP, Edmond MB. Infection control: the case for horizontal rather than vertical interventional programs. Int J Infect Dis. 2010;14(Suppl 4):S3–5.
25. Maslow JN, Glaze T, Adams P, Lataillade M. Concurrent outbreak of multidrug-resistant and susceptible subclones of Acinetobacter baumannii affecting different wards of a single hospital. Infect Control Hosp Epidemiol. 2005;26:69–75.
26. ECDC. Antimicrobial resistance surveillance in Europe 2016. Annual report of the European antimicrobial resistance surveillance network (EARS-net). Stockholm: European Centre for Disease Prevention and Control; 2017.
27. Remschmidt C, Schneider S, Meyer E, Schroeren-Boersch B, Gastmeier P, Schwab F. Surveillance of antibiotic use and resistance in intensive care units (SARI). Dtsch Arztebl Int. 2017;114:858–65.
28. Maragakis LL, Perl TM. Acinetobacter baumannii: epidemiology, antimicrobial resistance, and treatment options. Clin Infect Dis. 2008; 46:1254–63.
29. Higgins PG, Dammhayn C, Hackel M, Seifert H. Global spread of carbapenem-resistant Acinetobacter baumannii. J Antimicrob Chemother. 2010;65:233–8.
30. Cohen B, Cohen CC, Loyland B, Larson EL. Transmission of health care-associated infections from roommates and prior room occupants: a systematic review. Clin Epidemiol. 2017;9:297–310.
31. Marchaim D, Navon-Venezia S, Schwartz D, Tarabeia J, Fefer I, Schwaber MJ, et al. Surveillance cultures and duration of carriage of multidrug-resistant Acinetobacter baumannii. J Clin Microbiol. 2007;45:1551–5.
32. Warnke P, Johanna Pohl FP, Kundt G, Podbielski A. Screening for gram -negative bacteria: impact of preanalytical parameters. Sci Rep. 2016;6:30427.
33. Tankovic J, Legrand P, De Gatines G, Chemineau V, Brun-Buisson C, Duval J. Characterization of a hospital outbreak of imipenem-resistant Acinetobacter

baumannii by phenotypic and genotypic typing methods. J Clin Microbiol. 1994;32:2677–81.

34. Kochanek M, Boll B, Shimabukuro-Vornhagen A, Michels G, Barbara W, Hansen D, et al. Staffing needs of an intensive care unit in consideration of applicable hygiene guidelines--an exploratory analysis. Dtsch Med Wochenschr. 2015;140:e136–41.
35. Deurenberg RH, Bathoorn E, Chlebowicz MA, Couto N, Ferdous M, Garcia-Cobos S, et al. Application of next generation sequencing in clinical microbiology and infection prevention. J Biotechnol. 2017;243:16–24.
36. Willems S, Kampmeier S, Bletz S, Kossow A, Kock R, Kipp F, et al. Whole-genome sequencing elucidates epidemiology of nosocomial clusters of Acinetobacter baumannii. J Clin Microbiol. 2016;54:2391–4.

19

Prevalence and molecular characterization of *oqxAB* in clinical *Escherichia coli* isolates from companion animals and humans in Henan Province, China

Baoguang Liu[1†], Hua Wu[1†], Yajun Zhai[1†], Zhipei He[1], Huarun Sun[1], Tian Cai[1], Dandan He[1], Jianhua Liu[1], Shanmei Wang[2], Yushan Pan[1], Li Yuan[1] and Gongzheng Hu[1*]

Abstract

Background: The plasmid-encoded multidrug efflux pump *oqxAB* confers bacterial resistance primarily to olaquindox, quinolones, and chloramphenicol. The aims of this study were to investigate the prevalence of *oqxAB* among *Escherichia coli* isolates from dogs, cats, and humans in Henan, China and the susceptibilities of *E. coli* isolates to common antibiotics.

Methods: From 2012 to 2014, a total of 600 samples which included 400 rectal samples and 200 clinical human specimens were tested for the presence of *E. coli*. All isolates were screened for *oqxAB* genes by PCR and sequencing. The MICs of 11 antimicrobial agents were determined by the broth microdilution method. A total of 30 representative *oqxAB*-positive isolates were subjected to ERIC-PCR and MLST. Additionally, conjugation experiments and southern hybridizations were performed.

Results: Of 270 isolates, 58.5% (62/106) of the isolates from dogs, 56.25% (36/64) of the isolates from cats, and 42.0% (42/100) of the isolates from humans were positive for the *oqxAB*. Olaquindox resistance was found for 85.7%-100% of *oqxAB*-positive isolates. Of *oqxAB*-positive isolates from dogs, cats, and humans, ciprofloxacin resistance was inspected for 85.8%, 59.1%, and 93.8%, respectively. Several *oqxAB*-positive isolates were demonstrated by ERIC-PCR and MLST, and have high similarity. Phylogenetic analysis showed that *oqxAB*-positive isolates could be divided into 7 major clusters. *OqxAB*-positive conjugants were obtained, southern hybridization verified that the *oqxAB* gene complex was primarily located on plasmids.

Conclusion: In conclusion, *oqxAB*-positive isolates were widespread in animals and humans in Henan, China. Carriage of *oqxAB* on plasmids of *E. coli* isolates may facilitate the emergence of multidrug resistant and its transmission via horizontal transfer, and might pose a potential threat to public health.

Keywords: *OqxAB*, Multidrug efflux pump, Antimicrobial susceptibility, Southern hybridization, Conjugation experiments

Background

Nowadays, the growing frequency of antibiotic resistances is a universal problem. Antimicrobial resistance occurs through various mechanisms, such as drug efflux pumps [1, 2]. A novel multidrug efflux pump of Gram-negative bacteria, *oqxAB*, is a member of the root-nodulation-cell-division (RND) family and was first identified as being encoded by a plasmid-mediated gene that conferred resistance to olaquindox [3]. A number of studies have reported on the occurrence of *oqxAB* genes primarily in *Enterobacteriaceae*, including *Escherichia coli*, *Enterobacter cloacae*, and *Klebsiella pneumoniae* isolated from pigs, chickens, humans, and the environment [4–9]. However, the highest positive rates of *oqxAB* were found in surveys of animals in China [6, 7], and the primary reason might be the widespread use of olaquindox as a production animal growth enhancer [10]. It has been convincingly demonstrated that

* Correspondence: yaolilab@163.com
[†]Equal contributors
[1]College of Animal Husbandry and Veterinary Science, Henan Agricultural University, Zhengzhou 450002, China
Full list of author information is available at the end of the article

the genes *oqxAB* can be horizontally transferred among food-borne pathogens and confer antimicrobial resistance for a variety of antimicrobials, such as quinolones, and chloramphenicol [11, 12]. Because these antimicrobials are a significant part of drug therapy to some human bacterial infections, resistance to these drugs could ultimately pose a significant threat to human health. Thus, investigating prevalence of *oqxAB* genes in pathogenic *E. coli* isolates in China is paramount for establishing guidelines for veterinary and human clinical medication use.

Because of the close relationships between humans and their pets, an investigation of multidrug efflux pumps, especially those encoded by the identified *oqxAB* genes, would be of particular significance for medical science. The aim of this study was to investigate the prevalence of the *oqxAB* genes among *E. coli* isolates from companion animals and humans in Henan Province, China.

Methods

Sampling and bacterial isolates

From March 2012 to July 2014, a total of 400 rectal swab samples were recovered from 400 diseased pets (200 dogs and 200 cats) with symptoms of fever, diarrhea and respiratory diseases at three animal hospitals in Henan Agricultural University, ZhengZhou. A total of 200 blood specimens were recovered from adult humans with symptoms of fever, bacteraemia and diarrhea at Henan Provincial People's Hospital during October 2012 and August 2014. All samples were immediately transported to the laboratory under required preservation conditions (in a cooler with ice) within 6 h of collection, and processed within 2 h for samples to test the presence of *E. coli.* The samples were incubated in LB media (Beijing Land Bridge Technology Co., Ltd., Beijing, China) at 37 °C overnight for 16-20 h, and draw the line on MacConkey agar plateafter dipping the culture the next day. All presumptive *E. coli* colonies were identified using VITEK 2 compact automated identification system (BioMérieux, Marcy-I'Etoile, France).

Determination of *oqxAB* and insertion sequences

A total of 270 strains were screened for *oqxA* and *oqxB* genes by PCR using specific primers as described previously [5]. The amplicons obtained were confirmed by sequencing. The whole coding region of the *oqxAB* gene complex in representative strains isolated from three origins were amplified using primer pairs (producing a fragment of 5140 bp), as reported previously [6]. Then, a PCR product was ligated to a pUC18-T vector (TaKaRa Biotechnology, Dalian, China) and bi-directionally sequenced.

Additionally, the association of insertion sequences *ISEcp1* and *IS26* with *oqxA* were also investigated in all *oqxAB*-positive isolates by PCR using the forward primers *ISEcp1*-F (5'-GGCCACGTGCATTTTTTATT-3′) and *IS26*-F (5'-AGCGGTAAATCGTGGAGTGA-3′) and the reverse primer *oqxA*-R (5'-TCAGGTGAATGT TTCCCCAG-3′) located in *oqxA*, respectively. The PCR products were sequenced and analyzed with BLAST program to confirm correct amplification.

Antimicrobial susceptibility testing

The minimum inhibitory concentrations (MICs) of 11 antimicrobial agents (Additional file 1: Table S1) against the 270 *E. coli* strains, were determined by the broth microdilution method according to the recommendations of the Clinical and Laboratory Standards Institute (CLSI) [13]. *E. coli* ATCC 25922 was used as a reference strain for quality control in the MIC determinations. The MIC_{50} and MIC_{90} were determined which represent concentrations of the relevant antibiotics which inhibited growth of the bacteria by 50% or 90% respectively. The MIC breakpoints for most antimicrobial agents were in accordance with CLSI [13, 14]. The MIC breakpoints for olaquindox and mequindox were based on relevant references [3, 4]. But, if CLSI criteria were not available for some antibiotics, the results were interpreted according to criteria of the European Committee on Antimicrobial Susceptibility Testing (EUCAST) [15].

Molecular typing

A total of 30 representative *oqxAB*-positive *E. coli* strains (olaquindox-resistant and MIC≥128 μg/mL) selected randomly from humans, dogs and cats were subjected to Enterobacterial Repetitive Intergenic Consensus PCR (ERIC-PCR) using the primers [16]: ERIC-1, 5'-ATGTA AGCTCCTGGGGATTCAC-3′ and ERIC-2, 5'-AAGTAA GTGACTGGGGTGAGCG-3′. Template DNA was extracted using the conventional boiling method, the sample was heated in a thermocycler at 100 °C for 10 min. Immediately, the sample was incubated at − 20 °C for 15 min, and was centrifuged at 12000×g for 15 min. The size of the amplified fragments ranged from 300 to >3000 bp. A similarity coefficient greater than 80% was used to define the same subtype.

Multilocus Sequence Typing (MLST) of these 30 representatives was done by PCR and sequencing. Seven housekeeping genes (*aspC, clpX, fadD, icdA, lysP, mdh,* and *uidA*) were amplified and sequenced. The corresponding types (STs) were matched using the electronic database on the *E. coli* MLST website (http://www.mlst.net/). A phylogenetic tree for the 7 housekeeping gene sequences was constructed using Phylip 3.69 software and their affinity relationships were described.

The phylogenetic groups of the 30 isolates mentioned above were determined by the multiplex PCR-based method, as previously described [17].

Conjugation experiments

Conjugation experiments were done in LB broth or on filters with rifampicin-resistant *E. coli* C600 as the recipient [18]. Ten *oqxAB*-positive isolates were randomly selected among 30 *oqxAB*-positive strains and used as donor strains. Transconjugants were selected on LB agar or MacConkey plates containing olaquindox (64 μg/mL) and rifampicin (360 μg/mL). Antimicrobial susceptibility and detection of transferred *oqxAB* genes were performed for transconjugants.

Southern hybridization testing

Southern hybridizations were used to test for the plasmid location of *oqxAB*, according to the procedures as described previously [19]. Plasmid DNA from *E. coli* was extracted using a Plasmid Midi Kit (QIAGEN, Valencia, CA), according to the manufacturer's instructions. Plasmid DNA bands were then transferred and cross-linked onto a nylon membrane and were hybridised with digoxigenin (DIG) labeled *oqxAB* probes using the DIG high prime DNA labeling and detection starter kit (Roche, Mannheim, Germany).

Nucleotide sequencing and submission of *oqxAB* sequences

The complete nucleotide sequences of the *oqxAB* genes of *E. coli* strains Q63, M50, and H050 were submitted to GenBank and were given the accession numbers JX294475, JX412478, and JX469117, respectively.

Data and statistical analysis

The 270 isolated strains were categorized as sensitive (S), resistant (R) based on the MIC values and the CLSI interpretive criteria. For statistical analysis, we carried out chi-square test. A two-sided p-value ≤0.05 were considered to be statistically significant. SPSS 20.0 software (IBM, USA) was used for data analysis.

Results

Isolation and identification of *E. coli*

A total of 270 *E. coli* isolates were obtained, which included 106, 64, and 100 *E. coli* respectively collected from 200 rectal swab samples of dogs, 200 rectal swab samples of cats, and 200 clinical blood samples of humans.

Prevalence of *oqxAB*

As shown in Table 1, 58.5% (62/106) of the isolates from dogs, 56.25% (36/64) of the isolates from cats, and 42.0% (42/100) of the isolates from humans were positive for the *oqxAB*. Two common insertion sequences, *ISEcp1* and *IS26*, were investigated in all *oqxAB*-positive isolates. The whole coding region of the *oqxAB* genes were amplified and sequenced. *ISEcp1*, truncated by *IS26*, was also observed in some *oqxAB*-positive strains (77/140, 55.0%). Interestingly, most of the *oqxAB* cassettes of the *oqxAB*-positive strains (111/140, 79.3%) were also flanked by *IS26* similar to composite transposon *Tn6010* of *K. pneumoniae*, which suggested that the dissemination of *oqxAB* among different *E. coli* strains might be mediated by the mobile element. This genetic organization (*ISEcp1-IS26-oqxAB*) is almost identical to corresponding sequences of initially identified plasmid pOLA52 carrying *oqxAB* genes. The *ISEcp1* and *IS26* upstream sequences identified here was the first to be associated with the *oqxAB* genes in *E. coli* from companion animals in Henan Province, China.

Antimicrobial susceptibility testing

The MICs of 11 common antibiotics against the 270 *E. coli* isolates from dogs, cats, and humans are shown in Table 1. The MIC_{50} values of olaquindox for *oqxAB*-positive strains were 4 to 16-fold higher than those for *oqxAB*-negative strains ($p < 0.01$). The MIC_{50} (1-32 μg/mL) and MIC_{90} (4-128 μg/mL) values of mequindox were 2 to 8-fold lower than those for olaquindox against both *oqxAB*-positive and *oqxAB*-negative isolates. The MIC_{50} values of ciprofloxacin and florfenicol for *oqxAB*-positive isolates were all 2 to 16-fold higher than those for *oqxAB*-negative isolates from the three different origins. Importantly, the MIC_{50} values of ceftiofur and ceftriaxone were 4-128 μg/mL for both *oqxAB*-positive and *oqxAB*-negative isolates, which were much higher than the breakpoints (≤2 μg/mL) for susceptibility. By comparison, the MIC_{50} values of colistin were 0.125-0.5 μg/mL, which were much lower than the breakpoints (< 2 μg/mL) for susceptibility. Moreover, all isolates from companion animals were susceptible to colistin.

Among *oqxAB*-positive *E. coli* strains, resistance rates of ≥68.2% were found for six antibiotics (olaquindox, tetracycline, florfenicol, ceftiofur, doxycycline, and ciprofloxacin). The resistance rates of the *oqxAB*-positive isolates from dogs and humans to olaquindox were 85.7% and 90.6%. However, the resistance rates to tetracycline, olaquindox, ciprofloxacin, and gatifloxacin were significantly higher among *oqxAB*-positive isolates than among *oqxAB*-negative isolates ($p < 0.01$). Of a total of 270 *E. coli* strains, more than 59.1% strains were resistant at the same time to ceftiofur and ceftriaxone. However, there were no significant differences in the resistance rates between the *oqxAB*-positive and *oqxAB*-negative strains ($p > 0.05$).

ERIC-PCR, MLST, and phylogenetic analysis

A total of 13 genotypes were identified by ERIC-PCR homology analysis from 30 *oqxAB*-positive *E. coli* isolates. Eight isolates (26.7%) primarily belonged to genotype III, followed by genotypes I (7 strains; 23.3%), VI (5 strains; 16.7%), and VIII (4 strains; 13.3%). The remaining each genotypes were found in 1-3 isolates.

Table 1 Prevalence of *oqxAB* genes and susceptibility to 11 antimicrobial agents

Antibiotics[b]	Isolates from Dogs ($n = 106$)							Isolates from Cats ($n = 64$)							Isolates from Humans ($n = 100$)							Total *P*-value
	oqxAB-positive 58.5% (62//106)[a]			oqxAB-negative 41.5% (44//106)				oqxAB-positive 56.25% (36//64)[a]			oqxAB-negative 43.75% (28/64)				oqxAB-positive 42.0% (42//100)[a]			oqxAB-negative 58.0% (58/100)				
	MIC_{50}	MIC_{90}	R(%)	MIC_{50}	MIC_{90}	R(%)	*P*-value	MIC_{50}	MIC_{90}	R(%)	MIC_{50}	MIC_{90}	R(%)	*P*-value	MIC_{50}	MIC_{90}	R(%)	MIC_{50}	MIC_{90}	R(%)	*P*-value	
COL	0.25	1	0	0.25	1	0	–	0.125	0.25	0	0.03	0.25	0	–	0.25	8	15.6	0.5	4	11.1	0.505	0.674
TET	128	>256	95.2	32	64	72.7	0.054	64	256	100	16	64	80	0.091	32	64	100	16	64	72.2	0.004	6.63×10^{-5}
OLA	64	128	85.7	16	64	18.2	4.77×10^{-5}	64	256	100	2	64	20	0.008	64	128	90.6	4	32	11.1	2.69×10^{-8}	5.79×10^{-12}
MEQ	4	64	–	1	4	–	–	16	64	–	4	16	–	–	32	128	–	4	16	–	–	–
CEF	16	64	73.8	8	32	72.7	0.608	8	32	77.3	8	64	80	0.624	128	>512	96.9	128	>512	94.4	0.595	0.745
CIP	32	>512	85.8	<0.25	4	36.4	0.002	4	32	81.8	0.25	4	30	0.007	64	>512	93.8	8	256	66.7	0.019	1.57×10^{-6}
CRO	64	>512	73.8	8	32	63.6	0.375	4	32	59.1	8	64	70	0.427	64	>512	90.6	128	>512	94.4	0.544	0.704
DOX	64	>128	88.1	8	16	54.5	0.023	32	>128	81.8	4	16	70	0.376	16	128	93.8	16	64	88.9	0.456	0.039
GAT	8	64	57.5	0.5	4	18.2	0.021	2	8	59.1	<0.25	8	30	0.127	16	64	87.5	8	64	44.4	0.001	2.47×10^{-4}
AMK	32	>512	61.9	16	512	81.8	0.191	0.25	8	13.6	2	16	30	0.264	256	512	84.4	256	>512	88.9	0.505	0.144
FFC	16	128	78.6	4	128	63.6	0.257	4	16	68.2	2	16	40	0.138	128	256	87.5	64	256	66.7	0.083	0.016

-, no statistical or not determined

[a]Rate of oqxAB-positive isolates; oqxAB-positive isolates/t total isolates

[b]*COL* colistin, *TET* tetracycline, *OLA* olaquindox, *MEQ* mequindox, *CEF* ceftiofur; *CRO* ceftriaxone, *DOX* doxycyclin, *CIP* ciprofloxacin, *GAT* gatifloxacin, *AMK* amikacin, *FFC* florfenicol

A total of 17 MLST types were identified among these 30 strains from different origins (Fig. 1). Nine novel sequence types (ST3081, ST3082, ST3092, ST3093, ST3094, ST3095, ST3097, ST3098 and ST3099) were detected in this study. The *E. coli* isolates from dogs, cats, and humans that exhibited identical ERIC-PCR patterns also showed coincident sequence types, for instance, M8 and Q26 (ST48), H029 and Q7 (ST10), Q1 and Q5 (ST155). As shown in Fig. 1, *oqxAB*-positive isolates could be divided into seven major clusters.

Phylogenetic analysis showed that 30 representative strains belonged to group A (23.3%), group B1 (30.0%), group B2 (26.7%), and group D (20.0%), respectively.

Transfer of antimicrobial resistance and the *oqxAB* genes

Eight transconjugants were successfully obtained from 10 *oqxAB*-positive isolates by conjugation experiments. Two isolates from dogs did not yield transconjugants. As shown in Table 2, the MICs of mequindox and olaquindox for all transconjugants were similar to those observed for the donors, but were about 8 to 64-fold higher than those observed for the recipients. The *oqxAB* genes in these 8 *oqxAB*-positive isolates and mequindox and olaquindox resistance were transferred in the conjugation experiments.

The MICs of florfenicol for the *oqxAB* transconjugants ranged from 2 to 32 μg/mL, which were about 2 to 32-

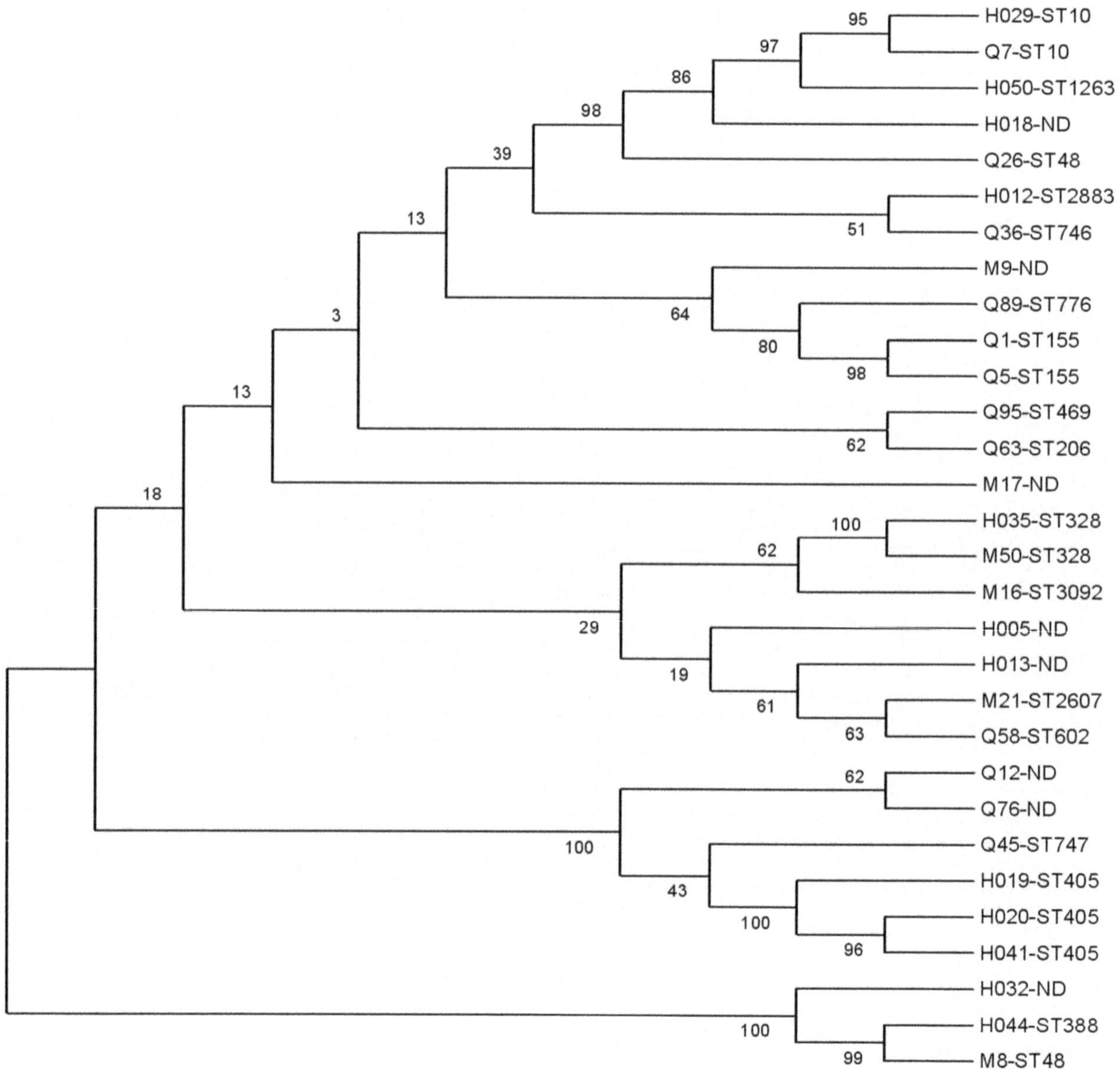

Fig. 1 Dendrogram showing the genetic relatedness of 30 *E. coli* strains (oqxAB-positive). A phylogenetic tree for the seven housekeeping gene sequences was constructed using Phylip 3.69 software and their affinity relationships were described. Notes: Number "M" strains isolated from cats; Number "Q" strains isolated from dogs; Number "H" strains isolated from humans; ND, not determined

Table 2 MICs for transconjugants and characterization of plasmids carrying *oqxAB*

Strains	Donors												Plasmid		Transconjugants							
	origin	MLST	ERIC-PCR	Phylogenetic group	MICs (μg/mL)								Amount	Size(kb)	MICs (μg/mL)							
					COL	OLA	MEQ	CEF	CIP	DOX	AMK	FFC			COL	OLA	MEQ	CEF	CIP	DOX	AMK	FFC
Q1	Dog	ST155	I type	A	0.5	512	32	<0.25	64	32	1	4	ND	ND	0.5	256	32	<0.25	4	2	1	4
M17	Cat	ST48	VI type	B1	0.5	256	64	32	8	32	256	64	1	54~ 108	0.5	256	32	32	1	16	4	8
Q63	Dog	ST206	II type	B2	0.25	256	16	8	1	8	64	128	2	54~ 108	0.5	256	16	<0.25	1	4	8	32
H050	Human	ST1263	VII type	A	0.125	256	64	256	64	16	512	128	2	54~ 108	0.25	512	64	32	8	32	64	16
H029	Human	ST10	V type	D	0.125	256	64	128	32	16	512	64	1	54~ 108	0.125	256	64	64	4	32	32	32
H035	Human	ST328	III type	B2	0.5	256	32	0.5	64	16	1	8	ND	ND	0.25	512	16	32	4	32	8	8
M50	Cat	ST328	III type	D	0.25	256	32	0.25	0.25	4	0.25	4	ND	ND	0.25	256	16	<0.25	<0.25	16	0.25	2
Q76	Dog	ND	IV type	B2	4	512	128	256	16	32	256	128	ND	ND	0.25	256	128	128	2	16	32	16
C600															0.25	4	4	0.06	0.03	0.25	0.5	1

ND **not determined,** ***COL*** **colistin,** ***OLA*** **olaquindox,** ***MEQ*** **mequindox,** ***CEF*** **ceftiofur,** ***DOX*** **doxycycline,** ***CIP*** **ciprofloxacin,** ***AMK*** **amikacin,** ***FFC*** **florfenicol**
C600, recipients in conjugation experiments

fold higher than those obtained for the recipients. The MICs of colistin, ceftiofur, and doxycycline for transconjugants (except of J-M50) and donors were all similar and showed distinct increases as compared to recipients.

Localization of the *oqxAB* genes

Southern hybridization results (Fig. 2b) indicated that *oqxAB* genes were primarily found in plasmids with sizes of approximately 54 kb, except one strain (Q1 isolated from dog). It was remarkable that the isolates Q63 (isolated from dog) and H050 (isolated from human) yielded two distinct signals located on two plasmids of approximately 54 kb and another unknown size (at least 108 kb), respectively.

Discussion

This is the first study to investigate the prevalence and dissemination of *oqxAB* in *E. coli* strains isolated from companion animals and from humans in Henan Province, China. It was surprising to find that there was a high prevalence of *oqxAB* in clinical isolates (51.85%), which was higher than those reported previously in Korea, Denmark, Sweden, Taiwan, and China from food animals and humans (0.06-46.3%) [3–7, 9, 11, 20, 21]. However, the prevalence of *oqxAB*-positive isolates in this study was lower than previously reported in Iran from urinary tract infections in humans (69.1%) [8]. The major reason may be that olaquindox has been extensively used as a growth promoter for food animals in China.

In agreement with previous studies [5, 11], 79.3% of the *oqxAB* cassettes of the *oqxAB*-positive isolates in this study were also flanked by *IS26* element similar to *Tn6010* of *K. pneumoniae*, suggesting that these mobile genetic elements are responsible for the dissemination of *oqxAB* genes [5, 22]. Interestingly, *ISEcp1* truncated by *IS26* was also observed in 55.0% of *oqxAB*-positive strains. This genetic organization (*ISEcp1-IS26-oqxAB*) is almost identical to corresponding sequences of initially identified plasmid pOLA52 carrying *oqxAB* genes [11]. This suggested that *IS26* was inserted in these strains at 3′ end of *ISEcp1* as a result of recombinatorial events.

However, this could not account for the significantly high prevalence of *oqxAB* in clinical isolates from humans, as olaquindox has not been overused for human clinical treatments in China. Probably, *oqxAB* genes were mostly located on transferable plasmids and could diffuse quickly between human and pet isolates through the food chain [5, 6, 11].

Mequindox, a new synthetic quinoxaline 1,4-dioxide (QdNO) derivative, was developed and widely used in China during the 1990s [10]. It has the same effects as olaquindox as a common animal feed additive to increase the economic benefits of breeding industry. In Table 1, the MIC_{50} values of mequindox were much lower than those for olaquindox, which differed from a previous report from China [6], and may have been due to its rare use in pets and its limited use in humans.

Excessive antimicrobial use in animals is considered to be the most important contributor to the selection of resistant bacteria [23]. Recently, the use of colistin should be limited in food and companion animals due to reduce the occurrence of *MCR*-1-harboring strains [24, 25]. Moreover, the use of olaquindox and mequindox also should be limited in food animals due to the high prevalence of the *oqxAB* gene that we found in China [16]. However, this study demonstrates that *oqxAB*-positive isolates were not all resistant to olaquindox, which is inconsistent with previous reports [4–7]. This is most probably related to the regulation of *oqxAB* genes expression. Additionally, it is possible that the *oqxAB* genes are either poorly expressed or not expressed in these isolates.

The diverse ERIC-PCR patterns among certain *oqxAB*-positive strains from different origins implied that the

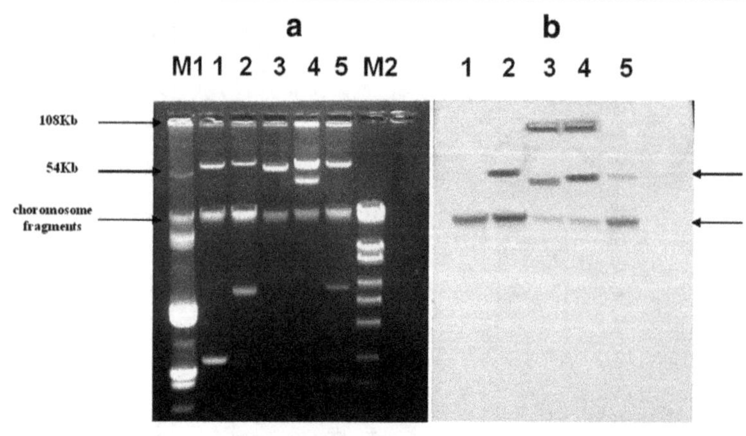

Fig. 2 Agarose gel electrophoresis (**a**) and Southern hybridization (**b**) results for plasmid DNA preparations. Notes: Lanes M1, plasmid Marker V517; 1 to 5, *E. coli* Q1, M17, Q63, H050, and H029, respectively; M2, Marker 5000. Upper arrow in (**b**) indicates plasmid DNA; lower arrow in (**b**) indicates the location of chromosomal DNA and/or sheared plasmid DNA

horizontal transmission of *oqxAB* was a possible determinant rather than the direct clonal dissemination between pets and humans, which is consistent with previous reports [26]. A total of 17 MLST types were identified among these 30 *oqxAB*-positive *E. coli* isolates from different origins, the same STs of *E. coli* strains from different origins suggested clonal dissemination of *oqxAB*-positive strains. Previously, a high prevalence of *oqxAB* in *E. coli* isolates associated with predominantly ST238 was reported [27]. However, recent reports showed that the *oqxAB*-positive *E. coli* isolates in all belonged to ST533 [28]. In view of this, further studies are needed to investigate the possible transmission of *oqxAB* genes by either the food chain or by co-infection.

Conjugation experiments and Southern blotting indicated that *oqxAB* genes were primarily located on plasmids (except of one strain Q1), which is consistent with previous reports [3–7, 11, 29]. However, in this study it was remarkable that there were two hybridization signals found on two plasmids (Fig. 2b) for one isolate from dog and one from human, which indicated they could simultaneously exist on plasmids of different sizes. Meanwhile, *oqxAB* conferred not only resistance to quinoxalines and chloramphenicol, but also reduced susceptibility to other antimicrobials such as florfenicol and fluoroquinolones. Carriage of *oqxAB* on plasmids of *E. coli* isolates may facilitate the emergence of multi-antibiotc resistance and its transmission via horizontal transfer, might pose a potential threat to public health and need for vigilant monitoring these isolates at the human-animal interface.

Conclusion

In conclusion, *oqxAB*-positive isolates were widespread in pets and humans in Henan Province, China, and the prevalence of *oqxAB* genes were significantly higher than what was previously found in other countries or areas. Carriage of *oqxAB* on plasmids of *E. coli* isolates may facilitate the emergence of multidrug resistant and its transmission via horizontal transfer. The same STs of *E. coli* strains from different origins suggested clonal dissemination of *oqxAB*-positive strains. Probably, *oqxAB* genes were mostly located on transferable plasmids and could diffuse quickly between human and pet isolates through the food chain, this needs to further strengthen supervision and resistance detection. More attention should be paid to the transmission of *oqxAB* genes in the future.

Abbreviations

CLSI: Clinical and laboratory standards institute; EUCAST: European committee on antimicrobial susceptibility testing; MICs: Minimum inhibitory concentrations; MLST: Multilocus sequence typing

Acknowledgements

We thank Ling Yang (South China Agricultural University, CHINA) for reading this manuscript and providing helpful feedback, and key laboratory for animal-derived food safety of Henan Province.

Funding

This study was supported by the National Natural Science Foundation of China (Grant no. 31372481) and the Innovative Support Program for Young Teachers in Universities of Tibet (Grant no. QC2015-77).

Authors' contributions

BGL and GZH participated in study conception, design and prepared the manuscript. BGL, YJZ, ZPH, TC, HRS and SMW participated in sample collection and performed the experiments. BGL and HW performed most of the experiments, and reviewed the manuscript. DDH, JHL and YSP analyzed result and reviewed the manuscript. LY and GZH revised the manuscript and coordinated the whole project. All authors read and reviewed the final manuscript. All authors read and approved the final manuscript.

Ethics approval

With regards to our study's use of animals, this study protocol was reviewed and approved by the Henan Agriculture University animal ethics committee, and the experiment was performed in accordance with the regulations and guidelines established by this committee. For experiments involving human participants, this study was approved by the Chinese Academy of Sciences human ethics committee, and was carried out strictly in accordance with the approved guidelines. Informed consent was obtained from the hospital.

Consent for publication

Not applicable.

Competing interests

The authors declare that they have no competing interests.

Author details

[1]College of Animal Husbandry and Veterinary Science, Henan Agricultural University, Zhengzhou 450002, China. [2]Medical Microbiology Laboratory, Henan Provincial People's Hospital, Zhengzhou 450002, China.

References

1. Adewoye L, Topp E, Li XZ. Antimicrobial drug efflux genes and pumps in bacteria of animal and environmental origin. In: Li XZ, Elkins C, Zgurskaya H, editors. Efflux-mediated antimicrobial resistance in bacteria. Adis, Cham: Springer International Publishing; 2016. p. 561–93.
2. Shafaati M, Boroumand M, Nowroozi J, Amiri P, Kazemian H. Correlation between *qacE* and *qacE*Δ*1* efflux pump genes, antibiotic and disinfectant resistant among clinical isolates of *E. coli*. Recent Pa Antiinfec Drug Discov. 2016;11:189–95.
3. Hansen LH, Johannesen E, Burmølle M, Sørensen AH, Sørensen SJ. Plasmid-encoded multidrug efflux pump conferring resistance to olaquindox in *Escherichia coli*. Antimicrob Agents Chemother. 2004;48:3332–7.
4. Hansen LH, Sørensen SJ, Jorgensen HS, Jensen LB. The prevalence of the *OqxAB* multidrug efflux pump amongst olaquindox-resistant *Escherichia coli* in pigs. Microb Drug Resist. 2005;11:378–82.
5. Hong BK, Wang M, Chi HP, Kim EC, Jacoby GA, et al. *OqxAB* encoding a multidrug efflux pump in human clinical isolates of *Enterobacteriaceae*. Antimicrob Agents Chemother. 2009;53:3582–4.
6. Zhao JJ, Chen ZL, Chen S, Deng YT, Liu YH, et al. Prevalence and dissemination of *oqxAB* in *Escherichia coli* isolates from animals, farm workers, and the environment. Antimicrob Agents Chemother. 2010;54:4219–24.
7. Yuan JY, Xu XG, Guo QL, Zhao X, Ye XY, et al. Prevalence of the *oqxAB* gene complex in *Klebsilla pneumoniae* and *Escherichia coli* clinical isolates. J Antimicrob Chemother. 2012;67:1655–9.

8. Tayebi Z, Heidari H, Kazemian H, Ghafoori SM, Boroumandi S, et al. Comparison of quinolone and beta-lactam resistance among *Escherichia coli* strains isolated from urinary tract infections. Infez Med. 2016;24:326–30.
9. Kao CY, Wu HM, Lin WH, Tseng CC, Yan JJ, et al. Plasmid-mediated quinolone resistance determinants in quinolone-resistant *Escherichia coli* isolated from patients with bacteremia in a university hospital in Taiwan, 2001-2015. Sci Rep. 2016;6:32281.
10. Huang XJ, Ihsan A, Wang X, Dai MH, Wang YL, et al. Long-term dose-dependent response of Mequindoxon aldosterone, corticosterone and five steroidogenic enzyme mRNAs in the adrenal of male rats. Toxicol Lett. 2009;191:167–73.
11. Norman A, Hansen LH, She Q, Sørensen SJ. Nucleotide sequence of pOLA52: a conjugative IncX1 plasmid from *Escherichia coli* which enables biofilm formation and multidrug efflux. Plasmid. 2008;60:59–74.
12. Hansen LH, Jensen LB, Sørensen HI, Sørensen SJ. Substrate specificity of the *oqxAB* multidrug resistance pump in *Escherichia coli* and selected enteric bacteria. J Antimicrob Chemother. 2007;60:145–7.
13. Clinical and Laboratory Standards Institute. Performance standards for antimicrobial disk and dilution Suseptibility tests for bacteria isolated from animals; approved standard-Fouth edition. CLSI document VET01-A4. Wayne, PA: CLSI; 2013.
14. Clinical and Laboratory Standards Institute. Performance standards for antimicrobial susceptibility testing; twenty-six informational supplement. CLSI document M100-S26. Wayne, PA: CLSI; 2016.
15. The European Committee on Antimicrobial Susceptibility Testing (EUCAST). Breakpoint tables for interpretation of MICs and zone diameters. Version 7.0. 2017. [updated 2017.1.1]. Available from: http://www.eucast.org/clinical_breakpoints/.
16. Li XZ, Nikaido H. Efflux-mediated drug resistance in bacteria. Drugs. 2004;64:159–204.
17. Clermont O, Bonacorsi S, Bingen E. Rapid and simple determination of the *Escherichia coli* phylogenetic group. Appl Environ Microbiol. 2000;66:4555–8.
18. Chen L, Chen ZL, Liu JH, Zeng ZL, Ma JY, et al. Emergence of *RmtB* methylase-producing *Escherichia coli* and *Enterobacter cloacae* isolates from pigs in China. J Antimicrob Chemother. 2007;59:880–5.
19. Liu BT, Wang XM, Liao XP, Sun J, Zhu HQ, et al. Plasmid-mediated quinolone resistance determinants *oqxAB* and *aac(6')-Ib-cr* and extended-spectrum-β-lactamase gene $bla_{CTX\text{-}M\text{-}24}$ co-located on the same plasmid in one *Escherichia coli* strain from China. J Antimicrob Chemother. 2011;66:1638–9.
20. Ciesielczuk H, Hornsey M, Choi V, Woodford N, Wareham DW. Development and evaluation of a multiplex PCR for eight plasmid-mediated quinolone-resistance determinants. J Med Microbiol. 2013;62:1823–7.
21. Liu BT, Liao XP, Yang SS, Wang XM, Li LL, et al. Detection of mutations in the *gyrA* and *parC* genes in *Escherichia coli* isolates carrying plasmid-mediated quinolone resistance genes from diseased food-producing animals. J Med Microbiol. 2012;61:1591–9.
22. Jacoby GA, Strahilevitz J, Hooper DC. Plasmid-mediated quinolone resistance. Microbiol Spectr. 2014;2:207–10.
23. Thomas MG, Smith AJ, Tilyard M. Rising antimicrobial resistance: a strong reason to reduce excessive antimicrobial consumption in New Zealand. New Zeal Med J. 2014;127:72–84.
24. Huang XH, Yu LF, Chen XJ, Zhi CP, Yao X, et al. High prevalence of Colistin resistance and *mcr-1* gene in *Escherichia coli* isolated from food animals in China. Front Microbiol. 2017;8:562.
25. Liu YY, Wang Y, Walsh TR, Yi LX, Zhang R, et al. Emergence of plasmid-mediated colistin resistance mechanism *MCR-1* in animals and human beings in China: a microbiological and molecular biological study. Lancet Infect Dis. 2016;16:161–8.
26. Macedo NR, Oliveira SR, Lage AP, Santos JL, Araújo MR, et al. ERIC-PCR genotyping of Haemophilus parasuis isolates from Brazilian pigs. Vet J. 2011;188:362–4.
27. Dotto G, Giacomelli M, Grilli G, Ferrazzi V, Carattoli A, et al. High prevalence of *oqxAB* in *Escherichia coli* isolates from domestic and wild lagomorphs in Italy. Microb Drug Resist. 2014;20:118–23.
28. Chen Y, Sun J, Liao XP, Shao Y, Li L, et al. Impact of enrofloxacin and florfenicol therapy on the spread of *oqxAB* gene and intestinal microbiota in chickens. Vet Microbiol. 2016;192:1–9.
29. Fang LX, Li XP, Li L, Li SM, Liao XP, et al. Co-spread of metal and antibiotic resistance within ST3-IncHI2 plasmids from *E. coli* isolates of food-producing animals. Sci Rep. 2016;6:25312.

20

Environmental colonization and onward clonal transmission of carbapenem-resistant *Acinetobacter baumannii* (CRAB) in a medical intensive care unit: the case for environmental hygiene

Deborah H. L. Ng[1], Kalisvar Marimuthu[1,2*], Jia Jun Lee[1], Wei Xin Khong[1], Oon Tek Ng[1*], Wei Zhang[3], Bee Fong Poh[3], Pooja Rao[4], Maya Devi Rajinder Raj[4], Brenda Ang[1,2] and Partha Pratim De[4]

Abstract

Background: In May 2015, we noticed an increase in carbapenem-resistant *Acinetobacter baumannii* (CRAB) infections in the Medical Intensive Care Unit (MICU). To investigate this, we studied the extent of environmental contamination and subsequent onward clonal transmission of CRAB.

Methods: We conducted a one-day point prevalence screening (PPS) of the patients and environment in the MICU. We screened patients using endotracheal tube aspirates and swabs from nares, axillae, groin, rectum, wounds, and exit sites of drains. We collected environmental samples from patients' rooms and environment outside the patients' rooms. CRAB isolates from the PPS and clinical samples over the subsequent one month were studied for genetic relatedness by whole genome sequencing (WGS).

Results: We collected 34 samples from seven patients and 244 samples from the environment. On the day of PPS, we identified 8 CRAB carriers: 3 who screened positive and 5 previously known clinical infections. We detected environmental contamination in nearly two-thirds of the rooms housing patients with CRAB. WGS demonstrated genetic clustering of isolates within rooms but not across rooms. We analysed 4 CRAB isolates from clinical samples following the PPS. One genetically-related CRAB was identified in the respiratory sample of a patient with nosocomial pneumonia, who was admitted to the MICU five days after the PPS.

Conclusion: The extensive environmental colonization of CRAB by patients highlights the importance of environmental hygiene. The transmission dynamics of CRAB needs further investigation.

Keywords: Colonization, Carbapenem-resistant *Acinetobacter baumannii*, Intensive care unit, Whole genome sequencing

Background

Carbapenem-resistant *Acinetobacter baumannii* (CRAB) has been emerging as a healthcare threat in recent years, owing to its ability to survive in the environment for prolonged periods and to acquire multiple antibiotic resistance mechanisms [1, 2]. There is a high prevalence of *A. baumannii* in the Asia-Pacific region, with hospitals reporting rates of CRAB infection from 50% to over 90% in countries such as Vietnam and Singapore [3]. A survey of multidrug-resistant organisms (MDROs) across public hospitals in Singapore in 2006 found that the incidence density of all CRAB isolates was 0.59 per 1000 inpatient-days, while the incidence density in the intensive care unit (ICU) increased more than 4-fold to 2.78 per 1000 ICU inpatient-days [4]. More recently, Cai et al. reported that 71.9% of all *Acinetobacter* spp. implicated in healthcare-associated infections were carbapenem non-susceptible [5].

* Correspondence: kalisvar_marimuthu@ttsh.com.sg; Oon_Tek_Ng@ttsh.com.sg
[1]Institute of Infectious Diseases and Epidemiology, Tan Tock Seng Hospital, 11 Jalan Tan Tock Seng, Singapore 304833, Singapore
Full list of author information is available at the end of the article

Point-prevalence studies have been useful in investigating the extent of colonization with MDROs in various healthcare settings [6]. An investigation into an outbreak of *A. baumannii* in an ICU found that environmental colonization was present in 39.3% of swabs taken, of which 7.1% had similar antibiotic sensitivity profiles to the outbreak strain [7]. Another study investigating an outbreak of *Pseudomonas aeruginosa* in a neonatal ICU demonstrated that although majority of the clinical isolates were identical, the additional use of whole genome sequencing (WGS) demonstrated that some of the isolates were not in fact related to the outbreak strain despite having the same susceptibility pattern [8]. These studies highlight the limitation of using the phenotypic method in defining relatedness of isolates.

In May 2015, the prevalence of CRAB infections in the medical intensive care unit (MICU) of a teaching hospital in Singapore increased from a baseline rate of about 0.32 cases per 1000 patient days, to 0.55 cases per 1000 patient days. To investigate the surge, we conducted this study to (i) estimate the prevalence of CRAB among patients in the MICU, (ii) identify the level of environmental contamination within the unit and (iii) investigate the role of environmental contamination in horizontal transmission of CRAB.

Methods

Setting

We conducted a one-day point prevalence screening (PPS) and one-month surveillance of clinical cultures for CRAB in the MICU of Tan Tock Seng Hospital, a teaching hospital in Singapore. The hospital has 1500 beds and houses four intensive care units, namely the MICU, Surgical Intensive Care Unit, Neurological Intensive Care Unit and the Coronary Care Unit. The MICU contains a total of 6 high-dependency care beds and 12 single-room intensive care beds, of which 3 are negative-pressure rooms.

Study procedures

The study comprised two components: the first was a one-day PPS of patients who were in the MICU on the day of screening (23 July 2015); while the second component was a one-month surveillance of clinical cultures of CRAB isolated from patients within the MICU in the month of July 2015 (Fig. 1).

During the PPS, we collected patients' endotracheal tube (ETT) aspirates and swabs from their nares, axillae, groin, wounds and exit sites of drains, if any. Swabs were not taken from patients who had been in the MICU for less than 24 h or who were known CRAB carriers.

Environmental swabs were taken from all the patient rooms in the MICU, regardless of whether they were occupied by patients at the time. The following surfaces were swabbed: physiological monitor terminals, bedside rails, automatic door buttons, infusion pumps, resuscitation bags, ventilator panels, ventilator humidifiers, suction bottles, stethoscopes, patients' lockers, all-purpose tables, sink faucet openings, and sink drainage sites. Swabs were also taken from the MICU environment outside the patients' rooms. This included the computer keyboards and 'mice', cleaned ventilators, equipment carts and emergency carts.

We followed the PPS with a one-month surveillance for clinical cultures to detect onward clonal transmission. The Department of Laboratory Medicine cultured, identified and stored all CRAB isolates from existing and newly admitted MICU patients.

Clinical data collection

We investigated genetic linkage by collecting data from electronic medical records on ward movements of involved patients, overlap of healthcare workers caring for the patients during their stay in the MICU and sharing of any medical equipment.

Specimen collection and culture

All samples were collected by two microbiology doctors and eight infection control nurses who were trained and supervised by the microbiology doctors. Sterile cotton swabs were moistened with sterile water and were rolled over the surface five times. Each swab was collected in Amie's transport media. The samples were inoculated onto MacConkey agar and incubated at 37 °C for 48 h. A meropenem disc (10 µg, BD Diagnostics, USA) was placed on each plate to select for carbapenem-resistant organisms. Matrix-assisted laser desorption/ionization time-of-flight mass spectrometry (MALDI-TOF MS, Bruker Daltonics, GmbH, Germany) was performed on colonies growing next to the meropenem disc after overnight incubation to identify CRAB. Susceptibility testing was performed on all isolates of *A. baumannii* using the Kirby –Bauer method and those with a meropenem zone ≤14 mm were interpreted as resistant based on the Clinical Laboratory and Standards Institute criteria (M100- S22) [9].

Whole genome sequencing, species identification and strain typing

Sequencing libraries for each isolate were prepared according to the manufacturer's recommendation using the Illumina Nextera XT kit (Illumina Inc., USA). The Illumina FastQ files are in the process of being deposited into the GenBank database. De novo assembly of the Illumina reads was performed using SPAdes Genome Assembler [10]. Bacterial species were identified using Kraken [11]. Multilocus STs were identified using SRST2 [12]. Isolates with species discordance comparing phenotypic with genotypic speciation were excluded from further analysis.

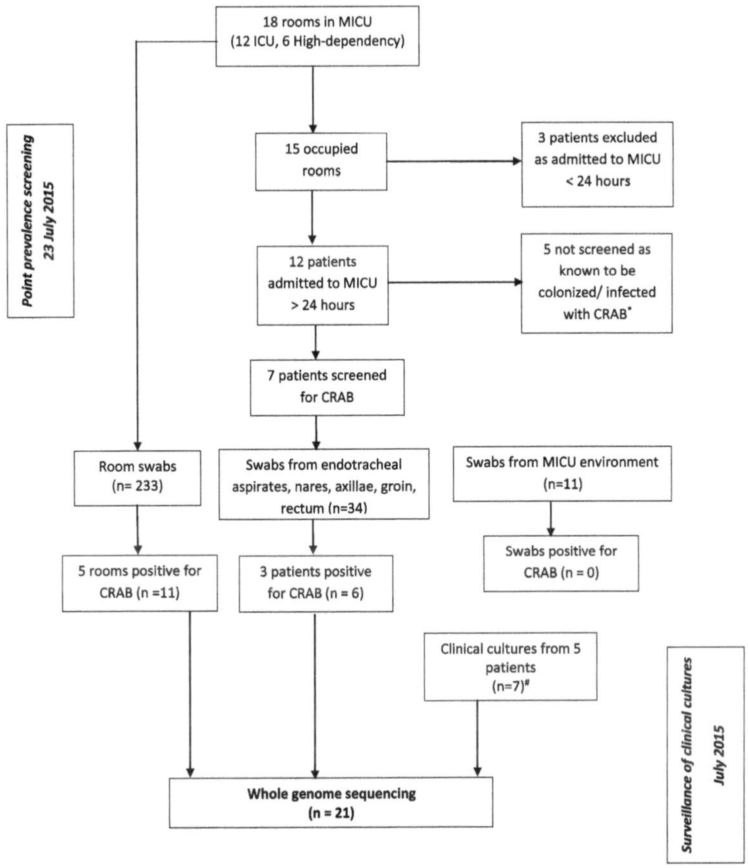

Fig. 1 Flowchart of swabs collected from the MICU. Legend: *MICU*, medical intensive care unit; *CRAB* carbapenem-resistant *Acinetobacter baumannii*, *PPS* point prevalence screening, *n* = number of swabs. *All isolates were not available for sequencing. #4 out of the 7 isolates were available for sequencing

Bacterial core genome analysis and determination of transmission clusters

The program Parsnp was used to generate core genome alignments (i.e. conserved orthologous regions present in all included genomes) for all isolates [13]. As previously described, Parsnp screens and excludes sequences based on a threshold MUMi distance. Input for this alignment was the de novo assemblies from the bacterial isolates, as well as a reference sequence available from GenBank (Accession Number: NC_009085.1). The core nucleotide alignments were used as input for Gubbins to exclude putative single-nucleotide polymorphisms (SNPs) arising from recombination [14]. Sequences were then aligned to be concatenated into an artificial 'genome assembly,' which was used to create a Maximum Likelihood phylogenetic tree with 100 replicates for bootstrap value calculation.

To determine transmission clusters of highest confidence, we defined transmission clusters as isolates that had pair-wise SNP distance less than the pair-wise SNP threshold [15]. The pair-wise SNP threshold was defined as the maximum intra-patient SNP count comparing all repeated isolates with identical species and strain type from the same patient [16]. The pair-wise SNP threshold implemented for this study based on the maximum pair-wise SNP count between CRAB isolates isolated from the same patient (excluding environmental samples) was equal or less than 11 SNP.

Results

There were fifteen patients in the MICU on the day of screening, with three unoccupied rooms. (Figure 2) Five patients were not swabbed as they were known to have CRAB, while another three were excluded from screening as they had been admitted to the MICU for less than 24 h. We collected 34 swabs from the remaining seven patients, 233 swabs from the environment of all 18 rooms in the MICU and 11 swabs from the external environment as demonstrated in Fig. 1.

Three of the 7 screened patients were found to be colonized with CRAB, identified from six surveillance swabs (1 ETT aspirate, 2 nasal swabs, 2 axillary swabs and 1 groin swab). All the patients who were colonised, infected or screened positive for CRAB were mechanically ventilated. Of the eight rooms occupied by patients colonized or infected with CRAB, there was environmental contamination present in 28% (5/18) of the rooms. None of the

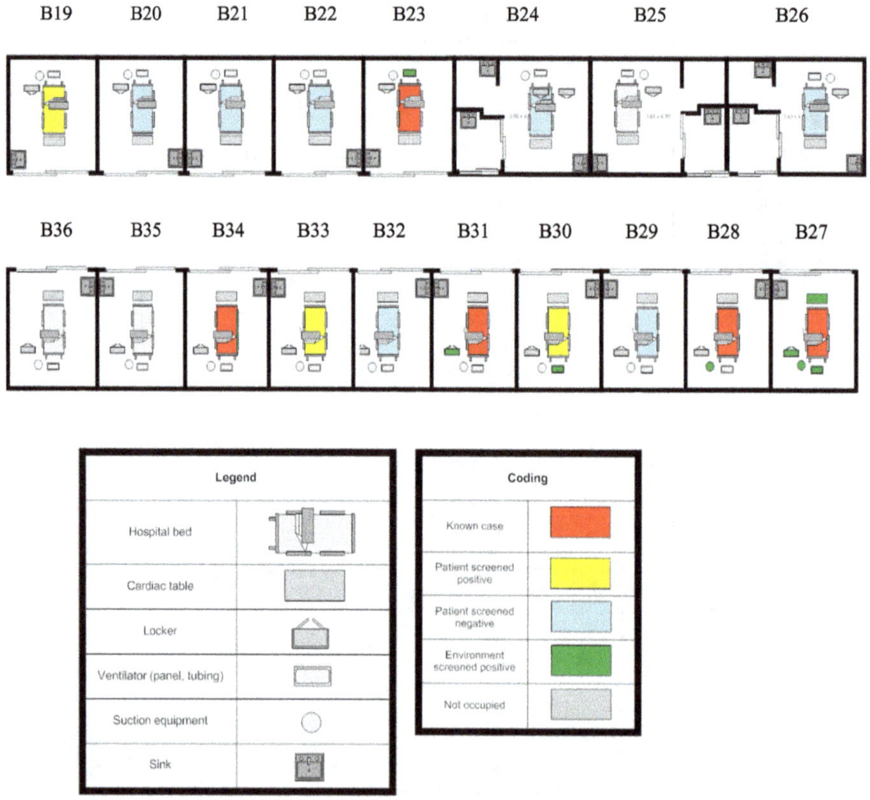

Fig. 2 Floor plan of the MICU showing the distribution patients and CRAB

swabs taken from door switches, sinks or faucet openings were positive for CRAB. The 17 positive screening swabs were sent for sequencing. All the swabs from the external environment were negative for CRAB.

Within the one-month period of PPS, CRAB was isolated from 7 clinical cultures from 5 patients. Of these, 4 isolates from 4 patients were available and sent for sequencing.

WGS results and clinical correlation

A total of 21 isolates were sent for WGS. Results of the WGS (Fig. 3) demonstrated that among patients whose rooms were colonised with CRAB, the isolates from the patient were clonal with their environment but differed between rooms. (Figure 2) Although isolates ACBA-6, 7 and 10 from bed (B) 27 showed intermediate susceptibility to ampicillin-sulbactam, while isolates ACBA-8 and 9 were pan-resistant, there was no other genotypic-phenotypic speciation discordance as shown by the antimicrobial susceptibility testing results in Table 1.

The pair-wise SNP threshold was as follows (Fig. 3):

B27: ACBA-6, ACBA-7, ACBA-8, ACBA-9, ACBA-10; 0–5 SNP.
B28: ACBA-12, ACBA-13; 4 SNP.
B30: ACBA-18, ACBA-20, ACBA-21, ACBA-22, ACBA-23; 0–11 SNP.

One of the 4 CRAB clinical isolates from B32 (ACBA-16) collected during the one-month surveillance revealed genetic relatedness with CRAB isolates from the patient and environment in B30, with a pair-wise SNP of one nucleotide. They had similar carbapenem resistance mechanisms (blaOXA-23). Further investigations showed that patient from B30 had been in the MICU for 54 days and was screened positive during the PPS. The other patient was admitted to the MICU after the screening and had been in the MICU for 3 days before developing pneumonia due to CRAB. These two patients were both in the MICU between 28 and 30 July 2015 but did not have previous admissions in the hospital that overlapped in time. Medical equipment were not shared between them; however, there was overlap of healthcare workers (two doctors and one nurse) who cared for both patients during this 3-day period.

Discussion

This one-day PPS found that the overall prevalence of CRAB in the MICU was 53% (8/15 patients). Environmental colonization was present in over a quarter of the room in the MICU, but only present in rooms occupied by patients with CRAB. We also found evidence for onward clonal transmission of CRAB; however, the exact mode of transmission needs further investigation.

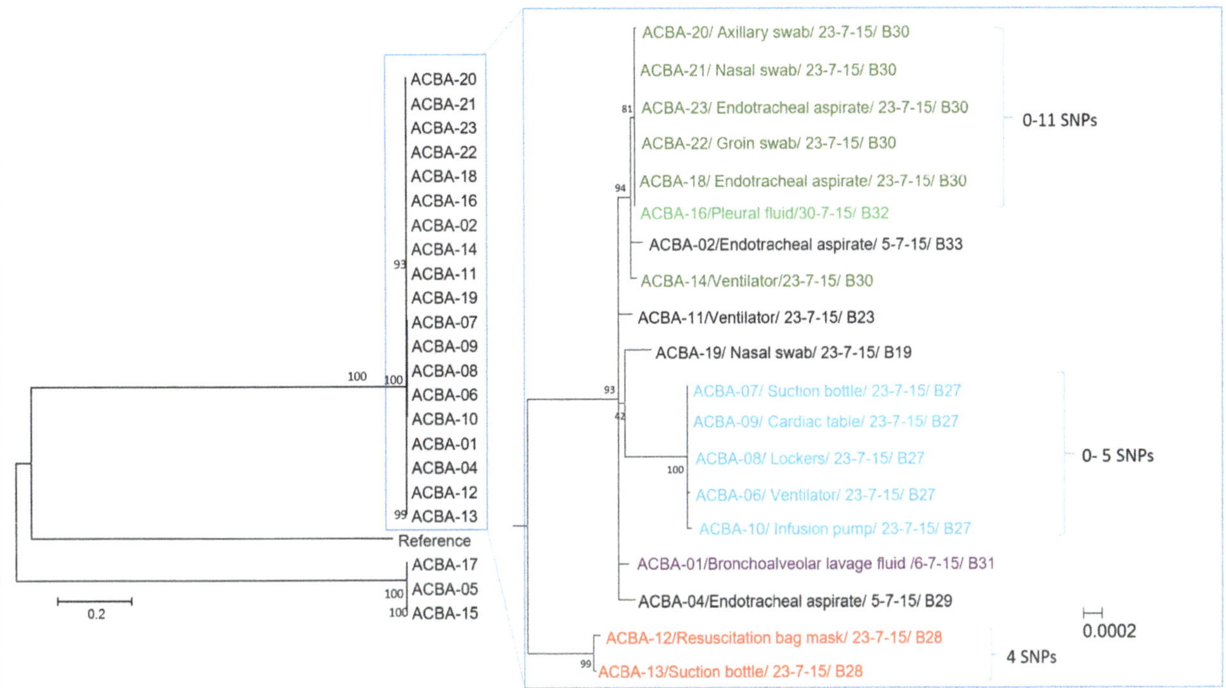

Fig. 3 Whole genome sequencing of clinical and screening isolates of CRAB. Labels were configured to represent: Specimen number/specimen type/date of collection/bed number. Legend: *ACBA Acinetobacter baumannii, SNPs* single nucleotide polymorphisms

There appears to be a correlation to the proximity of the equipment to the patient as items such as ventilators, control panels, infusion pumps and bedrails were more likely to be contaminated. This may be due to the fact that intubated patients may be undergoing aerosol-generating procedures or suctioning. A recent study also found that nebulized medication administration (NMA) and bronchoscope with NMA generated significantly higher levels of aerosols, compared to other activities such as bronchoscopy alone or non-invasive ventilation [17]. In contrast, door switches, sinks or faucet openings, which were situated further away from the head of the bed, were all negative for CRAB, as were the swabs from the external environment. In addition, the areas positive for CRAB were also high-touch surface areas, as defined by Carling et al [18]. All environmental surfaces are currently cleaned with granular sodium dichloroisocyanurate (NaDCC) diluted to 5000 ppm (ppm) as well as Mikro Quat® once a week. High-touch surface areas are cleaned on a daily basis while low-touch surface areas are cleaned when the patients are transferred out of the MICU. Reusable equipment such as infusion pumps and oximetry probes are wiped down with alcohol wipes after each patient use. As each patient has their own dedicated blood pressure cuff, they are cleaned with alcohol wipes after the patient is transferred out of the MICU.

According to local infection control policy, any staff member entering a patient's room is required to don personal protective equipment prior to entering and to doff prior to exiting the room, regardless of whether the patient is known to have colonization or infection with any MDR organisms. In the MICU, alcohol-based hand rub is placed at the foot of the patient's bed in close proximity to the exit, which facilitates the use of the hand rub prior to exiting the room. This may explain why the door switches and external environment were negative for CRAB. Staff are also encouraged to do hand hygiene with alcohol-based hand rub rather than water with disinfectant soap. Following the one-day PPS, strict contact precautions were enforced for patients known to be colonized or infected with CRAB. Surveillance rates of CRAB over the next 3 months reduced to the baseline average of 0.38 cases per 1000-patient days.

Although *A. baumannii* is ubiquitous in the environment, it is known to have a predilection for water sources [19]. A study conducted in an ICU in Japan reported that an outbreak of *A. baumannii* had been caused by tap water from sinks colonized with the organism and was transmitted through oral care using tap water [19]. In our study, all the swabs taken from sink faucet openings and drain holes were negative for CRAB. This may be due to local infection control procedures which prohibit staff from discarding body fluids or water that has been used for the patient down the sink. In the MICU, all contaminated fluid is disposed of in the sluice. However, compliance to local policies also

Table 1 Antibiotic susceptibility of isolates sent for WGS

	Swab	Ceftazidime	Cefepime	Ampicillin-sulbactam	Piperacillin-tazobactam	Meropenem	Gentamicin	Amikacin	Ciprofloxacin	Cotrimoxazole
ACBA 1	Locker	R	R	R	R	R	R	R	R	R
ACBA 2	Endotracheal tube aspirate	R	R	I	R	R	R	R	R	R
ACBA 4	Pleural fluid	R	R	R	R	R	R	R	R	R
ACBA 6	Ventilator panel	R	R	I	R	R	R	R	R	R
ACBA 7	Suction bottle connector	R	R	I	R	R	R	R	R	R
ACBA 8	Locker	R	R	R	R	R	R	R	R	R
ACBA 9	All-purpose table	R	R	R	R	R	R	R	R	R
ACBA 10	Infusion pump	R	R	I	R	R	R	R	R	R
ACBA 11	Heat and moisture exchanger	R	R	R	R	R	R	R	R	R
ACBA 12	Resuscitation bag-face mask connector valve	R	R	R	R	R	R	R	R	S
ACBA 13	Suction bottle connector	R	R	R	R	R	R	R	R	S
ACBA 16	Pleural fluid	R	R	R	R	R	R	R	R	R
ACBA 17	Axilla	R	R	R	R	R	R	R	R	R
ACBA 14	Ventilator panel	R	R	R	R	R	R	R	R	R
ACBA 18	Tracheal aspirate	R	R	R	R	R	R	R	R	R
ACBA 19	Nasal	R	R	R	R	R	R	R	R	R
ACBA 20	Axilla	R	R	R	R	R	R	R	R	R
ACBA 21	Nasal	R	R	R	R	R	R	R	R	R
ACBA 22	Groin	R	R	R	R	R	R	R	R	R
ACBA 23	Ventilator humidifier	R	R	R	R	R	R	R	R	R

need to be confirmed with audits of disposal methods and adherence to hand hygiene.

Similarly, our study also found that although antibiotic susceptibility of our isolates were all similar, WGS found that majority of them were not related across rooms. This shows that it is insufficient to rely on phenotypic patterns alone in determining relatedness of the isolates. WGS was instrumental in identifying one case of linked transmission between two patients in the MICU. The two patients did not share a room or medical equipment in the MICU. However, three healthcare workers had close contact with both patients. This occurred despite the background hand hygiene compliance rate averaging 72.5% and the mean compliance to contact precautions at 77.5% for the year of 2015. A CRAB outbreak investigation in a Korean ICU 10.9% of healthcare workers' hands were colonised with CRAB, suggesting that healthcare workers may inadvertently be responsible for horizontal transmission within the ICU [20]. Longitudinal studies, similar to those conducted by Price et al. [21] for MRSA, may help define the modes of transmission of CRAB and facilitate design of appropriate infection prevention and control measures.

This study demonstrates the limitations of a one-day PPS in investigating horizontal transmission, since the PPS only provides a snapshot of the extent of the spread of CRAB within the MICU. If the additional clinical isolate had not been sent for WGS, it would have likely been concluded that there was no horizontal transmission within the MICU. Further surveillance is required to understand the transmission dynamics and extent of horizontal transmission, as well as compliance rates to the use of personal protective equipment.

Another limitation of the study was the exclusion of patients who had been admitted for less than 24 h to the MICU which may have resulted in selection bias and underestimated the CRAB prevalence in the MICU by omitting patients who were admitted with CRAB. However, this is less likely to underestimate the rate of CRAB acquisition in the MICU as CRAB acquisition during such a short period of time would be rare.

One strength of the study is the large number of screening samples collected from each patient and the environment, with an average of five swabs collected from each patient. In a study of patients who were known to be carriers of multidrug-resistant *A.baumannii* and underwent screening for carriage from six sites (nostrils, pharynx, skin, rectum, wounds and endotracheal aspirates), the sensitivity of a single site and the sensitivity of six sites was only 55% [22]. Another study which surveyed 160 ICU patients who had at least one positive clinical culture found that a combination of four swabs from tracheal aspirates, rectum, sternal skin and urine identified up to 85% of patients known to have CRAB [23]. We also took nasal swabs from our patients, which were positive in two of the three patients screened to be positive for CRAB, suggesting that this may also be an important screening site. As an additional 20% of patients were found to be carriers of CRAB from this one-day surveillance screening alone, our findings also suggest that there may be a need to carry out regular screening of patients on admission and discharge from the MICU to identify any ongoing transmission.

Conclusion

In conclusion, this study demonstrates that in a setting where CRAB is endemic, environmental contamination is common if patients are also colonized or infected with CRAB. Furthermore, longitudinal screening of patients in an environment where patients are at high risk for acquisition of CRAB, combined with WGS can be a powerful tool in discerning nosocomial CRAB transmission and informing infection control decisions. We are currently piloting the use of real-time WGS combined with epidemiological linkage analysis to track the transmission of CRAB as they emerge, to allow for early institution of infection control measures and reducing further transmission.

Abbreviations

B: Bed; CRAB: Carbapenem-resistant *Acinetobacter baumannii*; ETT: Endotracheal tube; ICU: Intensive Care Unit; MDRO: Multi-drug resistant organisms; MICU: Medical Intensive Care Unit; NaDCC: sodium dichloroisocyanurate; NMA: Nebulised medication administration; ppm: parts per million; PPS: Point prevalence screening; SNP: Single-nucleotide polymorphism; WGS: Whole genome sequencing

Funding

Grant support was provided by the Seed Funding by CDC centre grant, NMRC Clinician-Scientist Individual Research Grant (NMRC/CIRG/1463/2016), MOE Tier 2: New Delhi Metallo-Beta-Lactamase: A global multi-centre, whole-genome study (MOE2015-T2-2-096) and NMRC Collaborative Grant: Collaborative Solutions Targeting Antimicrobial Resistance Threats in Health Systems (CoSTAR-HS) (NMRC CGAug16C005). Ng OT was supported by the NMRC Clinician Scientist Award (NMRC/CSA-INV/0002/2016). The funders had no role in study design, data collection and analysis, decision to publish, or preparation of the manuscript.

Authors' contributions

KM, BA and PD conceived the presented idea. WZ, BP, PR, MR collected the data and samples. PR and MR also processed the samples collected. JL and WK were responsible for analysis and sequencing of the samples. DN wrote the manuscript with support from KM and NOT. All authors read and approved the final manuscript.

Competing interests

The authors report no conflict of interest relevant to this article.

Author details
[1]Institute of Infectious Diseases and Epidemiology, Tan Tock Seng Hospital, 11 Jalan Tan Tock Seng, Singapore 304833, Singapore. [2]National University of Singapore, 21 Lower Kent Ridge Road, Singapore 119077, Singapore. [3]Infection Control Unit, Tan Tock Seng Hospital, 11 Jalan Tan Tock Seng, Singapore 304833, Singapore. [4]Department of Laboratory Medicine, Tan Tock Seng Hospital, 11 Jalan Tan Tock Seng, Singapore 304833, Singapore.

References

1. Hota B. Contamination, disinfection, and cross-colonization: are hospital surfaces reservoirs for nosocomial infection? Clin Infect Dis. 2004 Oct 15; 39(8):1182–9.
2. Towner KJ. *Acinetobacter*: an old friend, but a new enemy. J Hosp Infect. 2009 Dec;73(4):355–63.
3. Suwantarat N, Carroll KC. Epidemiology and molecular characterisation of multidrug-resistant gram-negative bacteria in Southeast Asia. Antimicrob Resist Infect Control. 2016;5:15. https://doi.org/10.1186/s13756-016-0115-6.
4. Hsu L-Y, Tan T-Y, Jureen R, et al. Antimicrobial drug resistance in Singapore hospitals. Emerg Inf Dis. 2007;13(12):1944–7.
5. Cai Y, Venkatachalam I, Tee NW, et al. Prevalence of healthcare-associated infections and antimicrobial use among adult inpatients in Singapore acute-care hospitals: results from the first national point prevalence survey. Clin Inf Dis. 2017;64(2):S61–7.
6. Lim CJ, Cheng AC, Kennon J, et al. Prevalence of multidrug-resistant organisms and risk factors for carriage in long-term care facilities: a nested case-control study. J Antimicrob Chemother. 2014;69(7):1972–80.
7. Aygun G, Demirkiran O, Utku T, et al. Environmental contamination during a carbapenem-resistant *Acinetobacter baumannii* outbreak in an intensive care unit. J Hosp Inf. 2002;52(4):259–62.
8. Davis RJ, Jensen SO, Van Hal S, et al. Whole genome sequencing in real-time investigation and management of a *Pseudomonas aeruginosa* outbreak on a neonatal intensive care unit. Infection Control & Hospital Epidemiology. 2015;36(9):1058–64. https://doi.org/10.1017/ice.2015.133.
9. Clinical and Laboratory Standards Institute. Performance standards for antimicrobial susceptibility testing; CLSI publication M100-S22. Wayne, PA: CLSI; 2012.
10. Bankevich A, Nurk S, Antipov D, et al. SPAdes: a new genome assembly algorithm and its applications to single-cell sequencing. J Comput Biol. 2012;19(5):455–77.
11. Wood DE, Salzberg SL. Kraken: ultrafast metagenomic sequence classification using exact alignments. Genome Biol. 2014;15(3):R46.
12. Inouye M, Dashnow H, Raven LA, et al. SRST2: rapid genomic surveillance for public health and hospital microbiology labs. Genome medicine. 2014; 6(11):90.
13. Treangen TJ, Ondov BD, Koren S, et al. The harvest suite for rapid core-genome alignment and visualization of thousands of intraspecific microbial genomes. Genome Biol. 2014;15(11):524.
14. Croucher NJ, Page AJ, Connor TR, et al. Rapid phylogenetic analysis of large samples of recombinant bacterial whole genome sequences using Gubbins. Nucleic Acids Res. 2015;43(3):e15.
15. Khong WX, Marimuthu K, Teo J, et al. Tracking inter-institutional spread of NDM and identification of a novel NDM-positive plasmid, pSg1-NDM, using next-generation sequencing approaches. J Antimicrob Chemother. 2016;71(11):3081–9.
16. Eyre DW, Cule ML, Wilson DJ, et al. Diverse sources of *C. difficile* infection identified on whole-genome sequencing. N Engl J Med. 2013;369(13):1195–205.
17. O'Neil CA, Li J, Leavey A, et al. Characterisation of aerosols generated during patient care activities. Clin Inf Dis. 2017;65(8):1342–8.
18. Carling PC, Parry MF, Von Beheren SM, et al. For the healthcare environmental hygiene study group. Identifying opportunities to enhance environmental cleaning in 23 acute care hospitals. Infect Control Hosp Epidemiol. 2008;29:1–7.
19. Umezawa K, Asai S, Ohshima T, et al. Outbreak of drug-resistant *Acinetobacter baumannii* ST 219 caused by oral care using tap water from contaminated hand hygiene sinks as a reservoir. Am J Infect Control. 2015;43(11):1249–51. https://doi.org/10.1016/j.ajic.2015.06.016.
20. Choi WS, Kim SH, Jeon EG, et al. Nosocomial outbreak of carbapenem-resistant *Acinetobacter baumannii* in intensive care units and successful outbreak control program. J Korean Med Sci. 2010;25:999–1004.
21. Price JR, Cole K, Bexley A, et al. Transmission of *Staphylococcus aureus* between health-care workers, the environment, and patients in an intensive care unit: a longitudinal cohort study based on whole-genome sequencing. Lancet Infect Dis. 2017;17:207–14.
22. Marchaim D, Navon-Venezia S, Schwartz D, et al. Surveillance cultures and duration of carriage of multidrug-resistant *Acinetobacter baumannii*. J Clin Microbiol. 2007;45(5):1551–5.
23. Apisarnthanarak A, Warren DK. Screening for Carbapenem-resistant *Acinetobacter baumannii* colonization sites: an implication for combination of horizontal and vertical approaches. Clin Inf Dis. 2013;56:1057–9.

Nudge to better care - blood cultures and catheter-related bloodstream infections in Germany at two points in time (2006, 2015)

Florian Salm[1,2,3*], Frank Schwab[2,3], Michael Behnke[2,3], Frank M. Brunkhorst[4,5,6], André Scherag[4,7], Christine Geffers[2,3] and Petra Gastmeier[2,3]

Abstract

Background: Blood cultures (BCs) are the gold standard for diagnosing sepsis and are prerequisite for a targeted antibiotic treatment and essential for patient outcomes. Aim of the study was to analyze the frequency of BCs, the rate of central line-associated bloodstream infections (CLABSIs) and to study the association between both parameters on intensive care units in Germany over time.

Methods: Cross-sectional studies at two points in time (2006, 2015) on ICUs participating in the German hospital infection surveillance system. CLABSIs were defined according to the Center for Disease Control and Prevention (CDC). Univariable and multivariable analyses were performed using generalized linear models.

Results: A total of 639 ICUs participated in 2006 or 2015 and 90 ICUs (*"core group"*) in both years. Overall, 2,427,921 patient days from 644,575 patients were analyzed. In the ICU core group the frequency of BCs per 1000 patient days doubled from 57.8 (interquartile range [IQR] 29.8–101.2; 2006) to 128.2 (IQR 71.6–183.2; 2015). In the same time, the pooled median CLABSI rate decreased from 0.8 (IQR 0–1.9; 2006) per 1000 central-line catheter days to 0.2 (IQR 0–0.9; 2015).

Conclusions: From 2006 to 2015 the frequency of BCs increased on ICUs in Germany and is now within the recommended 100 to 200 BCs sets per 1000 patient days.

Keywords: Infection control, Bloodstream infections, Sepsis, Blood cultures, Surveillance, Healthcare associated infections

Background

Early and sufficient diagnostics to identify the causative pathogen is prerequisite for a timely therapy start, a targeted antibiotic treatment and most importantly for the patient outcome. It is essential to become aware of the pathogen and potential antibiotic resistances [1, 2]. Sufficient diagnostic with BC can reduce mortality, length of stay on the intensive care unit and furthermore hospital expense [3, 4]. A targeted antimicrobial therapy can shorten the use of antibiotics and lower the selection pressure and the development of antibiotic resistances, it is one of the core elements of antibiotic stewardship approaches [5]. A range of 100–200 BC sets per 1000 patient days is recommended [6–8], especially because BSI detection rate depends on the frequency of the performance of BCs. Low performers have lower BSI rates compared to wards with a higher frequency in BC diagnostics [8, 9]. Therefore, the frequency of BCs per ward is an important quality indicator if BSI rates are compared. Over the last decade there were a lot of approaches to improve patient safety in critically ill patients by reducing the prevalence of central line-associated bloodstream infections (CLABSIs) [10–13] and by increasing the frequency of performing BCs when there is a suspicion of a BSI [14–16].

The goal of this investigation was to evaluate the frequency of BCs and the influence on the detection rate of CLABSIs and the association between both

* Correspondence: florian.salm@uniklinik-freiburg.de
[1]Institute for Infection Prevention and Hospital Epidemiology, Medical Center – University of Freiburg, Faculty of Medicine, Freiburg, Germany
[2]Institute of Hygiene and Environmental Medicine, Charité – Universitätsmedizin, Berlin, Germany
Full list of author information is available at the end of the article

parameters on ICUs in Germany at two points in the year 2006 and 2015.

Methods

In Germany, the majority of acute care hospitals participate voluntary in the German hospital infection surveillance system (KISS, "Krankenhaus-Infektions-Surveillance-System") which is a surveillance system with confidential data feedback [17, 18]. Data were included from ICUs participating in KISS. The surveillance in this module includes invariable different indicator infections like infections of the lower respiratory system (pneumonia and bronchitis), urinary tract infection and (laboratory-confirmed) BSIs. BSIs are defined according to the Center for Disease Control and Prevention (CDC) [19]. A BSI is central catheter-associated (CLABSI) when on the day with the first symptoms of the infection ("infection day") the patient had a catheter for at least 3 days. It must be mentioned, that the CDC definitions for CLABSI with coagulase-negative staphylococci (CNS) changed. Since 2011, at least two positive BCs with CNS are necessary to meet the criteria of a CNS-BSI. Before 2011, it was sufficient if at least one BC was positive with CNS and the attending physicians started an antimicrobial therapy. Therefore, all CLABSIs with CNS as a pathogen were excluded from the analysis. The CLABSI rate is calculated as the quotient of total BSI of patients with a central-line catheter divided by the total per 1000 central-line days (for more detail please see: nrz-hygiene.de). One BC is defined as a blood collection with no matter how many bottles but at least with one pair of aerobe und anaerobe BC bottles.

The German National Reference Center for Surveillance of Nosocomial Infections provides reference data for each healthcare-associated infection and works with social norm feedback. Mean, median and the 75th percentile are core parameters. Values within the upper quartile are highlighted. For selected infections and particular wards (e.g. neonatal intensive care units) a *Standardized Infection Ratio* (SIR) is provided and is calculated by the number of observed infections divided by the number of expected infections. The SIR is a parameter to help estimate whether the value is higher than in other wards with same characteristics. In addition, the data are graphically processed as a distribution curve and as funnel plots. Outlier values are also highlighted in the graphical representation.

2006 and 2015 a cross-sectional survey among the KISS participants was carried out to collect the blood culture density (BCD). BCD is defined as frequency of BCs per 1000 patient days per ICU. The method of the cross-sectional study conducted in the year 2006, is described in detail elsewhere [9]. Ten years later, in 2015, a cross-sectional study was carried out using the same methods as in the first investigation. Within the participants from 2006 ($n = 223$) and 2015 ($n = 506$), 90 ICUs provided data in both years and will be called *core-group* in the following.

Statistical analysis

In the descriptive analysis we calculate pooled mean, median and interquartile range (IQR) in total and stratified by year, type of hospital and hospital size (</> 600 beds), type of ICU, the device use, the invasive ventilation rate and length of stay. Differences between categories were tested by Chi-squared test. The rates of the years 2006 and 2015 in the core-group were tested by Wilcoxon test for paired samples and in the entire cohort by Wilcoxon-Mann-Whitney test for unpaired samples.

To investigate the association between the incidences of CLABSI and the frequency of BC univariable and multivariable analysis were performed using generalized linear models (GLM). In the models, we used negative-binomial distribution as probability distribution and the logarithm of central venous catheter (CVC) days was treated as offset parameter. To adjust for confounding the following variables were considered in the regression analysis: type and size of hospital, type and size of ICU, device use of CVC, ventilation and urinary tract catheter and length of stay. In the univariable analyses incidence rate ratios (IRR) were calculated for the individual factors. In the multivariable analyses, adjusted IRRs for BC density categories were calculated and all variables with $p < 0.1$ in the univariable analyses were included following a stepwise backward variable selection (excluding a variable from the model if $p > 0.05$ in the type III test).

All analyses were performed using SPSS [IBM SPSS statistics, version 23, Somer, NY, USA] and SAS 9.4 [SAS Institute, Cary, NC, USA].

Ethical approval

All data were anonymous and collected in accordance with the German recommendation for good epidemiological practice with respect to data protection [20]. As a federal law, the German Protection against Infection Act ("Infektionsschutzgesetz" §23) regulates the prevention and management of infectious diseases in humans. All hospitals are obliged to continuously collect and analyse healthcare-associated infections and drug-resistant pathogens [21]. These data are reported regularly to the National Reference Centre for the Surveillance of nosocomial infections. Ethical approval and informed consent were therefore not required.

Results

A total of 639 ICUs participated in 2006 or 2015 and 90 ICUs in both years. Overall, 2,427,921 patient days from 644,575 patients were analyzed. Over 1352 CLABSIs with no CNS as pathogen and 343,388 BCs were reported.

Wards characteristics can be seen in Table 1. In the ICU core group the BCD doubled from 57.8 (interquartile range [IQR] 29.8–101.2; 2006) to 128.2 (IQR 71.6–183.2; 2015, see Fig. 1a). In the same time, the pooled median CLABSI rate decreased from 0.8 (IQR 0–1.9; 2006) per 1000 central-line catheter days to 0.2 (IQR 0–0.9; 2015, see Table 1 and Fig. 1b). The crude and adjusted incidence rate ratios for the BCD categories compared to 50–99 BC per 1000 patient days can be found in Table 2 and Fig. 2. Wards with 100–199 BC per 1000 patient days did not detect significantly more CLABSIs compared to those wards with 50–99 BC per 1000 patient days. ICUs with more than 250 BCs per 1000 patient days had a 1.50 (95% confidence interval [CI] 1.07–2.11) higher risk to detect CLABSIs compared to ICUs with a low frequency of BCs (50–99- BCs per 1000 patient days). The adjusted IRR for the outcome CLABSI increased with higher frequency of BCs, length of stay and decreased significantly comparing the years 2006 and 2015 (IRR 0.74, 95%CI 0.60–0.92).

Discussion

We conducted 2006 and 2015 cross-sectional surveys on, in total, 639 intensive care units in Germany. We found an increase in the frequency of BCs and a significant decrease of catheter-related primary bloodstream infections. An important question is what has caused the strong increase in the BC performance?

In 2007, the German DRG- (Diagnosis Related Groups) reimbursement system changed and for sepsis, a new diagnosis code (R.65) was implemented. It became mandatory to perform at minimum two sets of BCs

Table 1 Intensive care units (ICU) characteristics – data from all ICUs ($n = 639^{**}$) and from the core group ($n = 90$) from two time points year 2006 and year 2015

Characteristics/ Outcomes	Total ICUs ($n = 639^{**}$)		Core Group ($n = 90$)		Core group ($n = 90$)	
	2006 ($n = 223$)	2015 ($n = 506$)	2006 ($n = 90$)	2015 ($n = 90$)	Diff. 2015–2006	p-value*
Size of ICU						
ICU beds, median (IQR)	11 (8–14)	12 (9–16)	11 (9–14)	11 (9–14)	–	–
ICU > =12 beds, N (%)	100 (44.8)	285 (56.3)	50 (55.6)	50 (55.6)		
Type of ICU, N (%)						
Surgical	40 (17.9)	77 (15.2)	15 (16.7)	15 (16.7)		
Interdisciplinary	108 (48.4)	285 (56.3)	41 (45.6)	41 (45.6)		
Medical	47 (21.1)	73 (14.4)	21 (23.2)	21 (23.2)		
Neurosurgical	4 (1.8)	9 (1.8)	2 (2.2)	2 (2.2)		
Neurological	4 (1.8)	11 (2.2)	2 (2.2)	2 (2.2)		
Pediatric	7 (3.1)	9 (1.8)	3 (3.3)	3 (3.3)		
other[a]	13 (5.8)	42 (8.3)	6 (6.7)	6 (6.7)		
Size of hospital						
Hospital beds, median (IQR	490 (274–841)	431 (270–724)	511 (289–890)	511 (289–890)	–	–
Hospital > = 600 beds, N (%)	85 (38.5)	174 (34.4)	36 (40.0)	36 (40.0)		
Type of hospital						
Tertiary hospital, N (%)	67 (30.0)	130 (25.7)	41 (45.6)	41 (45.6)		
Patients, median (IQR)	741 (506–1036)	814.5 (492–1191)	763.5 (489–1053)	722 (434–1112)	–	–
Patient days, median (IQR)	2744 (1854-3643)	3245 (2183-4365)	2744 (1915-3624)	3028 (2153-4215)	–	–
CLABSI rate[c], median (IQR)	0.6 (0.0–1.3)	0.5 (0.0–1.2)	0.8 (0–1.9)	0.2 (0–0.9)	– 0.01 (– 1.14–0.02)	0.001
Blood culture density[a], median (IQR)	60.0 (32.6–107.9)	115.4 (67.6–177.4)	57.8 (29.8–101.2)	128.2 (71.6–183.2)	54.8 (1.6–119.1)	0.001
Length of stay, median (IQR)	3.6 (2.7–5.2)	3.8 (3–5.5)	3.6 (2.8–5.5)	4.2 (2.9–6.2)	0.3 (–0.5–1.3)	0.025
CVC use[b], median (IQR)	67.3 (49.5–82.1)	66.6 (52.9–80.4)	70.8 (54.2–83.7)	69.0 (57.7–82.7)	0.6 (–6.3–8)	0.672
Invasive ventilation use [b], median (IQR)	34.1 (22.7–49.9)	36.8 (26.1–50.4)	35.3 (21.9–52.0)	37.1 (26.5–55.6)	3.1 (– 6.4–10.3)	0.078
Urinary tract catheters use [b], median (IQR)	81.3 (70.5–91.5)	85.4 (75.5–92.0)	83.7 (71.6–93.0)	86.7 (78.2–92.4)	2.5 (–2.8–10.0)	0.003

Abbreviations: *Diff* difference, *IQR* interquartile range, *CVC* central venous catheter, *CLABSI* central-line-associated bloodstream infection
*Wilcoxon-rank-sum test for paired sample; ** 90 ICUs collected data in 2006 and 2015
[a]per 1000 patient days
[b]per 100 patient days
[c]per 1000 CVC-days

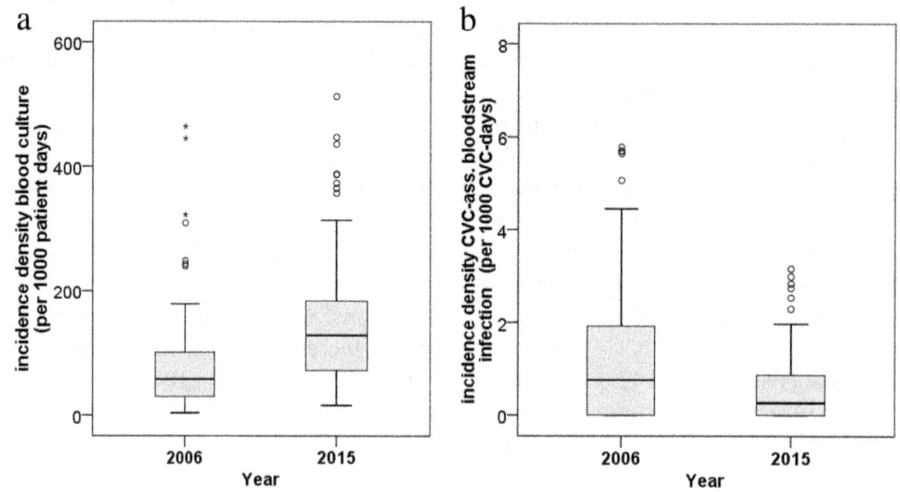

Fig. 1 **a** Incidence densitiy of blood cultures in the core group ($n = 90$), **b** Incidence densitiy of central line-associated bloodstream infection in the core group ($n = 90$)

Table 2 Results from the univariable and multivariable regressions analysis using generalized linear models[a] with the outcome central line-associated bloodstream infection

Parameter		Univariable Analysis			Multivariable Analysis		
	Category /unit	IRR	95%CI	*p*-value	IRR	95%CI	*p*-value
blood culture density (per 1000pd)	< 50	1.07	0.81–1.41	0.639	1.00	0.76–1.32	0.996
	100–149	1.07	0.81–1.4	0.637	1.14	0.87–1.50	0.343
	150–199	1.18	0.87–1.6	0.283	1.26	0.93–1.71	0.139
	200–249	1.38	0.91–2.09	0.127	1.48	0.98–2.23	0.061
	> = 250	1.46	1.04–2.05	0.029	1.50	1.07–2.11	0.019
	50–99	1 = reference			1 = reference		
Length of stay (days)	per day	1.05	1.02–1.08	0.001	1.05	1.02–1.08	0.001
Year (compared to year 2006)	2015	0.83	0.68–1.02	0.079	0.74	0.60–0.92	0.006
Invasive ventilation use (per 100 pd)	per 1%	1.01	1–1.01	0.004			
CVC use (per 100 pd)	per 1%	1	0.99–1	0.143			
Urinary tract catheter use (per 100 pd)	per 1%	0.99	0.99–1	0.013			
type of ICU	medical	1.49	1.15–1.94	0.002			
	surgical	1.17	0.9–1.51	0.239			
	neurosurgical	1.27	0.62–2.61	0.514			
	neurological	1.26	0.61–2.57	0.534			
	pediatric	1.27	0.6–2.66	0.533			
	other[a]	1.81	1.27–2.58	0.001			
	interdisciplinary	1 = reference					
Size of ICU	> 12 beds	1.11	0.91–1.34	0.306			
type of hospital	tertiary	1.59	1.24–2.03	<.001			
size of hospital	> 600 beds	1.37	1.13–1.65	0.001			

IRR incidence rate ratio, *CI* confidence interval, *pd* patient days, *CVC* central venous catheter, *ICU* intensive care unit

[a]The generalized linear models (GLM) with the outcome CLABSI and negative-binomial distribution as probability distribution and the logarithm of CVC days as offset parameter analyzed 729 yearly observations from 639 different ICUs in the years 2006 and 2015

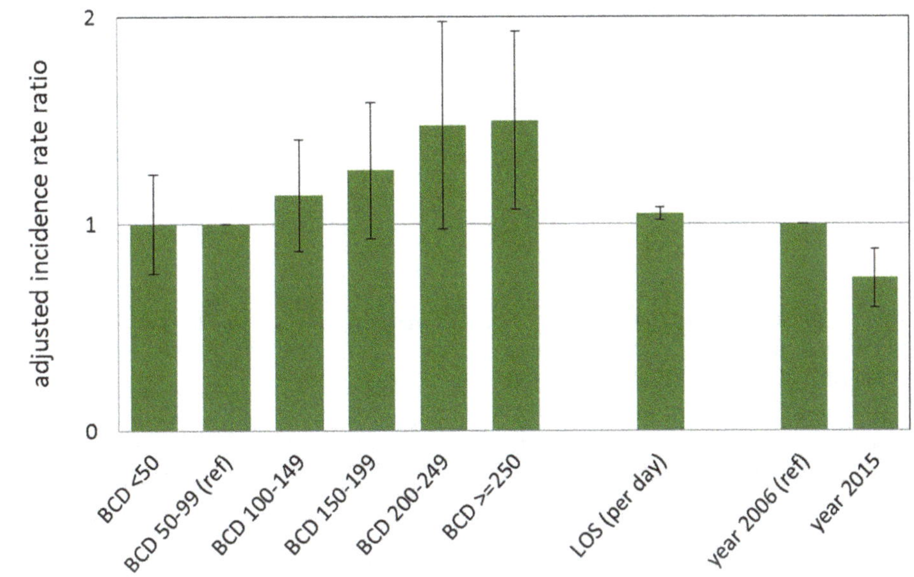

Fig. 2 Adjusted incidence rate ratios for blood culture density categories with the outcome central line-associated bloodstream infection (per 1000 CVC days), results of the multivariable regression analysis of 639 wards, 2006 & 2015. Whiskers represent 95% confidence interval. BCD, blood culture density per 1000 patient days; ref., reference in the model; LOS, length of stay

for the reimbursement of a R.65 patient case [22]. It can be assumed that the change in the DRG-reimbursement system influenced the BCD. Furthermore, several projects addressed this issue over the last years and tried to increase guideline adherence and the implementation of evidence-based diagnostic standard in the care of patients with suspicion of a bloodstream infections [15, 23]. It is well described that higher frequency of BCs are associated with a higher detection rate of BSIs [8, 9]. After a linear trend between culturing rates and the detection of BSIs with higher frequency of BCs a saturation effect can be found, but the optimal frequency of BCs is not well described yet [24]. Focusing on used DRG codes (R.65) for sepsis and sepsis shock, the clinical correlates of BSI, the annual number rose significantly between 2007 to 2013 [25]. In contrast, the CLABSI rate decreased enormously from 2006 to 2015. Potentially, the CLABSI rate decreased due to the different infection and control measures to improve patient safety in critically ill patients by implementing intervention bundles focusing on proper insertion techniques and managing of the CVCs over the last decade [10–13]. In the United States there are approaches to reduce preventable health-care associated infections with *Pay for Performance* policy [26, 27]. Some authors emphasize that reduced payments for CLABSIS did not influence the overall CLABSI rate [27]. On the other hand, from 2008 to 2014 the rate of CLABSIs decreased about 50% in the United States [28], while the BC rate declined from 2008 to 2010 [26]. Calderwood and colleagues highlighted that after implementation of the *Pay for Performance* policy the CLABSI rates decreased in hospitals operating at a financial loss, but in those operating at a financial profit the CLABSI rate was not affected by the policy [29]. In summary, the impact of the *Pay for Perfomance* system on the CLABSI rate in the United States is still unclear.

Nevertheless, considering that in Germany we found a similar decrease in the CLABSI rate without reimbursement penalties, we must critically scrutinize *Pay for Performance* approaches, especially when the outcome can be influenced by diagnostic methods.

However, the burden of health-care associated bloodstream infection is very high with estimated 160.000 cases and a number of about 25.000 attributable deaths in Europe per year [30]. Some investigations pointed out that German inpatient care physicians still have deficits concerning the knowledge of BC sampling; however, the results of this study suggest a positive upward trend in the frequency of BC sampling [31, 32]. Raupach-Rosin et al. reported that the majority of the physicians do not adhere to diagnostic guideline recommendations (two sets of BC from two different sites) [31].

The results are limited by the point that the 1976 reported BSI occurred after the 3rd day according to the surveillance protocol and are only primary BSIs. In contrast, the 343,388 reported BCs are from 1st day until discharge. It must be also considered that the median length of stay on the ICU per patient was less than 4 days. In this investigation, it remains unclear how many BCs were done due to primary and how many due to secondary BSI diagnosis. Nevertheless, from 2006 to 2015 the BCD increased enormously on ICUs and is now within the recommended range for BC of 100 to 200 BCs sets per 1000 patient days [6]. While the large number of observed ICUs ($n = 639$) with over two million patient days under surveillance is a strength of this study, the temporal comparison was limited to the core group of 90 ICUs. However, this core group had consistent ward characteristics over the 10-year period.

Conclusion

In conclusion, we must assume that many of the BC diagnostics are associated with secondary BSIs. Despite the expected parallel increase of BSI rates a decrease of primary BSI was observed. This underlines our observations of a decreasing trend of BSI rates in ICUs participating in the German hospital infection surveillance system [17].

Abbreviations

BC: Blood culture; BCD: Blood culture density; BSI: Bloodstream infection; CLABSI: Central line-associated bloodstream infection; CNS: Coagulase-negative; CVC: Central venous catheter; GLM: Generalized linear models; ICU: Intensive care unit; IQR: Interquartile range; IRR: Incidence rate ratios; SIR: Standardized infection ratio

Acknowledgements

Not applicable.

Funding

The study was not funded.

Authors' contributions

FSa, CG and PG led initial study design and development. MB, FSc and PG led the data collection. FSc and FSa led the analysis with input from FMB and AS, who also helped to draft the manuscript. All authors have made essential contributions to the interpretation of the data and to the preparation of the manuscript. All authors approved the final version of the manuscript.

Consent for publication

Not applicable, because all data were surveillance based data which were obtained within the German Law on Protection against Infection ("Infektionsschutzgesetz").

Competing interests

The authors declare that they have no competing interests.

Author details

[1]Institute for Infection Prevention and Hospital Epidemiology, Medical Center – University of Freiburg, Faculty of Medicine, Freiburg, Germany. [2]Institute of Hygiene and Environmental Medicine, Charité – Universitätsmedizin, Berlin, Germany. [3]National Reference Center for the Surveillance of Nosocomial Infections, Berlin, Germany. [4]Center for Sepsis Control and Care, Jena University Hospital, Jena, Germany. [5]Center for Clinical Studies, Jena University Hospital, Jena, Germany. [6]Department of Anesthesiology and Intensive Care Medicine, Jena University Hospital, Jena, Germany. [7]Institute of Medical Statistics, Computer Sciences and Documentation, Jena University Hospital, Jena, Germany.

References

1. Liu VX, Fielding-Singh V, Greene JD, Baker JM, Iwashyna TJ, Bhattacharya J, et al. The timing of early antibiotics and hospital mortality in Sepsis. Am J Respir Crit Care Med. 2017;196:856–63.
2. Singer M, Deutschman CS, Seymour CW, Shankar-Hari M, Annane D, Bauer M, et al. The third international consensus definitions for Sepsis and septic shock (Sepsis-3). JAMA. 2016;315:801–10.
3. Berild D, Mohseni A, Diep LM, Jensenius M, Ringertz SH. Adjustment of antibiotic treatment according to the results of blood cultures leads to decreased antibiotic use and costs. J Antimicrob Chemother. 2006; 57:326–30.
4. Adrie C, Garrouste-Orgeas M, Ibn Essaied W, Schwebel C, Darmon M, Mourvillier B, et al. Attributable mortality of ICU-acquired bloodstream infections: impact of the source, causative micro-organism, resistance profile and antimicrobial therapy. J Inf Secur. 2017;74:131–41.
5. Barlam TF, Cosgrove SE, Abbo LM, MacDougall C, Schuetz AN, Septimus EJ, et al. Implementing an antibiotic stewardship program: guidelines by the Infectious Diseases Society of America and the Society for Healthcare Epidemiology of America. Clin Infect Dis Off Publ Infect Dis Soc Am. 2016;62:e51–77.
6. Seifert H, Abele-Horn M, Fätkenheuer G, Glück T, Jansen B, Kern WV, et al. Blutkulturdiagnostik: sepsis, endokarditis, katheterinfektionen. DGHM DGfHuM Ed Mikrobiol-Infekt Qual MiQ Elsevier. 2007:74–5.
7. Baron EJ, Weinstein MP, Dunne WM Jr, Yagupsky P, Welch DF, Wilson DM. Cumitech 1C, blood cultures IV, p 1–16, 23–25 coordinating ed, baron EJ, editor. Washington, DC: ASM Press; 2005.
8. Karch A, Castell S, Schwab F, Geffers C, Bongartz H, Brunkhorst FM, et al. Proposing an empirically justified reference threshold for blood culture sampling rates in intensive care units. J Clin Microbiol. 2015;53:648–52.
9. Gastmeier P, Schwab F, Behnke M, Geffers C. Less blood culture samples: less infections? Anästhesist. 2011;60:902–7.
10. Gavin NC, Webster J, Chan RJ, Rickard CM. Frequency of dressing changes for central venous access devices on catheter-related infections. Cochrane Database Syst Rev. 2016;2:CD009213.
11. Lai NM, Lai NA, O'Riordan E, Chaiyakunapruk N, Taylor JE, Tan K. Skin antisepsis for reducing central venous catheter-related infections. Cochrane Database Syst Rev. 2016;7:CD010140.
12. Sutcliffe KM, Paine L, Pronovost PJ. Re-examining high reliability: actively organising for safety. BMJ Qual Saf. 2017;26:248–51.
13. Pronovost P, Needham D, Berenholtz S, Sinopoli D, Chu H, Cosgrove S, et al. An intervention to decrease catheter-related bloodstream infections in the ICU. N Engl J Med. 2006;355:2725–32.
14. Karch A, Schmitz RP, Rißner F, Castell S, Töpel S, Jakob M, et al. Bloodstream infections, antibiotic resistance and the practice of blood culture sampling in Germany: study design of a Thuringia-wide prospective population-based study (AlertsNet). BMJ Open. 2015;5:e009095.
15. Weis S, Hagel S, Schmitz RPH, Scherag A, Brunkhorst FM, Forstner C, et al. Study on the utility of a statewide counselling programme for improving mortality outcomes of patients with Staphylococcus aureus bacteraemia in Thuringia (SUPPORT): a study protocol of a cluster-randomised crossover trial. BMJ Open. 2017;7:e013976.
16. Schmitz RP, Keller PM, Baier M, Hagel S, Pletz MW, Brunkhorst FM. Quality of blood culture testing-a survey in intensive care units and microbiological laboratories across four European countries. Crit Care. 2013;17:R248.
17. Schröder C, Schwab F, Behnke M, Breier A-C, Maechler F, Piening B, et al. Epidemiology of healthcare associated infections in Germany: nearly 20 years of surveillance. Int J Med Microbiol. 2015;305:799–806.
18. German hospital infection surveillance system > KISS (Krankenhaus-Infektions-Surveillance-System). [cited 2017 May 22]. Available from: nrz-hygiene.de/surveillance/kiss/
19. Horan TC, Andrus M, Dudeck MA. CDC/NHSN surveillance definition of health care–associated infection and criteria for specific types of infections in the acute care setting. Am J Infect Control. 2008;36:309–32.
20. Deutsche Gesellschaft für Epidemiologie. Leitlinien und Empfehlungen zur Sicherung von Guter Epidemiologischer Praxis (GEP). 2004. BMBF

Gesundheitsforschung URL https://dgepi.de/assets/Leitlinien-und-Empfe hlungen/6074a4e7b8/Leitlinien-fuer-Gute-Empidemiologische-Praxis.pdf. Accessed 24 Jan 2017. WebCite Cache ID 6nlBtZZZO. 2016.

21. Gesetz zur Verhuetung und Bekaempfung von Infektionskrankheiten beim Menschen (Infektionsschutzgesetz - IfSG). 2017. BGBl. I S. 2615. Available from: https://www.gesetze-im-internet.de/ifsg/
22. Brunkhorst FM, Seifert H, Kaasch A, Welte T. Leitliniengerechte Blutkulturdiagnostik bei Sepsis und schweren Organinfektionen in der Intensivmedizin–ein unterschätztes Defizit. Dtsch Ärzte-Verl. 2010:1–8.
23. Scheer CS, Fuchs C, Kuhn S-O, Vollmer M, Rehberg S, Friesecke S, et al. Quality improvement initiative for severe Sepsis and septic shock reduces 90-day mortality: a 7.5-year observational study. Crit Care Med. 2017;45:241–52.
24. Laupland KB, Niven DJ, Pasquill K, Parfitt EC, Steele L. Culturing rate and the surveillance of bloodstream infections: a population-based assessment. Clin Microbiol Infect. 2018;24:910.e1–4.
25. Fleischmann C, Thomas-Rueddel DO, Hartmann M, Hartog CS, Welte T, Heublein S, et al. Hospital incidence and mortality rates of Sepsis. Dtsch Arzteblatt Int. 2016;113:159–66.
26. Kadri S, Hohmann S, Zhang F, O'Grady N, Klompas M. 24: impact of penalties for central line-associated bloodstream infections on blood culture ordering. Crit Care Med. 2016;44:92 Available from: https://journals.lww.com/ccmjournal/Fulltext/2016/12001/24___IMPACT_OF_PENALTIES_FOR_CENTRAL.27.aspx.
27. Lee GM, Kleinman K, Soumerai SB, Tse A, Cole D, Fridkin SK, et al. Effect of nonpayment for preventable infections in U.S. hospitals. N Engl J Med. 2012; 367:1428–37.
28. Centers for Disease Control and Prevention. Current HAI Progress Report - 2016 National and State Healthcare-Associated Infections Progress Report. Atlanta: CDC. p. 2016. Available from: https://www.cdc.gov/hai/progress-report/index.html
29. Calderwood MS, Vaz LE, Kawai AT, Jin R, Rett MD, Grant PS, et al. Impact of hospital operating margin on central line–associated bloodstream infections following Medicare's hospital-acquired conditions payment policy. Infect Control Hosp Epidemiol. 2016;37:100–3.
30. Cassini A, Plachouras D, Eckmanns T, Abu Sin M, Blank H-P, Ducomble T, et al. Burden of six healthcare-associated infections on European population health: estimating incidence-based disability-adjusted life years through a population prevalence-based modelling study. PLoS Med. 2016;13:e1002150.
31. Raupach-Rosin H, Duddeck A, Gehrlich M, Helmke C, Huebner J, Pletz MW, et al. Deficits in knowledge, attitude, and practice towards blood culture sampling: results of a nationwide mixed-methods study among inpatient care physicians in Germany. Infection. 2017;45:433–41.
32. She RC, Alrabaa S, Lee SH, Norvell M, Wilson A, Petti CA. Survey of physicians' perspectives and knowledge about diagnostic tests for bloodstream infections. PLoS One. 2015;10:e0121493.

22

In vitro studies of the antibacterial activity of *Copaifera* spp. oleoresins, sodium hypochlorite, and peracetic acid against clinical and environmental isolates recovered from a hemodialysis unit

Rosimara Gonçalves Leite Vieira[1], Thaís da Silva Moraes[1], Larissa de Oliveira Silva[1], Thamires Chiquini Bianchi[1], Rodrigo Cassio Sola Veneziani[1], Sérgio Ricardo Ambrósio[1], Jairo Kenupp Bastos[2], Regina Helena Pires[1] and Carlos Henrique Gomes Martins[1*]

Abstract

Background: Patients submitted to hemodialysis therapy are more susceptible to infection, especially to infection by Gram-positive bacteria. Various research works have attempted to discover new antimicrobial agents from plant extracts and other natural products.

Methods: The present study aimed to assess the antibacterial activities of *Copaifera duckei*, *C. reticulata*, and *C. oblongifolia* oleoresins; sodium hypochlorite; and peracetic acid against clinical and environmental isolates recovered from a Hemodialysis Unit. The Minimum Inhibitory Concentration and the Fractionated Inhibitory Concentration Index were determined; the ability of the tested compounds/extracts to inhibit biofilm formation was evaluated by calculating the $MICB_{50}$ and IC_{50}.

Results: *C. duckei* was the most efficient among the assayed *Copaifera* species, and its oleoresin was more effective than peracetic acid and sodium hypochlorite. *Copaifera* oleoresins and disinfectants did not act synergistically at any of the tested combinations. Certain of *C. duckei* oleoresin, peracetic acid, and sodium hypochlorite concentrations inhibited biofilm formation and eradicated 50% of the biofilm population.

Conclusion: *C. duckei* oleoresin is a potential candidate for disinfectant formulations. Based on these results and given the high incidence of multi-resistant bacteria in hemodialysis patients, it is imperative that new potential antibacterial agents like *C. duckei* oleoresin, which is active against *Staphylococcus*, be included in disinfectant formulations.

Keywords: *Copaifera*, Antibacterial activity, Hemodialysis water, Biofilm, Peracetic acid, Sodium hypochlorite

Background

During End Stage Renal Disease (ESRD), characterized by progressive kidney function loss, the glomerular filtration rate is below 15 mL/min/1.73 m^2. The kidney can no longer regulate the internal environment, and the patient requires support therapies like hemodialysis, peritoneal dialysis, and kidney transplantation to sustain life. Such support therapies are denominated Renal Replacement Therapies (RRT), being hemodialysis the most widely applied RRT [1–3].

Pontoriero et al. [4] have reported that hemodialysis patients are exposed to 400 L of water used to produce dialysis fluids every week. Despite interposition of a semi-permeable artificial membrane, this water comes into direct contact with the bloodstream. Therefore, knowing and monitoring the dialysis water chemical and microbiological purity is important.

* Correspondence: carlos.martins@unifran.edu.br
[1]Nucleus of Research in Sciences and Technology, Laboratory of Research in Applied Microbiology, University of Franca, Avenida Armando Salles de Oliveira, 201, Franca - São Paulo 14404-600, Brazil
Full list of author information is available at the end of the article

Although dialysis fluid quality depends on a complex chain of devices and procedures and on the implemented quality control procedure, the best strategy to ensure patient safety is to prevent contamination in each dialysis process phase. Water constitutes 95% of the dialysate, and tubes, tanks, and taps represent potential reservoirs for microorganisms to form biofilms, which are extremely hard to eradicate by chemical or mechanical means [5, 6].

Several procedures including physical, chemical, and physicochemical treatments are routinely used to disinfect hemodialysis monitors and the water treatment system [7]. Sodium hypochlorite and peracetic acid disinfectants are commonly applied during disinfection.

Antiseptics and disinfectants play an important role in controlling infection because they act to minimize the spread of microorganisms. However, continued use of these products in hospitals and other health services can trigger bacterial resistance, contributing to antimicrobial resistance development.

Given that bacterial resistance and the risks associated with the use of disinfectants pose a constant challenge, the search for new compounds with antibacterial activity and the development of new products with disinfectant action are crucial.

Effective medicinal plant use has contributed to disseminating information about their therapeutic importance and medicinal effects, validating therapeutic knowledge that has been accumulated for centuries. Nevertheless, the chemical constituents of medicinal plants are not yet fully known [8–12]. Identifying the active components of these plants should increase current knowledge about this inexhaustible natural source of medicinal compounds [13].

The economic and ecological relevance of the species belonging to the genus *Copaifera* has aroused researchers' interest. According to Leandro et al. [14] and Veiga Jr. and Pinto [15], *Copaifera* oleoresins contain mainly sesquiterpenes and diterpenes. The sesquiterpenes α-copaene, β-caryophyllene, β-bisabolene, α- and β-selinene, α-humulene, and δ- and γ-cadinene are worthy of note.

In vivo and in vitro evaluation has demonstrated that oils obtained from various *Copaifera* species have anti-inflammatory, healing, antiedematogenic, antitumor, trypanocidal, and bactericidal activities [16, 17].

Investigating natural products is clearly essential to the search for new molecules with antibacterial activity. In this sense, this work shall significantly contribute to research into the potential use of *Copaifera* species oleoresins against bacterial strains involved in hemodialysis.

Methods

Copaifera species oleoresins: Collection and chemical characterization

C. duckei and *C. reticulata* oleoresins were both collected in Mosqueiro and Brasil Novo, respectively, located in Pará State, Brazil. Plant materials were identified by Silvane Tavares Rodrigues at "Herbário da Embrapa de Belém", where the voucher specimens NID:96/2012 and NID:03/2013 were stored. *C. oblongifolia* oleoresin was collected in Pirajuba, Minas Gerais State, Brazil. A voucher specimen (NID 14437) was identified by Prof. Dr. Milton Groppo Júnior and deposited at the SPFR herbarium (Faculdade de Filosofia, Ciências e Letras-USP). Chemical characterization of these oleoresins was carried out by HPLC-MS/MS (Fig. 1) and had been previously reported by Santiago et al. [18], Bardaji et al. [19], and Moraes et al. [20]. Collection of the oleoresins used in this study was authorized by the Environment Ministry (MMA, Brazil) and the Chico Mendes Institute for Biodiversity Conservation (ICMBio, Brazil), Number: 35,143–3.

Bacteria used in the antibacterial assays

The bacteria used during the antibacterial assays had been previously obtained by the research group working in the Applied Microbiology Research Laboratory (LaPeMA) of the University of Franca. The bacteria had been recovered from the hydraulic system (environmental isolates) and from patients (clinical isolates) of a hospital hemodialysis unit and transported to LaPeMA for further isolation in the appropriate culture medium and identification by the commercial identification BBL Crystal Identification Systems (Becton & Dickinson, Sparks, MD, USA).

After identification, the microorganisms were kept in Brain Heart Infusion broth (BHI) containing glycerol at 20% (*v*/v), under cryopreservation (− 80 °C). The following microorganism isolates were used: twelve *Pseudomonas aeruginosa* isolates (water isolates), ten *Staphylococcus aureus* isolates (five isolates from Continuous Ambulatorial Peritoneal Dialysis (CAPD) dialysate, three isolates from hemoculture, one isolate from ascetic fluid, and one isolate from peritoneal liquid), three *Escherichia coli* isolates (water isolates), and nine *Staphylococcus epidermidis* isolates (water isolates).

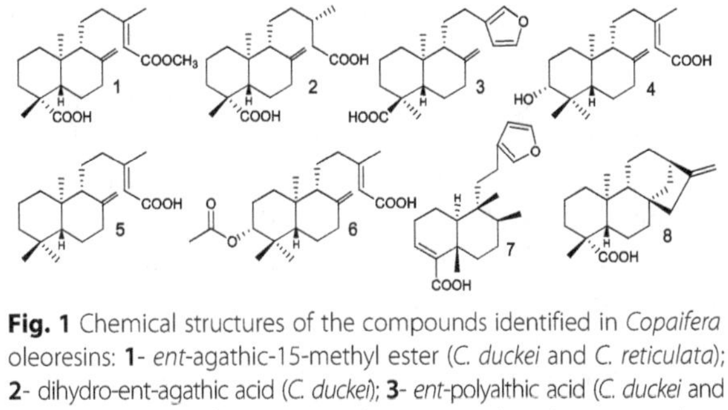

Fig. 1 Chemical structures of the compounds identified in *Copaifera* oleoresins: **1**- *ent*-agathic-15-methyl ester (*C. duckei* and *C. reticulata*); **2**- dihydro-ent-agathic acid (*C. duckei*); **3**- *ent*-polyalthic acid (*C. duckei* and *C. reticulata*); **4**- *ent*-3β-hydroxy-copalic acid (*C. multijuga*); **5**- *ent*-copalic acid (*C. multijuga, C reticulata and C. oblongifolia*); **6**- *ent*-3β-acetoxy copalic acid (*C. multijuga*); **7**- Hardwickiic acid (*C. oblongifolia*); and **8**- *ent*-kaurenoic acid (*C. oblongifolia*)

Copaifera species oleoresins: Minimum inhibitory concentration (MIC) determination

The microdilution method recommended by the Clinical and Laboratory Standards Institute (CLSI) [21], with some modifications, was used to determine MIC (Minimum Inhibitory Concentration). Experiments were conducted in triplicate. The oleoresins were dissolved in dimethylsulfoxide (DMSO; Merck, Darmstadt, HE, Germany) and diluted with Brain Heart Infusion broth (BHI; Difco Labs, Detroit, MI, USA). Then, twelve oleoresin concentrations ranging from 0.195 to 400 μg/mL were tested.

From a stock solution at 3.4%, the disinfectant peracetic acid was diluted in BHI broth and tested at twelve concentrations ranging from 0.000048 to 0.1%. For the disinfectant sodium hypochlorite, a stock solution at 12% was diluted in BHI broth, to obtain twelve concentrations ranging from 0.001464 to 3%.

The inocula were adjusted to give a cell concentration of 5×10^5 CFU/mL [21]. DMSO 5% (*v*/v) was used as negative control, and vancomycin and gentamicin (Sigma) were used as positive control for Gram-positive and Gram-negative bacteria, respectively, from 0.0115 to 5.9 μg/mL. An inoculum was included to monitor the ground for bacterial growth.

The 96-well microtiter plate containing microorganisms was incubated at 37 °C for 24 h in aerobic conditions. After incubation, 30 μL of aqueous resazurin (Sigma) solution at 0.02% was added to each well. Resazurin is an oxireduction probe that allows immediate observation of microbial growth. The blue and red colors represent the absence and the presence of microbial growth, respectively [22].

Synergistic antimicrobial activity

Checkerboard assays were carried out in triplicate as established by the CLSI [21] to investigate the antimicrobial efficacy of the disinfectants peracetic acid and sodium hypochlorite in association with *C. duckei* oleoresin. Checkerboard assays were performed according to the protocol previously described by Chaturvedi et al. [23]. Synergy tests were conducted in triplicate, and oleoresin and disinfectant concentrations were combined in standard MIC format against 5×10^5 CFU/mL for each bacterium. To evaluate synergism, Fractional Inhibitory Concentration (FIC) index values were calculated as previously established in the literature [23]. Index values were analyzed as follows: FIC index values ≤ 0.5, > 0.5 to < 1.0, ≥ 1.0 to < 4.0, and ≥ 4 corresponded to synergistic, additive, indifferent, and antagonistic effects, respectively [24].

C. duckei Oleoresin ability to inhibit biofilm formation as evaluated by the minimum inhibitory concentration of biofilm ($MICB_{50}$)

The Minimum Inhibitory Concentration of Biofilm ($MICB_{50}$) is defined as the minimum antimicrobial agent concentration that can inhibit biofilm formation by 50% or more [25]. $MICB_{50}$ was determined as described in the CLSI guidelines [21] with some modifications. To determine *C. duckei* oleoresin $MICB_{50}$, serial twofold dilutions were prepared in a 96-well polystyrene tissue culture plate (TPP, Trasadingen, Switzerland) containing BHI broth as described previously. The final *C. duckei* oleoresin concentrations ranged from 0.195 to 400 μg/mL. Vancomycin and gentamicin (Sigma) at concentrations between 0.0115 and 5.9 μg/mL were the positive control. The disinfectants peracetic acid and hypochlorite were tested at concentrations ranging from 0.48 to 1000 μg/mL and from 58.59 to 120,000 μg/mL, respectively. Bacterial strains in the absence of antibacterial agent were used as negative controls, and inocula were adjusted to give a cell concentration of 1×10^6 CFU/mL for each bacterium evaluated in the assay. The well contents were discarded after incubation at 37 °C for 24 h. Then, each well was washed three times with 150 μL of sterile Milli Q water and fixed with 150 μL of methanol for 20 min, and $MICB_{50}$ was determined in triplicate by optical density (OD) and by counting the number of microorganisms.

OD measurements aided biofilm formation quantification as described by Stepanovic et al. [26]. Briefly, 150 μL of crystal violet at 2% was added to the microtiter plate wells. After 15 min at room temperature, excess dye was removed by rinsing with tap water, which was followed by air-drying at room temperature. Then, 150 μL of glacial acetic acid at 33% was gently added to each well, to re-solubilize the dye bound to the cells. The microtiter plate was covered with the lid and kept at room temperature for at least 30 min, to minimize evaporation. The OD of each well was measured at 595 nm by using a microtiter plate reader. The percentage of inhibition was calculated by using the equation [25]:

$$(1 - At_{595}/Ac_{595}) \times 100,$$

where At_{595nm} and Ac_{595nm} are the absorbance values of the wells treated with *C. duckei* oleoresin and the control, respectively.

Antibiofilm activity was also measured by counting the number of microorganisms. Procedures were the same as the ones described above by Caetano da Silva et al. [27] and Moraes et al. [20], but they were conducted on another microplate. Experiments were performed in triplicate for all the assessed bacteria. After incubation, colonies were counted, and results were expressed as Log_{10} (CFU/mL). The best inoculum concentration and incubation time for the antibiofilm activity assay were selected by standardizing biofilm formation (data not shown).

C. duckei Oleoresin antimicrobial activity against pre-formed biofilms

The Minimum Biofilm Eradication Concentration (represented by IC_{50}) of *C. duckei* oleoresin, vancomycin, and disinfectants was determined by a microdilution method conducted in a 96-well microtiter plate as described by Polonio et al. [28], with some modifications. Adherent inoculum (1×10^6 CFU/mL) was incubated in a 96-well microtiter plate for 24 h. After incubation, the biofilm was rinsed, to remove the bacteria that did not adhere to the well.

After 24 h of biofilm growth, adherent biofilms were exposed to oleoresin or vancomycin ranging from 0.98 to 2000 μg/mL. The disinfectants peracetic acid and hypochlorite were tested at concentrations ranging from 0.48 to 1000 μg/mL and from 58.59 to 120,000 μg/mL, respectively. Incubation lasted 24 h.

Adherent bacteria were released and counted, and the percent killing of adherent bacteria was expressed as Log_{10} CFU/mL. Parallel assays were performed against adherent standard inoculum.

The effective concentration that inhibited growth by 50% (IC_{50}) was calculated with the GraphPad Prism 5.0 software. All the tests were carried out in triplicate.

Results

Copaifera species oleoresins: Minimum inhibitory concentration (MIC) determination

As reported previously, the compounds identified in the *Copaifera* oleoresins were as follows: *C. duckey*: *ent*-agathic-15-methyl ester (1), *ent*-agathic acid (2), and *ent*-polyalthic acid (3); *C. reticulata*: (1), (3), *ent*-copalic acid (4), and 3-(methyl)-5-(2,2,6-trimethyl-6-hydroxy-1-cyclohexyl)-pentanoic acid (5) [18, 19]; and *C. oblongifolia*: (4), Hardwickiic acid (6), and *ent*-kaurenoic acid (7) [20]. The MIC values obtained for the *Copaifera* species oleoresins against the tested bacteria varied from 25 to 400 μg/mL (Table 1).

MIC values determined for *C. duckei* oleoresin against the bacteria *P. aeruginosa* (all strains), *E. coli* (strains 1 and 3), and *S. epidermidis* (strains 60, 66, and 69); for *C. reticulata* oleoresin against the bacteria *P. aeruginosa* (all strains), *E. coli* (all strains), and *S. epidermidis* (60); and for *C. oblongifolia* oleoresin against the bacteria *P. aeruginosa* (all strains) and *S. aureus* (strains 2, 3, 4, 5, 7, 9, 13, 14, and 15) revealed lack of antibacterial action: MIC values were greater than 400 μg/mL. In contrast, *C. dukei* oleoresin provided promising results against *S. aureus* (strains 2, 3, 4, 5, 7, 9, 10, 13, 14, and 15) and *S. epidermidis* (strains 57 and 68). As for the control drugs gentamicin and vancomycin, they afforded MIC values of 0.7375 μg/mL against *P. aeruginosa* and *S. epidermidis*, 1.475 μg/mL against *S. aureus*, 2.95 μg/mL against *E. coli* strains 2 and 3, and 0.7375 μg/mL against *E. coli* strain 1 (Table 1). *C. reticulata* oleoresin displayed promising antibacterial activity against *S. epidermidis* strain 68 and all the *S. aureus* strains, except for strain 5 (Table 1).

Peracetic acid at concentrations between 0.97 and 3.90 μg/mL, 3.90 and 7.81 μg/mL, 7.81 and 15.62 μg/mL, and 3.90 a 7.81 μg/mL was active against *P. aeruginosa*, *S. aureus*, *E. coli*, and *S. epidermidis*, respectively (Table 1). *P. aeruginosa* and *E. coli* were the most sensitive and the most resistant to peracetic acid, respectively. All the tested strains were sensitive to peracetic acid at the concentration recommended by the manufacturer (1000 μg/mL, see Table 1). In the case of sodium hypochlorite, concentrations between 468.75 and 937.5 μg/mL were active against *P. aeruginosa* and *S. aureus* strains, while a concentration of 937.5 μg/mL was effective against all *E. coli* and *S. epidermidis* strains (Table 1).

Synergistic antimicrobial activity

The present study evaluated *C. duckei* oleoresin combined with the disinfectant peracetic acid against *S. aureus* strains 02, 03, 07, 09, 10, and 15 and *S. epidermidis* strains 57 and 68, to find an indifferent effect. When this combination was tested against *S. aureus* strains 13 and 14, interaction was antagonistic (Fig. 2). As for *C. duckei* oleoresin combined with the disinfectant sodium hypochlorite, interaction was indifferent for all the assessed strains (Fig. 2).

C. duckei Oleoresin ability to inhibit biofilm formation as determined by minimum inhibitory concentration of biofilm ($MICB_{50}$)

On the basis of the results listed in Table 2, *C. duckei* oleoresin had $MICB_{50}$ of 100, 50, 12.5, 6.25, 3.12, and 0.78 μg/mL against *S. aureus* (strain 13), *S. aureus* (strains 7 and 9), *S. epidermidis* (strains 57 and 68), *S. aureus* (strains 2 and 10), *S. aureus* (strain 3), and *S. aureus* (strains 14 and 15), respectively.

Regarding vancomycin, with standardized MIC values ranging from 0.5 to 2.0 μg/mL [21], results were similar: bacterial bioflm growth inhibition required higher vancomycin concentrations for the strains that were the most resistant to *C. duckei* oleoresin. $MICB_{50}$ varied from 1.475 to 0.0230 μg/mL for vancomycin (Table 2).

Concerning peracetic acid, $MICB_{50}$ was 1.95 and 0.97 μg/mL against *S. aureus* strains 2 and 13, respectively (Table 2), which were approximately 998 and 999 times lower than the concentration recommended by the manufacturer (1000 μg/mL) (Table 2). Among the other strains, the same effect required a range of different concentrations. *S. aureus* strain 9 was the most resistant - peracetic acid $MICB_{50}$ against this strain was 1000 μg/mL (Table 2).

The $MICB_{50}$ values obtained for sodium hypochlorite varied widely: concentrations spanning from 937.5 to 30,000 μg/mL were necessary to achieve the desired

Table 1 Minimum Inhibitory Concentration values (μg/mL) of *Copaifera* species oleoresins and disinfectants against bacterial isolates from a hemodialysis unit

Bacteria	Origin	*C. duckei* Oleoresin	*C. reticulata* Oleoresin	*C.oblongifolia* Oleoresin
P. aeruginosa (16)	Environmental-Water	> 400	> 400	> 400
P. aeruginosa (17)	Environmental-Water	> 400	> 400	> 400
P. aeruginosa (18)	Environmental-Water	> 400	> 400	> 400
P. aeruginosa (20)	Environmental-Water	> 400	> 400	> 400
P. aeruginosa (21)	Environmental-Water	> 400	> 400	> 400
P. aeruginosa (22)	Environmental-Water	> 400	> 400	> 400
P. aeruginosa (23)	Environmental-Water	> 400	> 400	> 400
P. aeruginosa (24)	Environmental-Water	> 400	> 400	> 400
P. aeruginosa (25)	Environmental-Water	> 400	> 400	> 400
P. aeruginosa (27)	Environmental-Water	> 400	> 400	> 400
P. aeruginosa (28)	Environmental-Water	> 400	> 400	> 400
S. aureus (2)	Clinical-CAPD dialysate	50	100	> 400
S. aureus (3)	Clinical-CAPD dialysate	50	100	> 400
S. aureus (4)	Clinical-Ascetic fluid	100	100	> 400
S. aureus (5)	Clínico-Peritoneal fluid	100	200	> 400
S. aureus (7)	Clinical-Hemoculture	50	100	> 400
S. aureus (9)	Clinical-CAPD dialysate	50	100	> 400
S. aureus (10)	Clinical-CAPD dialysate	25	50	400
S. aureus (13)	Clinical-Hemoculture	50	50	> 400
S. aureus (14)	Clinical-Hemoculture	50	100	> 400
S. aureus (15)	Clinical-CAPD dialysate	50	100	> 400
E. coli (1)	Environmental-Water	> 40	> 400	> 400
E. coli (2)	Environmental-Water	400	> 400	400
E. coli (3)	Environmental-Water	> 400	> 400	> 400
S. epidermidis (54)	Environmental-Water	400	400	> 400
S. epidermidis (57)	Environmental-Water	100	200	> 400
S. epidermidis (58)	Environmental-Water	400	400	> 400
S. epidermidis (60)	Environmental-Water	> 400	> 400	> 400
S. epidermidis (62)	Environmental-Water	400	400	> 400
S. epidermidis (66)	Environmental-Water	> 400	400	> 400
S. epidermidis (67)	Environmental-Water	400	400	> 400
S. epidermidis (68)	Environmental-Water	100	100	> 400
S. epidermidis (69)	Environmental-Water	> 400	400	> 400
Bacteria	Origin	Sodium Hypochlorite	Peracetic Acid	Positive Control
P. aeruginosa (16)	Environmental-Water	468.75	1.95	0.7375[a]
P. aeruginosa (17)	Environmental-Water	468.75	3.90	0.7375[a]
P. aeruginosa (18)	Environmental-Water	468.75	1.95	0.7375[a]
P. aeruginosa (20)	Environmental-Water	937.50	3.90	0.7375[a]
P. aeruginosa (21)	Environmental-Water	937.50	1.95	0.7375[a]
P. aeruginosa (22)	Environmental-Water	937.50	3.90	0.7375[a]
P. aeruginosa (23)	Environmental-Water	468.75	3.90	0.7375[a]
P. aeruginosa (24)	Environmental-Water	937.50	3.90	0.7375[a]
P. aeruginosa (25)	Environmental-Water	937.50	3.90	0.7375[a]

Table 1 Minimum Inhibitory Concentration values (µg/mL) of *Copaifera* species oleoresins and disinfectants against bacterial isolates from a hemodialysis unit *(Continued)*

Bacteria	Origin	*C. duckei* Oleoresin	*C. reticulata* Oleoresin	*C.oblongifolia* Oleoresin
P. aeruginosa (27)	Environmental-Water	937.50	3.90	0.7375[a]
P. aeruginosa (28)	Environmental-Water	468.75	0.97	0.7375[a]
S. aureus (2)	Clinical-CAPD dialysate	937.50	7.81	1.475[b]
S. aureus (3)	Clinical-CAPD dialysate	937.50	7.81	1.475[b]
S. aureus (4)	Clinical-Ascetic fluid	937.50	3.90	1.475[b]
S. aureus (5)	Clínico-Peritoneal fluid	937.50	3.90	1.475[b]
S. aureus (7)	Clinical-Hemoculture	937.50	3.90	1.475[b]
S. aureus (9)	Clinical-CAPD dialysate	937.50	3.90	1.475[b]
S. aureus (10)	Clinical-CAPD dialysate	468.75	7.81	1.475[b]
S. aureus (13)	Clinical-Hemoculture	937.50	3.90	1.475[b]
S. aureus (14)	Clinical-Hemoculture	937.50	3.90	1.475[b]
S. aureus (15)	Clinical-CAPD dialysate	937.50	3.90	1.475[b]
E. coli (1)	Environmental-Water	937.50	7.81	0.7375[a]
E. coli (2)	Environmental-Water	937.50	15.62	2.95[a]
E. coli (3)	Environmental-Water	937.50	7.81	2.95[a]
S. epidermidis (54)	Environmental-Water	937.50	3.90	0.7375[a]
S. epidermidis (57)	Environmental-Water	937.50	7.81	0.7375[a]
S. epidermidis (58)	Environmental-Water	937.50	3.90	0.7375[a]
S. epidermidis (60)	Environmental-Water	937.50	3.90	0.7375[a]
S. epidermidis (62)	Environmental-Water	937.50	3.90	0.7375[a]
S. epidermidis (66)	Environmental-Water	937.50	3.90	0.7375[a]
S. epidermidis (67)	Environmental-Water	937.50	7.81	0.7375[a]
S. epidermidis (68)	Environmental-Water	937.50	7.81	0.7375[a]
S. epidermidis (69)	Environmental-Water	937.50	3.90	0.7375[a]

[a] Gentamicin
[b] Vancomycin
CAPD Continuous Ambulatorial Peritoneal Dialysis

effect (Table 2). Hence, biofilm formation inhibition was lower for all the tested bacteria.

S. aureus (strains 14 and 15), *S. aureus* (strain 15), *S. aureus* (strain 13), and *S. epidermidis* (strain 68) were the most sensitive to *C. duckei* oleoresin, vancomycin, peracetic acid, and sodium hypochlorite, respectively.

C. duckei Oleoresin antimicrobial activity on pre-formed biofilms

Table 3 lists the results achieved after pre-formed biofilms were exposed to the antimicrobials. The lowest IC_{50} values were 21.85 µg/mL for *C. duckei* oleoresin against *S. aureus* strain 15; 69.85 µg/mL for vancomycin against *S. epidermidis* strain 68; 8.47 µg/mL for peracetic acid gainst *S. epidermidis* strain 68; and 608.7 µg/mL for sodium hypochlorite against *S. aureus* strain 10 (Table 3).

Discussion

Given that *Copaifera* oleoresins contain many easily deprotonable acid terpenes [15, 18], the presence of this class of compounds in the oleoresins might contribute to the antibacterial activity observed in this study.

Plants are a source of great chemical and functional diversity, which has allowed investigations into an array of drugs for therapeutic use [29]. *Copaifera* species oleoresins are produced by exudation of trunks from trees belonging to the genus *Copaifera*. Studies have not evidenced that these oleoresins are cytotoxic to mammalian cells, induce behavioral changes, or cause lesions or hemorrhage in the stomach of rats treated with these extracts [30, 31]. Therefore, determining the sensitivity of bacteria, especially Gram-positive organisms, to *Copaifera* species oleoresins could prove a useful tool to combat these microorganisms [32].

Gram-positive bacteria underlie community-acquired infections as well as hospital-acquired infections [33]. Patients undergoing dialysis, mainly through venous access, are at 100 times higher risk of bacteremia than patients that do not require hemodialysis [34]. Most of the times, the etiological agent of such infections is *S.*

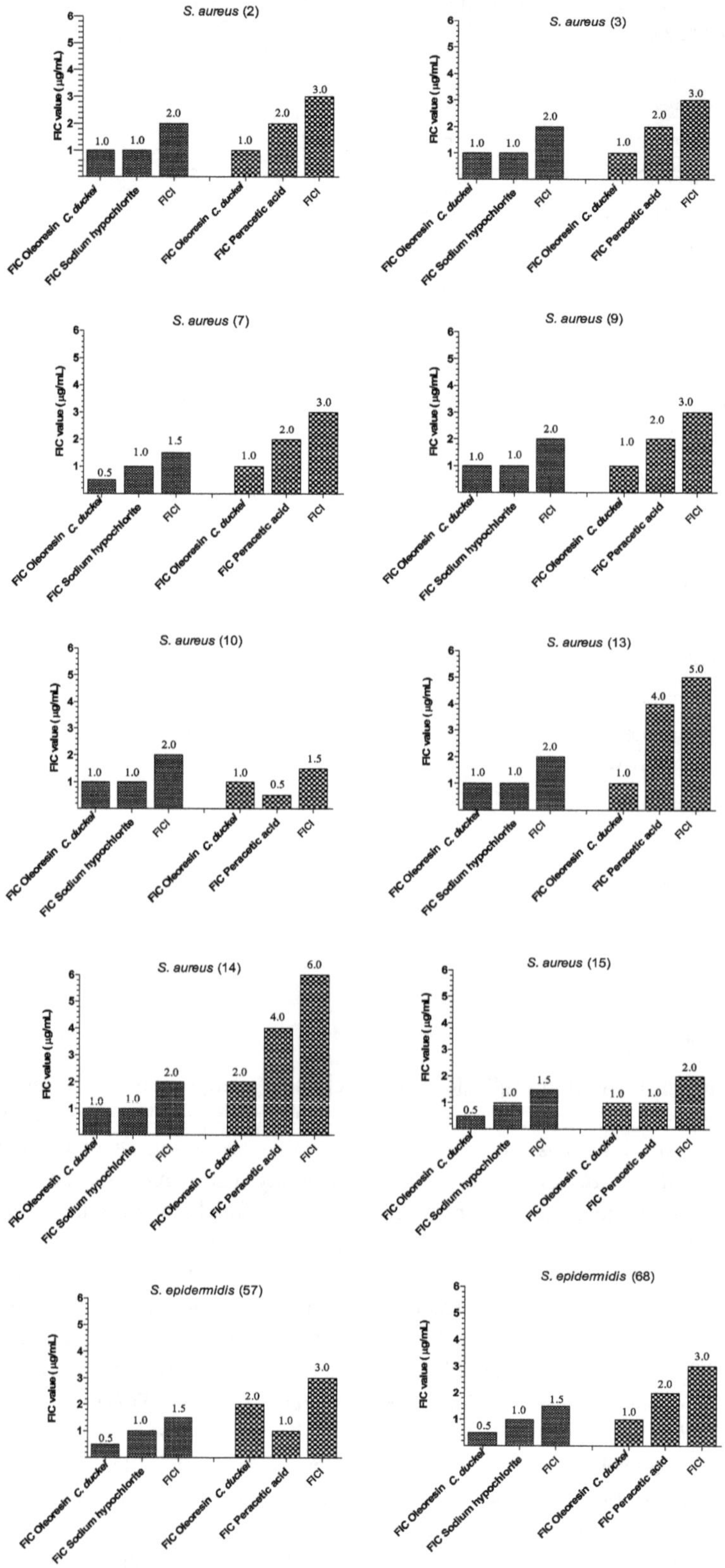

Fig. 2 Fractional inhibitory concentration (FIC) and fractional inhibitory concentration index (FICI) of a combination of *C. duckei* oleoresin alone and in combination with disinfectants (sodium hypochlorite or peracetic acid) against bacterial isolates recovered from a hemodialysis unit. FIC assays were performed in triplicate

Table 2 Antibiofilm activities of *C. duckei* oleoresin and disinfectants against bacterial isolates from a hemodialysis unit on the basis of $MICB_{50}$ (µg/mL)

Bacteria	*C. duckei* oleoresin	Peracetic acid	Sodium hypochlorite	Vancomycin
S. aureus (2)	6.25	1.95	30,000.0	0.7375
S. aureus (3)	3.12	15.62	30,000.0	0.0461
S. aureus (7)	50.0	31.25	30,000.0	1.475
S. aureus (9)	50.0	1000.0	15,000.0	1.475
S. aureus (10)	6.25	15.62	30,000.0	1.475
S. aureus (13)	100.0	0.97	15,000.0	1.475
S. aureus (14)	0.78	62.5	3.750	0.1844
S. aureus (15)	0.78	31.25	15,000	0.0230
S. epidermidis (57)	12.5	15.62	1.875	0.7375
S. epidermidis (68)	12.5	1000.0	937.5	0.7375

aureus [35]. In addition, the number of bacteria that are multiresistant to antimicrobial agents like beta-lactam antibiotics, fluoroquinolones, and macrolides has grown at an alarming rate [36]. This has motivated the search for new antimicrobial agents.

Resistance of some of the tested isolates to *C. duckei* oleoresin agrees with the report by Dos Santos et al. [37], who also observed that *E. coli*, *P. aeruginosa*, *S. aureus*, and *S. epidermidis* are resistant to this oleoresin. Moreover, Pacheco et al. [38] evaluated the antimicrobial activities of *Copaifera* species oleoresins against Gram-positive and Gram-negative bacteria, to find that these oleoresins inhibit Gram-positive bacteria at different levels, but they are inactive against Gram-negative bacteria (*E. coli* and *P. aeruginosa*), in agreement with the present study.

Our results are not satisfactory for any of the other tested bacteria and partly agree with the data reported by Santos et al. [39], who evaluated oleoresins obtained from three *Copaifera* species (*C. martii*, *C. officinalis*, and *C. reticulata*) against Gram-positive and Gram-negative bacteria as well as yeasts and dermatophytes. These authors found that *C. martii*, *C. officinalis*, and *C. reticulata* oleoresin concentrations between 31.3 and 62.5 µg/mL inhibit Gram-positive bacteria, including *Bacillus subtilis*, *Enterococcus faecalis*, *S. aureus*, *S. epidermidis*, and methicillin-resistant *Staphylococcus aureus* (MRSA).

Guissoni et al. [40] reported that the oleoresins extracted from two *Copaifera* species, *C. langsdorffii* and *C. reticulata*, can inhibit the growth of *E. coli*, *K. pneumoniae*, *S. marcescens*, *S. aureus*, including *S. aureus* isolates (MRSA). According to these authors, *C. langsdorffii* oleoresin presents MIC of 5000 µg/mL against all the tested bacteria, except for *E. coli*, for which MIC is 620 µg/mL. In the present study, the MIC values determined for *C. reticulata* oleoresin are not satisfactory against any of the assayed bacterial strains.

Papers on the antibacterial activity of *C. oblongifolia* are rare, but *Copaifera* species have been described to be efficient antibacterial agents. Masson et al. [41] assessed the *C. langsdorffii* oleoresin antibacterial activity against standard *S. aureus*, *Streptococcus pyogenes*, *E. faecalis*, *P. aeruginosa*, and *E. coli* strains in vitro, to detect a broad

Table 3 Antibiofilm activities of *C. duckei* oleoresin, disinfectants, and vancomycin against bacterial isolates from a hemodialysis unit on the basis of IC_{50} (µg/mL), after 24 h of incubation

Bacteria	*C. duckei* oleoresin	Peracetic acid	Sodium hypochlorite	Vancomycin
S. aureus (2)	> 2000	65.4	> 120,000	> 2000
S. aureus (3)	330.2	480.7	1048	> 2000
S. aureus (7)	> 2000	464.6	10,616	> 2000
S. aureus (9)	258.6	28.94	> 120,000	> 2000
S. aureus (10)	1042	13.85	608.7	> 2000
S. aureus (13)	1565	30.84	> 120,000	343.3
S. aureus (14)	191.4	213.5	4750	> 2000
S. aureus (15)	21.85	56.56	2471	> 2000
S. epidermidis (57)	> 2000	8473	910.0	> 2000
S. epidermidis (68)	112.7	18.70	896.0	69.85

inhibition spectrum for Gram-positive bacteria only. According to these authors, MIC values are 200, 400, and 1100 μg/mL against *S. aureus*, *S. pyogenes*, and *E. faecalis*, respectively. Our MIC values against *S. aureus* are more promising.

In contrast to Gram-negative bacteria, Gram-positive microorganisms are more sensitive to certain compounds. Antimicrobials act on the cell wall, and the different cell wall composition of these classes of bacteria may account for these results. In fact, Gram-positive bacteria present a thick cell wall consisting mainly of peptidoglycan, whereas Gram-negative bacteria display a stratified cell wall consisting of an outer membrane and a thin peptidoglycan layer [42–44]. The unique structural cell wall properties of Gram-negative bacteria may have prevented *Copaifera* species oleoresins from penetrating the cell wall; the external membrane contains lipopolysaccharides, which determine surface properties and alter cell permeability and susceptibility to the investigated oleoresins [45].

Dialysis units have to follow a range of guidelines to disinfect the water distribution system. Among the various disinfecting agents employed in Brazil, sodium hypochlorite and peracetic acid are the most satisfactory [46]. In this context, the present study aimed to evaluate the sodium hypochlorite and peracetic acid activities. Our results corroborate with data from a previous investigation [47] reporting that 58% of the hemodialysis units that conduct disinfection use peracetic acid-based disinfectants. Here, disinfection occurs in 36% of the surveyed units every month, and these units follow the same guidelines followed in the unit where we collected the bacterial isolates for this work.

Compared to the usually recommended concentration of between 25,000 and 45,000 μg/mL [48], we found that all the assayed strains are sensitive to sodium hypochlorite. This has been the standard disinfectant for water treatment and distribution systems in hemodialysis units. Nevertheless, events of bacteremia caused mainly by Gram-negative bacteria in dialysis patients have pointed out that this procedure is inadequate [49–52].

Oliveira et al. [53] tested disinfectants like quaternary ammonium salts; sodium hypochlorite at 0.5%, 1%, and 2%; glutaraldehyde at 2%; Lysoform®; aqueous ethanol solution at 70%; peracetic acid at 2%; and vinegar at 100% against 32 *S. aureus* isolates carried by insects within hospitals, to verify that the bacteria are only resistant to ethanol at 70% and vinegar.

The results we obtained for the assayed *Copaifera* species oleoresins and disinfectants against selected *Staphylococcus* strains show that *Copaifera* oleoresin 100 μg/mL, peracetic acid 7.81 μg/mL, and sodium hypochlorite 937.5 μg/mL inactivate all the bacteria. A comparative analysis reveals that *C. duckei* oleoresin is 12.8 times less efficient than peracetic acid but 9.37 times more efficient than sodium hypochlorite.

Interaction between compounds with antimicrobial activity has been used to reduce minimum inhibitory concentrations and to improve antimicrobial agent efficiency, once participating antimicrobials may act on different bacterial cell sites. Interactions are calculated on the basis of a mathematical equation and are defined as synergistic, additive, indifferent, or antagonist as compared to each isolated antimicrobial MIC [54].

According to the criteria established by Rios and Recio [55] and Gibbons [56], MIC values of 100 μg/mL or lower are promising. Hence, just *C. duckei* oleoresin presents antibacterial potential, and we only assayed this oleoresin in further tests.

The literature does not describe interaction between the *Copaifera* oleoresins and the disinfectants tested herein, but there are some papers on the sysnergism between plant compounds and these same disinfectants against bacteria. One example is the report by Zago et al. [57], who evaluated the synergistic potential of essential oils [(cinnamon (*Cinnamomum zeylanicum Blume Lauraceae*), lemon grass (*Cymbopogon citratus* (DC.) Stapf, Poaceae), peppermint (*Mentha piperita L. Lamiaceae*), ginger (*Zingiber officinale Roscoe Zingiberaceae*), clove (*Caryophillus aromaticus L. Myrtaceae*), and rosemary (*Rosmarinus officinalis L. Lamiaceae*)] combined with eight antimicrobial drugs (chloramphenicol, gentamicin, cefepime, tetracycline, sulfazotrim, cefalotin, ciprofloxacin, and rifampicin) against 12 *S. aureus* strains and 12 *E. coli* human isolates, to demonstrate that *S. aureus* is the most susceptible to interaction between drugs and essential oils, and synergism occurs between lemon grass essential oil and eight of the tested drugs as well as between peppermint essential oil and seven of the tested drugs. In the case of *E. coli*, synergism emerges only between rosemary essential oil and three of the tested drugs and between lemon grass essential oil and two of the tested drugs.

Moraes et al. [20] assessed the synergistic antimicrobial action of *C. oblongifolia* oleoresin with chlorhexidine dihydrochloride against bacteria that cause oral infections. Regarding chlorhexidine dihydrochloride combined with *C. oblongifolia* oleoresin against *S. mutans* (ATCC 25175), *L. casei* (ATCC 11578), *P.gingivalis* (ATCC 33277), and *P. micros* (clinical isolate), the authors found that the effect is indifferent. As for *S. mitis* (ATCC 49456) and *A. actinomycetemcomitans* (ATCC 43717), the effect is additive.

Olmedo et al. [58] examined the synergistic action between sodium hypochlorite and hydrogen peroxide, to observe that the combination of these compounds inactivates planktonic cells and inhibits biofilm formation by *E. coli*, *Salmonella* enterica subsp. enterica, *Klebsiella pneumonia*, and *S. aureus* standard strains as well as *S.* Enterica, *K. oxytoca*, and *E. coli* clinical isolates.

Previous hospitalization, access type during dialysis, comorbidities, gender, time elapsed since the beginning of treatment with dialysis, and previous use of antibiotics contribute to *S. aureus* colonization in dialysis patients [59]. Hence, introducing new compounds with potential antibacterial action in disinfecting solutions is mandatory, especially to combat infection with *S. aureus*.

Despite the development of some research into active combinations of conventional antibiotics, the scientific community has focused on identifying new antibacterial molecules, especially molecules of plant origin, to act as antibiofilm compounds and thus prevent biofilm formation [60].

$MICB_{50}$ is defined as the lowest antibacterial agent concentration that can inhibit biofilm formation by approximately 50% [25]. Moraes et al. [20] investigated *C. oblongifolia* oleoresin antibiofilm activity against bacteria that cause oral infections, to verify that this oleoresin inhibits 50% biofilm formation for the bacteria *Lactobacillus casei* (ATCC 11578) and *Peptostreptococcus micros* (clinical isolate) at 400 µ/mL, *Streptococcus mutans* (ATCC 25175) and *Aggregatibacter actinomycetemcomitans* (ATCC 43717) at 200 µ/mL, and *S. mitis* (ATCC 49456) and *Porphyromonas gingivalis* (ATCC 33277) at 100 µ/mL.

Leandro et al. [61] evaluated the antibiofilm effect of the hydroalcoholic extract of *Copaifera trapezifolia* rich in phenolic compounds against endodontic bacteria, to verify that the oleoresin at 200 µg/mL inhibits *P. gingivalis* (ATCC 33277) and *P. micros* (clinical isolate) biofilm formation by at least 50%.

Alencar et al. [62] reported the *C. langsdorffii* essential oil and oleoresin activities against *Staphylococcus*, *Pseudomonas*, and *Candida* (resistant to azo compounds) and showed that a nanostructured suspension based on *C. langsdorffii* essential oil or oleoresin presents efficient antibiofilm action.

Both sodium hypochlorite and peracetic acid have been tested against *S. aureus*. However, comparison between studies is difficult due to lack of standardized methodologies and concentrations that act on biofilms. Many methodologies have been proposed to probe the microbiocidal action of various disinfectants. Das et al. [63] were one of the first to pioneer the use of microplate methodology to report on the antimicrobial inhibitory effects of certain compounds on planktonic growth and adhered bacteria. These methodologies are based on visual alterations in color or on turbidimetric/colorimetric changes measured by spectrophotometric readings at a specific wavelength. A linear relationship is established between the inoculum size ($10–10^7$ CFU/mL) and the exposure time for individual wells, to obtain turbidity between 0.1 and 0.3 OD units within a certain time interval, generally between 1 and 24 h [64]. Several dyes, such as crystal violet, have been proposed to verify microorganism growth after treatment [65]. Another methodological possibility is plating in agar followed by incubation of bacterial inoculum aliquots before and after cell exposure [66, 67].

Svidzinski et al. [68] described that both peracetic acid and sodium hypochlorite at 0.1% (1000 µg/mL) act against MRSA staphylococcus, which agrees with our results demonstrating sodium hypochlorite activity at concentrations as low as 937.5 µg/mL. These authors also found that *S. aureus* strain 15 is approximately 999 times more sensitive to peracetic acid.

Guimarães et al. [69] studied how biocides (hydrogen peroxide at 7% combined with peracetic acid at 0.2%, sodium hypochlorite with 1% active chlorine, ethanol at 70% in aqueous solution and in gel, chlorhexidine digluconate at 0.5%, and povidone iodine at 10%) impact *S. aureus* MRSA biofilm formation, to show that povidone iodine, sodium hypochlorite, and hydrogen peroxide combined with peracetic acid can reduce bacterial film formation by 90%.

Concerning sodium hypochlorite antibacterial activity, our results agree with the data reported by Silva et al. [70], who developed *S. aureus* and *P. aeruginosa* biofilms on polyvinyl chloride (PVC) disks and treated them for 5 min with (a) aqueous chlorhexidine gluconate solution or (b) aqueous sodium hypochlorite solution at 3% and compared them with biofilm growth in buffer solution, to find that all the tested antimicrobials significantly reduce biofilm formation by both microorganisms. Cabeça et al. [71] also evaluated the efficiency of disinfectants like iodine tincture (0.20% *w*/*v*), biguanide (0.50% w/v), quaternary ammonium compounds (0.50% w/v), peracetic acid (0.50% *v*/v), and sodium hypochlorite (1.50% v/v) against planktonic cells (10^8 CFU/mL) and biofilms formed over sterile stainless steel disks of *Listeria monocytogenes*, *S. aureus*, and *E. coli* reference strains, to verify that planktonic cells of all the organisms are sensitive to all the assayed antimicrobials. Biofim treatment with the disinfectants decreases the number of viable sessile cells. Sodium hypochlorite is the most effective agent, as corroborated by our results.

Toté et al. [72] analyzed 12 disinfectants, including sodium hypochlorite at 1% (10,000 µg/mL) and peracetic acid at 0.3% (3000 µg/mL) diluted in water, against *S. aureus* (ATCC 6538) and *P. aeruginosa* (ATCC 700928) in the planktonic and biofilm growth modes. Samples were treated for 1, 5, 15, 30, and 60 min. The authors found that *P. aeruginosa* planktonic cells are as sensitive as *S. aureus* planktonic cells. Most biocides are effective after 1 min of contact with the microorganisms. Hydrogen peroxide and sodium hypochlorite are the most active biocides against sessile cells: they affect cell viability and diminish biofilm matrix, as also demonstrated herein.

Ueda and Kuwabara [73] investigated *E. coli* O:157, *Salmonella enteritidis*, and *S. aureus* biofilm sensitivities to various disinfectants and sanitizers, to verify that none of the disinfectants (acid, neutral, or alkaline) eliminate sessile cells effectively, all the sanitizers fail to inactivate the biofilm cells completely, and the most effective agent – sodium hypochlorite – still gives colony countings of 25 to 200 microorganisms/mL after treatment at concentrations recommended by the manufacturers. At the studied concentrations, the authors found that bezalkonium chloride, alkyl diaminoethylglycine hydrochloride, chlorhexidine digluconate, and polyhexamethylene biguanide inactivate most of the *E. coli* and *S. enteritidis* cells but not the *S. aureus* cells. The authors concluded that *S. aureus* is the most resistant microorganism evaluated in their study.

Królasik et al. [74] assessed the efficiency of commercially available hydrogen peroxide- and peracetic acid-based disinfecting agents against *Listeria innocua*, *Pseudomonas putida*, *Micrococcus luteus*, and *Staphylococcus hominis* biofilms grown on stainless steel disks, to find that the disinfectants at 0.5% (5000 μg/mL) are ineffective against the bacterial biofilms after 10 min. However, the authors reported that after 30 min at 1% (10,000 μg/mL), *M. luteus* counting reduces by 5 Log UFC/mL in the presence of the disinfectants. Given the results, the concentrations recommended by the manufacturers are ineffective against the assayed bacteria. In our assays, biofilm treatment with the recommended peracetic acid concentration of 0.1% (1000 μg/mL) for 24 or 48 h provides colony countings reduced by 11 Log UFC/mL in the case of the initial inocula of *S. aureus* strains 2, 3, 9, 10, 13, and 15 and *S. epidermidis* strains 57 and 68.

Gilbert et al. [75] simultaneously evaluated five disinfectants diluted in culture medium containing peracetic acid (Proxitane 4002, Solvay Interox Ltd., Warrington, UK) against *E. coli* and *S. epidermidis* planktonic and biofilm cells. Disinfectant concentrations varied from 0 to 100 nanomoles (nmol)/L. Analyses considered the planktonic/biofilm cell ratio corresponding to 95% of dead cells within 30 min of exposure. The authors demonstrated that biofilm age affects results very little, but data heavily depend on the tested microorganism and disinfectant. They also showed that peracetic acid is the most effective agent against planktonic cells and significantly decreases biofilm cell activity at similar concentrations. One of the explanations for data dependence on concentration is that antimicrobial agents, especially agents that interfere in the membrane potential (for example, oxidizing agents such as peracetic acid), operate in many sites and through several mechanisms. Our results agree with the results of Gilbert et al. [75] in the case of planktonic cells. However, we verified that sodium hypochlorite is more efficient against biofilm cells: IC_{50} is 57.425% as compared to 33.060% achieved for peracetic acid.

In conclusion, MIC determination showed that *C. duckei* oleoresin is the most effective among the evaluated *Copaifera* species oleoresins: it inhibits the growth of *S. aureus* and *S. epidermidis* strains. Interaction between *Copaifera* oleoresins and disinfectants does not result in synergism. All the investigated strains form biofilms in the assayed conditions. Overall, the capacity of disinfectants to inhibit biofilm formation varies widely, and very low *C. duckei* oleoresin, vancomycin, peracetic acid, and sodium hypochlorite concentrations are necessary to achieve this effect. On the basis of the Minimum Biofilm Erradication Capacity, represented by IC_{50}, sodium hypochlorite is the most effective antimicrobial tested herein.

Conclusions

In general, *C. duckei* oleoresin is as active as peracetic acid in terms of *S. aureus* biofilm cell eradication. Therefore, this oleoresin is potentially useful in formulations that aim at *S. aureus* disinfection even when the microorganism grows in the biofilm mode, with possible application in dialysis settings.

Abbreviations

BHI: Brain heart infusion broth; CAPD: Continuous ambulatorial peritoneal dialysis; CLSI: Clinical and laboratory standards institute; FIC: Fractional inhibitory concentration; MIC: Minimum inhibitory concentration; $MICB_{50}$: Minimum inhibitory concentration of biofilm; OD: Optical density

Acknowledgements

Vieira R.G.L thanks University of Franca for a PhD scholarship. The authors are grateful to Conselho Nacional de Desenvolvimento Científico e Tecnológico (CNPq) for the granted fellowships.

Funding

This work was supported by São Paulo Research Foundation (FAPESP), Grant number: 2011/13630-7 and 2012/25237-0.

Authors' contributions

RGLV, TSM (PhD student), and RHP evaluated the biological activities, ran the laboratory work, analyzed data, drafted the paper, and were major contributors to the manuscript. LOS (undergraduate) and TCB (PhD student) contributed during the biological assays. RCSV contributed with critical reading of the manuscript. SRA contributed with compound isolation and identification s. JKB and CHGM designed the study, analyzed and interpreted the data, and supervised the laboratory. All the authors read and approved the final manuscript.

Consent for publication

All the authors approve the publication of this work.

Competing interests

The authors declare that they have no competing interests.

Author details
[1]Nucleus of Research in Sciences and Technology, Laboratory of Research in Applied Microbiology, University of Franca, Avenida Armando Salles de Oliveira, 201, Franca - São Paulo 14404-600, Brazil. [2]School of Pharmaceutical Sciences of Ribeirão Preto, University of São Paulo, Avenida do Café, s/n, Ribeirão Preto - São Paulo 14040-903, Brazil.

References

1. Romão D Jr. Doença Renal Crônica: Definição, Epidemiologia e Classificação. J Bras Nefrol. 2004;26(Supp 1):1-3.
2. Hoenich N, Thijssen S, Kitzler T, Levin R, Ronco C. Impact of water quality and dialysis fluid composition on dialysis practice. Blood Purif. 2008;26:6–11.
3. Bastos MG, Bregman R, Kirsztajn GM. Doença renal crônica: frequente e grave, mas também prevenível e tratável. Rev Assoc Med Bras. 2010;56:248–53.
4. Pontoriero G, Pozzoni P, Andrulli S, Locatelli F. The quality of dialysis water. Nephrol Dial Transplant. 2003;18:21–5.
5. Montanari LB, Sartori FG, Cardoso MJ, Varo SD, Pires RH, Leite CQ, Prince K, Martins CH. Microbiological contamination of a hemodialysis center water distribution system. Rev Inst Med Trop. 2009;51:37–43.
6. Coulliette AD, Arduino MJ. Hemodialysis and water quality. Semin Dial. 2013;26:427–38.
7. Cappelli G, Riccardi M, Perrone S, Bondi M, Ligabue G, Albertazzi A. Water treatment and monitor disinfection. Hemodial Int. 2006;10:13–8.
8. Moreira RRD, Martins GZ, Botelho VT, Santos LE, Cavaleiro C, Salgueiro L, Andrade G, Martins CHG. Composition and activity against oral pathogens of the essential oil of *Melampodium divaricatum* (rich.) DC. Chem Biodivers. 2014;11:438–44.
9. Severino VGP, Felixa MA, Silva MFGF, Lucarini R, Martins CHG. Chemical study of *Hortia superba* (Rutaceae) and investigation of the antimycobacterial activity of crude extracts and constituents isolated from *Hortia* species. Quím Nova. 2015;38:42–5.
10. Bardaji DK, Reis EB, Medeiros TC, Lucarini R, Crotti AE, Martins CH. Antibacterial activity of commercially available plant-derived essential oils against oral pathogenic bacteria. Nat Prod Res. 2015;13:1–4.
11. Newman DJ, Cragg GM. Natural products as sources of new drugs from 1981 to 2014. J Nat Prod. 2016;79:629–61.
12. Suleimen E, Ibataev ZH, Iskakova ZH, Ishmuratova M, Ross S, Martins CHG. Constituent composition and biological activity of essential oil from *Artemisia terrae*-albae. Chem Nat Compd. 2016;52:173–5.
13. Maciel MAM, Pinto AC, Veiga VF Jr. Plantas Medicinais: A necessidade de estudos multidisciplinares. Quim Nova. 2002;25:429–38.
14. Leandro LM, Vargas FS, Barbosa PCS, Neves JKO, Silva JA, Veiga-Junior VF. Chemistry and biological activities of Terpenoids from copaiba (*Copaifera* spp.) oleoresins. Molecules. 2012;17:3866–89.
15. Veiga Junior VF, Pinto ACO. Gênero Copaifera L. Quim Nova. 2002;25:273–86.
16. Mendonça DE, Onofre SB. Atividade antimicrobiana do óleo-resina produzido pela copaiba – *Copaifera multijuga* Hayne (Leguminosae). Rev Bras Farm. 2009;19:577–81.
17. Abrão F, Costa LDA, Alves JM, Senedese JM, Castro PT, Ambrósio SR, Veneziani RCS, Bastos JK, Tavares DC, Martins CHG. *Copaifera langsdorffii* oleoresin and its isolated compounds: antibacterial effect and antiproliferative activity in cancer cell lines. BMC Complement Altern Med. 2015;15:443.
18. Santiago KB, Conti BJ, Andrade BFMT, da Silva JJM, Rogez HLG, Crevelin EJ, Moraes LAB, Veneziani RCS, Ambrósio SR, Bastos JK, Sforcin JM. Immunomodulatory action of *Copaifera* spp oleoresins on cytokine production by human monocytes. Biomed Pharmacother. 2015;70:12–8.
19. Bardaji DK, da Silva JJ, Bianchi TC, de Souza ED, de Oliveira PF, Leandro LF, Rogez HL, Venezianni RC, Ambrosio SR, Tavares DC, Bastos JK, Martins CHG. *Copaifera reticulata* oleoresin: chemical characterization and antibacterial properties against oral pathogens. Anaerobe. 2016;40:18–27.
20. Moraes TS, Leandro LF, de Oliveira SL, Santiago MB, Souza AB, Furtado RA, Tavares DC, Veneziani RC, Ambrósio SR, Bastos JK, Martins CHG. *In vitro* evaluation of *Copaifera oblongifolia* oleoresin against bacteria causing oral infections and assessment of its cytotoxic potential. Curr Pharm Biotechnol. 2016;17:894–904.
21. Clinical and Laboratory Standards Institute. Methods for dilution antimicrobial susceptibility tests for bacteria that grow aerobically. In: Approved standard M7-A9. Wayne, Pensilvânia 32: CLSI; 2012.
22. Sarker SD, Nahar L, Kumarasamy Y. Microtitre platebased antibacterial assay incorporating resazurin as an indicator of cell growth, and its application in the in vitro antibacterial screening of phytochemicals. Methods. 2007;42:321–4.
23. Chaturvedi V, Ramani R, Ghannoum MA, Killian SB, Holliday N, Knapp C, Ostrosky-Zeichner L, Messer SA, Pfaller MA, Igbal NJ, Arthington-Skaggs BA, Vazquez JA, Sein T, Rex JH, Walsh TJ. Multilaboratory testing of antifungal combinations against a quality control isolate of *Candida krusei*. Antimicrob Agents Chemother. 2008;52:1500–2.
24. Lewis RE, Diekema DJ, Messer SA, Pfaller MA, Klepser ME. Comparison of Etest, chequerboard dilution and time-kill studies for the detection of synergy or antagonism between antifungal agents tested against *Candida* species. J Antimicrob Chemother. 2002;49:345–51.
25. Wei GX, Campagna AN, Bobek LA. Effect of MUC7 peptides on the growth of bacteria and on *Streptococcus mutans* biofilm. J Antimicrob Chemother. 2006;57:1100–9.
26. Stepanovic S, Vuković D, Hola V, Di Bonaventura G, Djukić S, Cirković I, Ruzicka F. Quantification of biofilm in microtiter plates: overview of testing conditions and practical recommendations for assessment of biofilm production by staphylococci. APMIS. 2007;115:891–9.
27. Caetano Da Silva SD, Souza MGM, Cardoso MJO, Moraes TS, Ambrosio SR, Veneziani RCS, Martins CHG. Antibacterial activity of *Pinus elliottii* against anaerobic bacteria present in primary endodontic infections. Anaerobe. 2014;30:146–52.
28. Polonio RE, Mermel LA, Paquette GA, Sperry F. Eradication of biofilm-forming *Staphylococcus epidermidis* (RP62A) by a combination of sodium salicylate and vancomycin. Antimicrob Agents Chemother. 2001;45:3262–6.
29. Shu Y. Recent natural products based drug development: a pharmaceutical industry perspective. J Nat Prod. 1998;61:1053–71.
30. Gomes NM, Rezende CM, Fontes SP, Matheus ME, Fernandes PD. Antinociceptive activity of Amazonian copaiba oils. J Ethnopharmacol. 2007; 12:486–92.
31. Veiga Junior VF, Rosasc EC, Carvalho MV, Henriques MGMO, Pinto AC. Chemical composition and anti-inflammatory activity of copaiba oils from *Copaifera cearensis* Huber ex Ducke, *Copaifera reticulata* Ducke and *Copaifera multijuga* Hayne - a comparative study. J Ethnopharmacol. 2007;112:248–54.
32. Alves EG, Vinholis AHC, Casemiro LA, Furtado NAJC, Silva MLA, Cunha WR, Martins CHG. Estudo comparativo de técnicas de screening para avaliação da atividade antibacteriana de extratos brutos de espécies vegetais e de substâncias puras. Quim Nova. 2008;31:1224–9.
33. Odakowska-Jedynak U, Paczek L, Krawczyk M, Zieniewicz K, Nyckowski P, Pawlak J, Patkowski W, Skwarek A, Paczkowska A. Resistence of gram-positive pathogens to antibiotic is a therapeutic challenge after liver transplantation: clinical experience in one center with linezolid. Transplant Proc. 2003;35:2304–6.
34. Collins AJ, Foley RN, Chavers B, Gilbertson D, Herzog C, Ishani A, Johansen K, Kasiske BL, Kutner N, Liu J, St Peter W, Guo H, Hu Y, Kats A, Li S, Li S, Maloney J, Roberts T, Skeans M, Snyder J, Solid C, Thompson B, Weinhandl E, Xiong H, Yusuf A, Zaun D, Arko C, Chen SC, Daniels F, Ebben J, Frazier E, Johnson R, Sheets D, Wang X, Forrest B, Berrini D, Constantini E, Everson S, Eggers P, Agodoa L. US Renal Data System Annual Data Report. Am J Kidney Dis. 2013;63:A7.
35. Chan KE, Warren HS, Thadhani RI, Steele DJ, Hymes JL, Maddux FW, Hakim RM. Prevalence and outcomes of antimicrobial treatment for *Staphylococcus aureus* Bacteremia in outpatients with ESRD. J Am Soc Nephrol. 2012;23:1551–9.
36. Zetola N, Francis JS, Nuermberger EL, Bishai WR. Community-acquired methicillin-resistant Staphylococcus Aureus: an emerging threat. Lancet Infect Dis. 2005;5:275–86.
37. Dos Santos ECG, Donnici CL, Camargos ER, Rezende AA, Andrade EH, Soares LA, Farias LM, Carvalho MAR, Almeida M. Effects of *Copaifera duckei* Dwyer oleoresin on the cell wall and cell division of *Bacillus cereus*. J Med Microbiol. 2013;62:1032–7.
38. Pacheco TARC, Barata LES, Duarte MCT. Antimicrobial activity of copaiba (*Copaifera* spp) balsams. Rev Bras Pl Med. 2006;8:123–4.
39. Santos AO, Ueda-Nakamura T, Dias Filho BP, Veiga Junior VF, Pinto AC, Nakamura CV. Antimicrobial activity of Brazilian copaiba oils obtained from different species of the *Copaifera* genus. Mem Inst Oswaldo Cruz. 2008;103:277–81.
40. Guissoni A, Souza K, Souza G, Santos L, Oliveira B, Vieira J, Silva H. Avaliação da Atividade antibacteriana de óleo-resina de *Copaiba* (Leguminosae, Caesalpinioideae). Rev Biotecnol Ciênc. 2015;4:1
41. Masson DS, Salvador SL, Polizello ACM, Frade MAC. Atividade antimicrobiana do óleo-resina de copaíba (*Copaifera langsdorffii*) em

bactérias de significância clínica em úlceras cutâneas. Rev Bras Pl Med. 2013; 15:664–9.

42. Beveridge TJ. Structures of gram-negative cell walls and their derived membrane vesicles. J Bacteriol. 1999;181:4725–33.
43. Navarre WW, Schneewind O. Surface proteins of Grampositive bacteria and mechanisms of their targeting to the cell wall envelope. Microbiol Mol Biol Rev. 1999;63:174–229.
44. Araújo EA, Andrade NJ, Carvalho AF, Ramos AM, Silva CAS, Silva LHM. Colloidal aspects of bacterial adhesion. Quim Nova. 2010;33:1940–8.
45. Leandro LF, Cardoso MJO, Silva SDC, Souza MGM, Veneziani RCS, Ambrosio SR, Martins CHG. Antibacterial activity of *Pinus elliottii* and its major compound, dehydroabietic acid, against multidrug-resistant strains. J Med Microbiol. 2014;63:1649–53.
46. Brasil. Ministério da Saúde. Agencia Nacional de Vigilância Sanitária. Curso básico de controle de infecção hospitalar. In: Caderno C métodos de proteção anti-infecciosa. Brasília: MS; 2000. p. 62.
47. Lindley EJ, Lopot F, Harrington M, Elseviers MM. Treatment of water for dialysis – a European survey. EDTNA ERCA J. 2000;26:22–7.
48. Ghezzi PM, Bonello M, Ronco C. Disinfection of dialysis monitors. Contrib Nephrol. 2007;154:39–60.
49. Pisani B, Simões M, Prandi MAG, Rocha MMM, Gonçalves CR, Vaz TMI, Irino K. Surto de bacteriemia por *Pseudomonas aeruginosa* na unidade de hemodiálise de um hospital de Campinas, São Paulo, Brasil. Rev Inst Adolfo Lutz. 2000;59:51–6.
50. Arvanitidou M, Vayona A, Spanakis N, Tsakris A. Occurrence and antimicrobial resistance of gram-negative bacteria isolated in haemodialysis water and dialysate of renal units: results of a Greek multicentre study. J Appl Microbiol. 2003;95:180–5.
51. Magalhães M, Doherty C, Govan JR, Vandamme P. Polyclonal outbreak of *Burkholderia cepacia* complex bacteraemia in haemodialysis patients. J Hosp Infect. 2003;54:120–3.
52. Borges CR, Lascowski KM, Filho NR, Pelayo JS. Microbiological quality of water and dialysate in a haemodialysis unit in Ponta Grossa-PR, Brazil. J Appl Microbiol. 2007;103:1791–7.
53. Oliveira PS, Souza SG, Campos GB, da Silva DC, Sousa DS, Araújo SP, Ferreira LP, Santos VM, Amorim AT, Santos AM, Timenetsky J, Cruz MP, Yatsuda R, Marques LM. Isolation, pathogenicity and disinfection of *Staphylococcus aureus* carried by insects in two public hospitals of Vitória da Conquista, Bahia, Brazil. Braz J Infect Dis. 2014;18:129–36.
54. Mitchell G, Lafrance M, Boulanger S, Séguin DL, Guay I, Gattuso M, Marsault E, Bouarab K, Malouin F. Tomatidine acts in synergy with aminoglycoside antibiotics against multiresistant *Staphylococcus aureus* and prevents virulence gene expression. J Antimicrob Chemother. 2012;67:559–68.
55. Rios JL, Récio MC. Medicinal plants and antimicrobial activity. J Ethnopharmacol. 2005;100:80–4.
56. Gibbons S. Phytochemicals for bacterial resistance – strengths, weaknesses and opportunities. Planta Med. 2008;74:594–602.
57. Zago JAA, Ushimaru PI, Barbosa LN, Fernandes JA. Sinergismo entre óleos essenciais e drogas antimicrobianas sobre linhagens de *Staphylococcus aureus* e *Escherichia coli* isoladas de casos clínicos humanos. Rev Bras Farmacogn. 2009;19:828–33.
58. Olmedo GM, Grillo-Puertas M, Cerioni L, Rapisarda VA, Volentini SI. Removal of pathogenic bacterial biofilms by combinations of oxidizing compounds. Can J Microbiol. 2015;61:351–6.
59. Karanika S, Zervou FN, Zacharioudakis IM, Paudel S, Mylonakis E. Risk factors for meticillin-resistant *Staphylococcus aureus* colonization in dialysis patients: a meta-analysis. J Hosp Infect. 2015;91:257–63.
60. Arciola CR, Campoccia D, Ravaioli S, Montanaro L. Polysaccharide intercellular adhesin in biofilm: structural and regulatory aspects. Front Cell Infect Microbiol. 2015;10:7.
61. Leandro LF, Moraes TS, de Oliveira PF, Alves JM, Senedese JM, Ozelin SD, Resende FA, De Grandis RA, Varanda EA, Bastos JK, Tavares DC, Martins CHG. Assessment of the antibacterial, cytotoxic and mutagenic potential of the phenolic-rich hydroalcoholic extract from *Copaifera trapezifolia* Hayne leaves. J Med Microbiol. 2016;65:937–50.
62. Alencar EN, Xavier-Júnior FH, Morais AR, Dantas TR, Dantas-Santos N, Verissimo LM, Rehder VL, Chaves GM, Oliveira AG, Egitol ES. Chemical characterization and antimicrobial activity evaluation of natural oil Nanostructured emulsions. J Nanosci Nanotechnol. 2015;15:880–8.
63. Das JR, Bhakoo M, Jones MV, Gilbert P. Changes in the biocide susceptibility of *Staphylococcus epidermidis* and *Escherichia coli* cells associated with rapid attachment to plastic surfaces. J Appl Microbiol. 1998;84:852–9.
64. Sabrah AH, Yassen GH, Gregory RL. Effectiveness of antibiotic medicaments against biofilm formation of *Enterococcus faecalis* and *Porphyromonas gingivalis*. J Endod. 2013;39:1385–9.
65. Mendoza-Olazarán S, Camacho-Ortiz A, Martínez-Reséndez MF, Llaca-Díaz JM, Pérez-Rodríguez E, Garza-González E. Influence of whole-body washing of critically ill patients with chlorhexidine on *Acinetobacter baumannii* isolates. Am J Infect Control. 2014;42:874–8.
66. Chojecka A, Wiercińska O, Röhm-Rodowald E, Kanclerski K, Jakimiak B. Effect of adaptation process of *Pseudomonas aeruginosa* to didecyldimethylammonium chloride in 2-propanol on bactericidal efficiency of this active substance. Rocz Panstw Zakl Hig. 2014;65:359–64.
67. Seier-Petersen MA, Nielsen LN, Ingmer H, Aarestrup FM, Agersø Y. Biocide susceptibility of *Staphylococcus aureus* CC398 and CC30 isolates from pigs and identification of the biocide resistance genes, qacG and qacC. Microb Drug Resist. 2015;21:527–36.
68. Svidzinski TIE, Svidzinski AE, Posseto I, de Pádua RAF, Tavares TR. Eficiência do Ácido Peracético no controle de *Staphylococcus aureus* Meticilina resistente. Cienc Cuid Saude. 2007;6:312–8.
69. Guimarães MA, Coelho LR, Souza RR, Ferreira-Carvalho BT, Figueiredo MAS. Impact of biocides on biofilm formation by methicillin-resistant *Staphylococcus aureus* (ST239-SCCmecIII) isolates. Microbiol Immunol. 2012;56:3–7.
70. Silva RC, Carver RA, Ojano-Dirain CP, Antonelli PJ. Efficacy of disinfecting solutions in removing biofilms from polyvinyl chloride tracheostomy tubes. Laryngoscope. 2013;123:259–63.
71. Cabeça TK, Pizzolitto AC, Pizzolitto EL. Activity of disinfectants against foodborne pathogens in suspension and adhered to stainless steel surfaces. Braz J Microbiol. 2012;43:1112–9.
72. Toté K, Horemans T, Vanden Berghe D, Maes L, Cos P. Inhibitory effect of biocides on the viable masses and matrices of *Staphylococcus aureus* and *Pseudomonas aeruginosa* biofilms. Appl Environ Microbiol. 2010;76:3135–42.
73. Ueda S, Kuwabara Y. Susceptibility of biofilm *Escherichia coli*, *Salmonella enteritidis* and *Staphylococcus aureus* to detergents and sanitizers. Biocontrol Sci. 2007;12:149–53.
74. Królasik J, Zakowska Z, Krepska M, Klimek L. Resistance of bacterial biofilms formed on stainless steel surface to disinfecting agent. Pol J Microbiol. 2010; 59:281–7.
75. Gilbert P, Das JR, Jones MV, Allison DG. Assessment of resistance towards biocides following the attachment of micro-organisms to, an growth on, surfaces. J Appl Microbiol. 2001;nn91:248–54.

Investigation of a Carbapenemase-producing *Acinetobacter baumannii* outbreak using whole genome sequencing versus a standard epidemiologic investigation

Chloe Bogaty[1*], Laura Mataseje[2], Andrew Gray[3], Brigitte Lefebvre[4], Simon Lévesque[4], Michael Mulvey[2] and Yves Longtin[5*]

Abstract

Background: The standard epidemiologic investigation of outbreaks typically relies on spatiotemporal data and pulsed-field gel electrophoresis (PFGE), but whole genome sequencing (WGS) is becoming increasingly used. This investigation aimed to characterize a carbapenemase-producing *Acinetobacter baumannii* (CPAb) nosocomial outbreak using WGS compared to a standard outbreak investigation.

Methods: The CPAb outbreak occurred in a single center between 2012 and 2014. The standard investigation used spatiotemporal data and PFGE to generate a chain of transmission. A separate WGS investigation generated a chain of transmission based solely on WGS and date of sampling and was blinded to all other spatiotemporal data and PFGE. Core single nucleotide variant (SNV) phylogenetic analysis was performed on WGS data generated using the Illumina MiSeq platform. The chains of transmission were compared quantitatively and qualitatively to assess the concordance between both methods.

Results: 28 colonized and infected cases were included. Of the 27 transmission events identified using the standard investigation, 12 (44%) were identical to the transmission events using WGS. WGS identified several transmission events that had not been detected by traditional method, and numerous transmission events that had occurred on different hospital wards than suspected by standard methods. The average number (standard deviation [SD]) of SNVs per transmission events was 1.63 (SD, 1.31) by traditional method and 0.63 (SD, 0.79) by WGS ($p = 0.001$) All isolates harbored the rare carbapenemase $bla_{\text{OXA-237}}$.

Conclusions: The traditional and WGS investigations had moderate concordance. When used alongside epidemiologic data and clinical information, WGS could help improve the mapping of transmission events.

Keywords: Outbreak investigations, Whole-genome sequencing, Acinetobacter baumannii, Carbapenemase-producing organisms, Single nucleotide variant analysis

* Correspondence: chloe.bogaty@gmail.com; yves.longtin@mcgill.ca
Presented in part at the 27th European Congress of Clinical Microbiology and Infectious Diseases (ECCMID), Vienna, Austria. April 2017. Abstract number 3737.
[1]University of Manitoba, Winnipeg, MB, Canada
[5]McGill University, Montreal, QC, Canada
Full list of author information is available at the end of the article

Background

Carbapenemase-producing *Acinetobacter baumannii* (CPAb) is of global concern [1]. Canada has had infrequent cases [2], but has not been spared from the occasional outbreak [3]. The most recent reported outbreak occurred from 2012 to 2014 in a primary and tertiary institution in Montreal (Canada) [4].

Control of CPAb outbreaks requires meticulous investigation. A standard epidemiologic investigation is a multi-step process including the creation of a chain of transmission [4]. Phenotypic characteristics such as biotypes, serotypes, and antimicrobial susceptibilities are used to infer pathogen inter-relatedness and is combined with spatiotemporal information to determine transmission events [5]. This information is sometimes combined with molecular typing methods (commonly pulsed-field gel electrophoresis (PFGE)). PFGE is usually considered the gold standard for its ability to detect differences across the entire genome [5, 6].

Whole genome sequencing (WGS) is increasingly being recognized as a powerful tool for epidemiologic studies. Its ability to distinguish strains that differ by single nucleotides provides high levels of resolution [7, 8]. WGS has been employed in outbreak investigations, both retrospectively to identify environmental sources [9] and additional cases [10], but also in real-time to confirm the existence of an outbreak [11] and track the emergence and spread of mutational resistance mechanisms [12]. However, only a few studies have compared standard epidemiologic outbreak investigations with investigations performed by WGS. Through the subsequent use of WGS, Kanamori et al observed that two epidemiologically unlinked outbreaks were in fact genetically connected [13]. In another study, WGS allowed for the identification of unexpected transmission routes not initially suggested by the epidemiologic data [14].

The aim of this study was to contrast the validity and accuracy of a standard epidemiologic outbreak investigation with one achieved using WGS. We retrospectively characterized the CPAb nosocomial outbreak that occurred in an academic institution in Montreal (Canada) using only WGS analysis and compared the predicted chain of transmission with an existing standard epidemiologic investigation.

Methods

Setting and definitions

A CPAb outbreak occurred in a 637-bed primary and tertiary care hospital between March 2012 and January 2014 [4]. A confirmed case was defined as any patient found to be colonized or infected during this period by the outbreak strain, as confirmed by pulsed-field gel electrophoresis interpretative criteria [15].

Standard epidemiologic investigation

Screening was performed using Acinetobacter-selective chromogenic agar (CHROMagar Acinetobacter, CHROMagar Microbiology, Paris, France). While initially carried out in patients who had shared hospital rooms with known cases, screening eventually evolved to include all patients sharing a ward with a case. Organism identification was conducted using matrix-assisted laser desorption/ionization time-of-flight mass spectrometry (MALDI-TOF MS, bioMérieux, Marcy l'Étoile, France) and antimicrobial susceptibility testing with disc diffusion and E-test following the Clinical and Laboratory Standards Institute breakpoints (2014 M100S). Strain clonality was confirmed by PFGE. Bacterial genomes were digested with *Apa*I restriction enzyme and samples were run on a CHEF-DR III system (Bio-Rad, Mississauga, ON, Canada). Banding patterns were analyzed using Tenover's criteria [15]. Detection of resistance genes was performed at the National Microbiology Laboratory in Winnipeg (Canada) [16]. Determining the chain of transmission followed a previously described approach, using a combination of spatiotemporal patient information, date of strain isolation, antibiogram results, and PFGE interpretations [4].

DNA extraction and whole genome sequencing

Total cellular deoxyribonucleic acid (DNA) was prepared using Epicentre MasterPure™ Complete kits (Mandel Scientific, Guelph, ON). Libraries were created with TruSeq Nano DNA HT sample preparation kits (Illumina, San Diego, CA). Paired-end, 301 bp indexed reads were generated on an Illumina MiSeq™ platform (Illumina, San Diego, CA). De novo assembly of Illumina reads were done using Spades v3.5. Assembled sequence data was analysed using the batch uploader mode at the Centre for Genomic Epidemiology website (https://cge.cbs.dtu.dk/services/) and data was produced from the ResFinder, PlasmidFinder, VirulenceFinder, and MLST tools.

Single nucleotide variant (SNV) analysis and creation of WGS-based chain of transmission

SNV analysis was conducted using a previously published pipeline [17]. The following parameters were added: map/base quality 30, alternate fraction 0.75, minimum read coverage of identification of variants 10, SNV density filtering of 2 SNVs within a 20-base pair window. The reference strain used was an assembled genome of one of the internal isolates to the outbreak (patient 29). Maximum likelihood phylogenetic trees were built using PhyML v3.1 using parameters "—quiet –b – 4 –m GTR –s BEST" [18]. Images were rendered in FigTree (v1.4.1) (http://tree.bio.ed.ac.uk/software/figtree).

A WGS-based chain of transmission was generated using only the sequencing data and the date of sampling to determine directionality, with complete blinding of the epidemiologic data. A cut-off of ≤2 SNV was selected to indicate a putative transmission event between patients. Also, when >1 potential source patient was plausible for a given transmission event, transmission events with a lower number of SNVs were considered more likely (e.g. 0 SNV more likely than 2 SNVs).

Comparison of the outbreak investigation methods

To compare the chains of transmission generated by standard epidemiologic investigation vs. WGS, four different strategies were used. Firstly, both chains of transmission were compared qualitatively. For each transmission event, epidemiologic data was revised to assess where patients had likely acquired the outbreak strain. Secondly, WGS was used to verify the plausibility of each transmission event determined by the standard investigation. Transmission events that remained unchanged were deemed to be supported by WGS, while those that differed were considered unsupported. Thirdly, quantitative SNV differences were calculated by comparing the mean number of SNVs per transmission event between the two investigation methods using the Student's T-test. Statistical significance was defined as a p-value of < 0.05. Finally, the WGS-generated data was compared to that obtained by PFGE for each isolate.

Results

Outbreak description

Twenty-eight cases were identified during the outbreak. The index case occurred in the intensive care unit in March 2012. Twenty-seven additional cases were detected up to 2014. Five cases developed CPAb bacteremia, and all died within 72 h of the first positive blood culture. These represented the only cases of infection, while the remaining 22 cases were only colonized. All isolates were resistant to penicillins, carbapenems, quinolones, and aminoglycosides. Four pulsovars were identified by PFGE. Further details on patient characteristics and the course of the outbreak have been reported previously [4].

Genomic analysis

By in silico sequence typing, all 28 isolates were found to be of sequence type (ST) 208. Resistant genes identified by WGS were consistent for all isolates. Carbapenem resistance was attributable to the presence of the acquired class D carbapenemase $bla_{OXA-237}$ as well as the intrinsic bla_{OXA-66}. Aminoglycoside resistance was attributable to the presence of *aadA1*, *aph(3')-Ia*, *armA*, *strA* and *strB*. Quinolone resistance was due to mutations in both GyrA (Ser-83-Leu) and ParC (Ser-80-Leu) [19, 20].

The total percentage of valid and included positions used for SNV analysis represented 96.8% of the total core genome. A total of 20 SNVs were used to generate phylogeny as they were identified across all outbreak strains. These 20 SNV loci were extracted and aligned for comparison (Table 1).

Comparison of epidemiologic investigations

Transmission events using a standard outbreak investigation [4] versus WGS-generated chain of transmission are found in Fig. 1. Of the 27 transmission events determined using a traditional investigation strategy, 12 (44.4%) were identical to transmission events predicted by WGS, while 15 (55.5%) were discordant (Fig. 1b).

In the standard investigation, patient 2 was predicted to be the central source for the two principal transmission

Table 1 Single nucleotide variant (SNV) differences between outbreak strains

Year	Identifier	PFGE Pulsovar	SNV Analysis	
			Pseudo-alignment	Difference in SNVs from Index Case
2012	1	A5-c	CGCAAGCTTCTGGTTTAACC	Index case
	2	A	C**A**CAAG**AC**TCTGGTT**C**AACC	4
	3	A5	CGCAAG**AC**TCTGGTTTAACC	2
	4	A4	CGC**C**AGCTTCTG**A**TTTAACC	2
2013	5	A5	CGCAAG**AC**TCTGGTTTAACC	2
	6	A5	CGCAAG**AC**TC**C**GGTTTAACC	3
	7	A5	CGCAAG**AC**TC**C**GGTTTAACC	3
	8	A5	CGCAAG**AC**TC**C**GGT**G**TAACC	4
	9	A5	CGCAAG**AC**TC**C**GGTTTA**G**CC	4
	10	A5	CGCAAG**AC**TC**C**GGTTTAACC	3
	11	A5	CGCAAG**ACC**CT**A**GTTTAACC	4
	12	A5	CGCAAG**AC**TC**C**GGTTTAACC	3
	13	A4	CGCA**TAAC**TC**C**GGTTTAACC	5
	14	A6	CGCAA**AAC**TC**C**GGTTTAACC	4
	15	A4	CGCA**TAAC**TC**C**GGTTTAACC	5
	16	A6	CGCA**TAAC**TC**C**GGTTTAACC	5
	17	A5	CGCAAG**AC**TCTGGTTTAACC	2
	18	A5	**T**G**T**AAG**AC**TCTGGTTTAACC	4
	19	A5-a	CGCAAG**AC**TCTGGTTTAACC	2
	20	A5-a	CGCAAG**AC**TCTGGTTTAACC	2
	21	A5-a	CGCAAG**AC**TCTGGTTTAACC	2
	22	A5-a	CGCAAG**AC**TCTGGTTTAACC	2
	23	A5-a	CGCAAG**AC**TCTGGTTTAACC	2
	24	A5	**T**G**T**AAG**AC**TCTGGTTTAACC	4
	25	A5	CGCAAG**AC**TCTGGTTTAA**T**C	3
	26	A5	**T**G**T**AAG**AC**TCTGGTTTAACC	4
	27	A5	**T**G**T**AAG**AC**TCTGGTTTAACC	4
2014	28	A6	CGCAAG**AC**TCTGG**A**TT**C**ACC	4

Bolded letters represent a SNV difference compared to the index case
Abbreviations: *SNV*, single nucleotide variants; *PFGE*, pulsed-field gel electrophoresis; *Q*, quarter

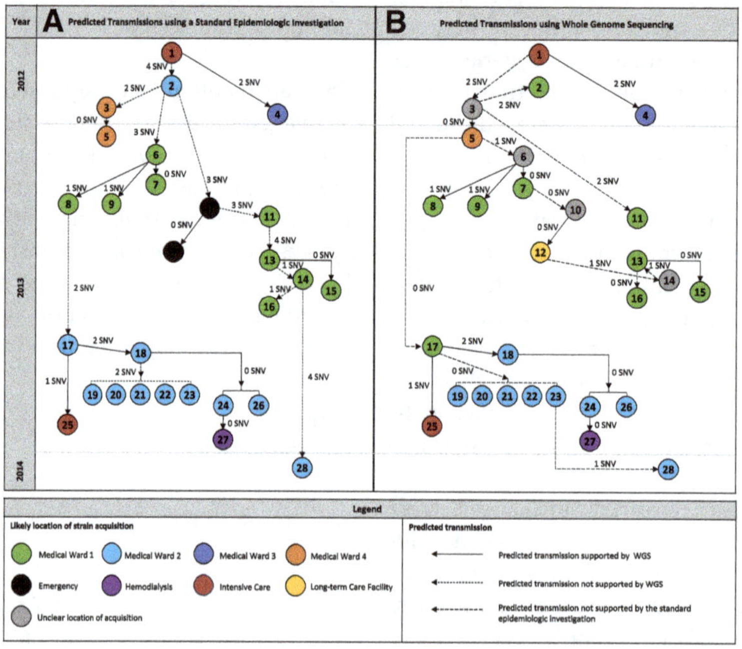

Fig. 1 Transmission of a carbapenemase-producing *Acinetobacter baumannii* during a hospital outbreak in Montreal, Canada (axis not to scale). (**a**) Standard epidemiologic investigation, where predicted transmissions were determined using spatiotemporal patient information, date of strain isolation, antibiogram results, and pulsed-field gel electrophoresis interpretation. (**b**) Whole genome sequencing investigation, where predicted transmissions were determined using single nucleotide variant analysis and the date of strain isolation. Colours indicate the case's location at the time of the predicted exposure. Dashed arrows indicate transmissions that were not supported by the other investigation method. SNV, single nucleotide variant

arms (Fig. 1a). The cluster of transmission that occurred on Medical Ward (MW) 1 in the first quarter of 2013 (patients 6–9) was believed to have been introduced by patient 2. WGS analysis, however, did not support this conclusion and suggested that the strain from patient 6 was more closely related to patient 5 than patient 2 (1 SNV vs 3 SNV, respectively). Similarly, the cluster on MW 2 in 2013 (patient 17–24, and 26) was initially believed to have originated from patient 8, whereas WGS suggested that the strain in this cluster was identical to the strain of patients 3 and 5 (0 SNV) and different from patient 8 (2 SNVs). Using WGS, patient 3 was deemed central to the outbreak, contributing both to clusters on MW 1 in early-to-mid 2013 and the cluster on MW 2 in late 2013 (Fig. 1b). On the other hand, the WGS-generated chain of transmission also incorrectly identified some transmission events. For example, the source of patient 17 was attributed to patient 5 by WGS and date of sampling, but considering that the strains of patients 3, 5 and 17 were identical, the source of patient 17 may have been patient 3 or an unknown intermediate case. In fact, spatiotemporal analysis indicated that patients 3 and 17 were both temporally located on MW 1 prior to patient 17 being transferred to MW 2 where the outbreak strain rapidly disseminated. Other notable discrepancies between both investigation methods included transmissions to patients 6, 10, 11, 13 and 28 (Fig. 1).

In the standard investigation, 26 of the 28 cases were found to have shared a ward with a potential source case. [4] In the WGS-generated chain of transmission, 23 of the 27 transmission events could be explained by patients sharing a ward with a known case, though acquisition of the outbreak strain occasionally occurred on a different ward than previously suspected (Fig. 1b).

Two discordant events differed only in terms of directionality. Using standard epidemiologic tools, patient 2 was thought to have transmitted the outbreak strain to patient 3, and patient 13 to 14. However, WGS suggested that the opposite had actually occurred, postulating that patients 3 and 14 had either acquired the outbreak strain at an earlier date than originally thought or that there were undetected carriers.

SNV differences between transmission events in the standard epidemiologic investigation ranged from 0 to 4 SNVs, while the range was from 0 to 2 SNVs in the WGS-generated chain of transmission. The largest SNV difference between the index case and a subsequent case was 19 SNVs in the standard investigation (index case and patient 28; Fig. 1a) compared to 5 SNVs in the WGS investigation (index case and patients 13, 15 and 16; Fig. 1b). The average number of SNVs (standard deviation) per transmission event was 1.63 (1.31) and 0.63 (0.79) for the standard vs. WGS-generated investigations, respectively ($p = 0.001$ by Student's T-test).

Comparison of conventional typing by PFGE and genomic analysis

Four pulsovars were identified by PFGE. By WGS, patients 3, 5, 17, and 19 to 23 had no SNV differences. However, PFGE established different band patterns, initially grouping the isolates into pulsovar A5 or A5-a. Examination of these sequences identified three small DNA segments unique to the earlier isolates, but none which explained the band variation seen on PFGE. It is suspected that a genetic event (insertion, deletion or recombination) occurred at or near the restriction site for *ApaI* causing different band numbers or shifting of band sizes. SNV analysis may not have detected this change as it may have occurred at a site of multiple events outside of our SNV parameters (i.e. 96.8% of core genome covered by WGS) or was a large event not captured by the SNV workflow. Similarly, PFGE grouped isolates 13 and 15 into pulsovar A4, and isolate 16 to pulsovar A6, but there were no SNV differences between these 3 strains by WGS.

Discussion

Outbreak investigations typically rely on spatiotemporal data and PFGE, but WGS is also becoming increasingly used. Our study compared the chains of transmission of a CPAb outbreak using a standard epidemiologic investigation and a WGS-based technique. Using qualitative and quantitative comparative strategies, our investigation identified many similarities between both investigations, but also major differences. Nearly 50% of the predicted transmissions were identical between both methods, and upon review of the epidemiologic data it was found that several transmissions had occurred on different hospital wards than previously assumed.

The extent of these differences was unexpected. Some discrepancies may be explained by the fact that transmission events in standard epidemiologic investigations are typically deduced based on commonality between a source and a case and are prone to missing transmission events between patients with little spatiotemporal commonality [5, 21]. The location where transmission occurred could not be identified for four patients from the WGS-generated chain after review of the epidemiologic data; these transmission events were at risk of being missed using traditional tools. Additionally, PFGE detected different band patterns among genetically related isolates by WGS, likely influencing some of the dissimilar epidemiologic predictions. Overall, the chain of transmission determined by WGS might be perceived as more accurate due to the close genetic relatedness of the strains. However, some WGS-generated transmission events may be incorrect: upon reviewing spatiotemporal data, the origin of patient 17 is probably patient 3 instead of patient 5.

Both chains did retain an important degree of concordance, which is noteworthy considering that the WGS-generated chain of transmission was fully blinded to any spatiotemporal information and to the PFGE typing results. It provides a glimpse of the potential for automated outbreak investigations. Some transmission events determined by traditional method were shown to be implausible by WGS given the high number of SNVs between the source and the recipient. However, it can be argued that some discrepancies are of minor importance, such as linking cases 19–23 to either patient 17 or 18. Knowing these differences would have changed little in terms of outbreak confinement measures.

Still, some observations suggested that WGS may have had practical value had it been available. Firstly, the WGS investigation suggests that infection control strategies around patient 3 had failed, leading to the cluster of cases on MW 2. Patients 3 and 17 had been hospitalized on the same ward prior to 17 being diagnosed with the outbreak strain, but this association was not captured in the original investigation. Had it been, there could have been efforts to understand why control measures were breached. Secondly, the SNV analysis suggested missed opportunities for earlier case findings. Real-time WGS-assisted investigation could have suggested the presence of additional unidentified cases. Finally, it was unclear where four cases acquired the outbreak strain. Had the connection between source and case been made in real-time, it might have assisted in generating hypotheses regarding transmission.

WGS is already used for public health surveillance in various jurisdictions [22–25], and has helped perform accurate contact tracing in health-care settings [11, 26, 27]. Our findings further support the potential role of WGS in hospital outbreak investigations, particularly as the technology becomes more affordable and accessible [6, 8, 28, 29].

Two additional observations are noteworthy. Firstly, our investigation demonstrated surprising discrepancies in the phylogenetic assessment of clonality between PFGE and WGS. While PFGE occasionally lacks discriminatory power with closely related bacterial strains [6, 30, 31], it seemed unusual for it to assign different pulsovars to strains that were found to have no SNV differences. However, *A. baumannii* can undergo significant horizontal gene transfer and genetic recombination, even over short time periods [32]. Other studies have observed low discriminatory powers of PFGE when applied to *A. baumannii* [27, 33]. With *A. baumannii*, PFGE may be too discriminatory between isolates and distort the interpretation of phylogenetic differences, essentially leading to "false-negative" results where WGS data may provide indistinguishable differences [7]. SNV analyses may be superior to PFGE for *A. baumannii* typing as it ignores changes due to horizontal gene transfers and genomic recombination.

Secondly, this study represents the third reported identification of the acquired class D carbapenemase $bla_{\text{OXA-237}}$, and its first identification in Canada. The $bla_{\text{OXA-235-like}}$ subclass, which includes $bla_{\text{OXA-237}}$, was first recognised from *A. baumannii* isolates in the United States and Mexico in 2013 [34] and was implicated in a multi-center outbreak in Oregon between 2012 and 2014 [35]. This resistance gene was located on a plasmid found in the most prominent *A. baumannii* clonal group, representing a potential for extensive dissemination [36].

Our study has some limitations. Due to its retrospective nature, it remains unknown whether performing WGS in real-time would have altered the outbreak progression. Despite all the discrepancies observed, the standard epidemiologic investigation was ultimately successful in controlling the outbreak. Also, review of the available epidemiologic data could not account for the method of CPAb acquisition in four cases. Subsequent epidemiologic investigation was not conducted to link these cases with a source. *A. baumannii* can contaminate the hospital environment, such that transmission through fomites or health care workers is possible [3, 27]. Neither investigation can account for the presence of additional unidentified colonized patients [37]. Finally, the lack of a standardized definition for "bacterial clones" in molecular epidemiology for *A. baumannii* also complicates WGS investigations [7, 33, 38–40]. Bacteria naturally undergo genomic diversification, and SNVs can accumulate at a rate of 2–10/year in most bacterial genomes [7, 27]. Still, our data demonstrates minimal genetic diversification between isolates, with no more than 5 SNV differences from the index case and some with 0 SNV changes over nearly a year.

Conclusion

This study suggests that an investigation based on WGS and date of sampling was able to create a transmission sequence that was in many aspects similar to a traditional outbreak investigation and that detected transmission events that had not been suspected using traditional tools. WGS may help improve the understanding of transmission during outbreaks when used alongside epidemiologic data and clinical information.

Abbreviations

CPAb: Carbapenemase-producing *Acinetobacter baumanii*; DNA: Deoxyribonucleic acid; MALDI-TOF MS: Matrix-assisted laser desorption/ionization time-of-flight mass spectrometry; MW: Medical ward; PFGE: Pulse-field gel electrophoresis; SNV: Single nucleotide variant; WGS: Whole genome sequencing

Acknowledgements

We thank all the members of the infection control unit and clinical microbiology laboratory for their dedication in controlling this outbreak.

Funding

This work was supported by institutional grants and by the Fonds de Recherche du Québec en Santé.

Availability of data and materials

The datasets used/or analyzed during the current study are available from the corresponding author on reasonable request.

Authors' contributions

CB and YL reviewed and analyzed the molecular data in comparison to the epidemiologic data, and equally contributed to the writing of the manuscript. APG collected and interpreted the epidemiologic data to generate the original outbreak tree. LM and MRM performed the genomic analysis of the outbreak strains using whole-genome sequencing and were major contributors in writing of the manuscript. BL and SL identified the different pulsovars using pulse-field gel electrophoresis and contributed to the epidemiologic investigation of this outbreak. All authors read and approved the final manuscript.

Ethics approval and consent to participate

Jewish General Hospital Research Review Office – # CODIM-MBM-CR18-05.

Consent for publication

Not applicable.

Competing interests

YL reported receiving research funding from Merck and Becton Dickinson. The authors declare that they have no competing interests.

Author details

[1]University of Manitoba, Winnipeg, MB, Canada. [2]National Microbiology Laboratory, Winnipeg, MB, Canada. [3]Northern Health, Prince George, BC, Canada. [4]Laboratoire de santé publique du Québec, Sainte-Anne-de-Bellevue, QC, Canada. [5]McGill University, Montreal, QC, Canada.

References

1. Peleg AY, Seifert H, Paterson DL. Acinetobacter baumannii: emergence of a successful pathogen. Clin Microbiol Rev. 2008;21:538–82.
2. Mataseje LF, Bryce E, Roscoe D, Boyd DA, Embree J, Gravel D, Katz K, Kibsey P, Kuhn M, Mounchili A, et al. Carbapenem-resistant gram-negative bacilli in Canada 2009-10: results from the Canadian nosocomial infection surveillance program (CNISP). J Antimicrob Chemother. 2012;67:1359–67.
3. Simor AE, Lee M, Vearncombe M, Jones-Paul L, Barry C, Gomez M, Fish JS, Cartotto RC, Palmer R, Louie M. An outbreak due to multiresistant Acinetobacter baumannii in a burn unit: risk factors for acquisition and management. Infect Control Hosp Epidemiol. 2002;23:261–7.
4. Gray AP, Allard R, Pare R, Tannenbaum T, Lefebvre B, Levesque S, Mulvey M, Maalouf L, Perna S, Longtin Y. Management of a hospital outbreak of extensively drug-resistant Acinetobacter baumannii using a multimodal intervention including daily chlorhexidine baths. J Hosp Infect. 2016;93:29–34.
5. Singh A, Goering RV, Simjee S, Foley SL, Zervos MJ. Application of molecular techniques to the study of hospital infection. Clin Microbiol Rev. 2006;19: 512–30.
6. Koser CU, Ellington MJ, Cartwright EJ, Gillespie SH, Brown NM, Farrington M, Holden MT, Dougan G, Bentley SD, Parkhill J, Peacock SJ. Routine use of microbial whole genome sequencing in diagnostic and public health microbiology. PLoS Pathog. 2012;8:e1002824.
7. Salipante SJ, SenGupta DJ, Cummings LA, Land TA, Hoogestraat DR, Cookson BT. Application of whole-genome sequencing for bacterial strain typing in molecular epidemiology. J Clin Microbiol. 2015;53:1072–9.

8. Robinson ER, Walker TM, Pallen MJ. Genomics and outbreak investigation: from sequence to consequence. Genome Med. 2013;5:36.
9. Reuter S, Harrison TG, Koser CU, Ellington MJ, Smith GP, Parkhill J, Peacock SJ, Bentley SD, Torok ME. A pilot study of rapid whole-genome sequencing for the investigation of a legionella outbreak. BMJ Open. 2013;3:e002175.
10. Butcher H, Elson R, Chattaway MA, Featherstone CA, Willis C, Jorgensen F, Dallman TJ, Jenkins C, Mc LJ, Beck CR, Harrison S. Whole genome sequencing improved case ascertainment in an outbreak of Shiga toxin-producing Escherichia coli O157 associated with raw drinking milk. Epidemiol Infect. 2016;144:2812–23.
11. Eyre DW, Golubchik T, Gordon NC, Bowden R, Piazza P, Batty EM, Ip CL, Wilson DJ, Didelot X, O'Connor L, et al. A pilot study of rapid benchtop sequencing of Staphylococcus aureus and Clostridium difficile for outbreak detection and surveillance. BMJ Open. 2012;2:e001124.
12. Otter JA, Doumith M, Davies F, Mookerjee S, Dyakova E, Gilchrist M, Brannigan ET, Bamford K, Galletly T, Donaldson H, et al. Emergence and clonal spread of colistin resistance due to multiple mutational mechanisms in carbapenemase-producing Klebsiella pneumoniae in London. Sci Rep. 2017;7:12711.
13. Kanamori H, Parobek CM, Juliano JJ, van Duin D, Cairns BA, Weber DJ, Rutala WA. A prolonged outbreak of KPC-3-producing Enterobacter cloacae and Klebsiella pneumoniae driven by multiple mechanisms of resistance transmission at a large academic burn center. Antimicrob Agents Chemother. 2017;61:e01516.
14. Snitkin ES, Zelazny AM, Thomas PJ, Stock F, Group NCSP, Henderson DK, Palmore TN, Segre JA. Tracking a hospital outbreak of carbapenem-resistant Klebsiella pneumoniae with whole-genome sequencing. Sci Transl Med. 2012;4:148ra116.
15. Tenover FC, Arbeit RD, Goering RV, Mickelsen PA, Murray BE, Persing DH, Swaminathan B. Interpreting chromosomal DNA restriction patterns produced by pulsed-field gel electrophoresis: criteria for bacterial strain typing. J Clin Microbiol. 1995;33:2233–9.
16. Woodford N, Ellington MJ, Coelho JM, Turton JF, Ward ME, Brown S, Amyes SG, Livermore DM. Multiplex PCR for genes encoding prevalent OXA carbapenemases in Acinetobacter spp. Int J Antimicrob Agents. 2006;27:351–3.
17. Petkau A, Mabon P, Sieffert C, Knox NC, Cabral J, Iskander M, Iskander M, Weedmark K, Zaheer R, Katz LS, et al. SNVPhyl: a single nucleotide variant phylogenomics pipeline for microbial genomic epidemiology. Microb Genom. 2017;3:e000116.
18. Guindon S, Dufayard JF, Lefort V, Anisimova M, Hordijk W, Gascuel O. New algorithms and methods to estimate maximum-likelihood phylogenies: assessing the performance of PhyML 3.0. Syst Biol. 2010;59:307–21.
19. Vila J, Ruiz J, Goni P, Marcos A, Jimenez de Anta T. Mutation in the gyrA gene of quinolone-resistant clinical isolates of Acinetobacter baumannii. Antimicrob Agents Chemother. 1995;39:1201–3.
20. Vila J, Ruiz J, Goni P, Jimenez de Anta T. Quinolone-resistance mutations in the topoisomerase IV parC gene of Acinetobacter baumannii. J Antimicrob Chemother. 1997;39:757–62.
21. Lesson 6: Investigating an outbreak. In: Principles of Epidemiology in Public Health Practice, Third edition: an introduction to applied epidemiology and biostatistics; 2012.
22. Inns T, Ashton PM, Herrera-Leon S, Lighthill J, Foulkes S, Jombart T, Rehman Y, Fox A, Dallman T, E DEP, et al. Prospective use of whole genome sequencing (WGS) detected a multi-country outbreak of Salmonella Enteritidis. Epidemiol Infect. 2016;145:1–10.
23. Joensen KG, Scheutz F, Lund O, Hasman H, Kaas RS, Nielsen EM, Aarestrup FM. Real-time whole-genome sequencing for routine typing, surveillance, and outbreak detection of verotoxigenic Escherichia coli. J Clin Microbiol. 2014;52:1501–10.
24. Agren EC, Wahlstrom H, Vesterlund-Carlson C, Lahti E, Melin L, Soderlund R. Comparison of whole genome sequencing typing results and epidemiological contact information from outbreaks of Salmonella Dublin in Swedish cattle herds. Infect Ecol Epidemiol. 2016;6:31782.
25. Mellmann A, Harmsen D, Cummings CA, Zentz EB, Leopold SR, Rico A, Prior K, Szczepanowski R, Ji Y, Zhang W, et al. Prospective genomic characterization of the German enterohemorrhagic Escherichia coli O104:H4 outbreak by rapid next generation sequencing technology. PLoS One. 2011;6:e22751.
26. Koser CU, Holden MT, Ellington MJ, Cartwright EJ, Brown NM, Ogilvy-Stuart AL, Hsu LY, Chewapreecha C, Croucher NJ, Harris SR, et al. Rapid whole-genome sequencing for investigation of a neonatal MRSA outbreak. N Engl J Med. 2012;366:2267–75.
27. Kanamori H, Parobek CM, Weber DJ, van Duin D, Rutala WA, Cairns BA, Juliano JJ. Next-generation sequencing and comparative analysis of sequential outbreaks caused by multidrug-resistant Acinetobacter baumannii at a large academic burn center. Antimicrob Agents Chemother. 2015;60:1249–57.
28. Didelot X, Bowden R, Wilson DJ, Peto TEA, Crook DW. Transforming clinical microbiology with bacterial genome sequencing. Nat Rev Genet. 2012;13: 601–12.
29. Kwong JC, McCallum N, Sintchenko V, Howden BP. Whole genome sequencing in clinical and public health microbiology. Pathology. 2015;47:199–210.
30. Leekitcharoenphon P, Nielsen EM, Kaas RS, Lund O, Aarestrup FM. Evaluation of whole genome sequencing for outbreak detection of Salmonella enterica. PLoS One. 2014;9:e87991.
31. Foley SL, Zhao S, Walker RD. Comparison of molecular typing methods for the differentiation of Salmonella foodborne pathogens. Foodborne Pathog Dis. 2007;4:253–76.
32. Valenzuela JK, Thomas L, Partridge SR, van der Reijden T, Dijkshoorn L, Iredell J. Horizontal gene transfer in a polyclonal outbreak of carbapenem-resistant Acinetobacter baumannii. J Clin Microbiol. 2007;45:453–60.
33. Fitzpatrick MA, Ozer EA, Hauser AR. Utility of whole-genome sequencing in characterizing Acinetobacter epidemiology and analyzing hospital outbreaks. J Clin Microbiol. 2016;54:593–612.
34. Higgins PG, Perez-Llarena FJ, Zander E, Fernandez A, Bou G, Seifert H. OXA-235, a novel class D beta-lactamase involved in resistance to carbapenems in Acinetobacter baumannii. Antimicrob Agents Chemother. 2013;57:2121–6.
35. Buser GL, Cassidy PM, Cunningham MC, Rudin S, Hujer AM, Vega R, Furuno JP, Marshall SH, Higgins PG, Jacobs MR, et al. Failure to communicate: transmission of extensively drug-resistant Bla OXA-237-containing Acinetobacter baumannii-multiple facilities in Oregon, 2012-2014. Infect Control Hosp Epidemiol. 2017;38:1–7.
36. Hujer AM, Higgins PG, Rudin SD, Buser GL, Marshall SH, Xanthopoulou K, Seifert H, Rojas LJ, Domitrovic TN, Cassidy PM, et al. Nosocomial outbreak of extensively drug-resistant Acinetobacter baumannii isolates containing blaOXA-237 carried on a plasmid. Antimicrob Agents Chemother. 2017;61: e00797.
37. Sheppard AE, Stoesser N, Wilson DJ, Sebra R, Kasarskis A, Anson LW, Giess A, Pankhurst LJ, Vaughan A, Grim CJ, et al. Nested Russian doll-like genetic mobility drives rapid dissemination of the Carbapenem resistance gene blaKPC. Antimicrob Agents Chemother. 2016;60:3767–78.
38. Willems S, Kampmeier S, Bletz S, Kossow A, Kock R, Kipp F, Mellmann A. Whole-genome sequencing elucidates epidemiology of nosocomial clusters of Acinetobacter baumannii. J Clin Microbiol. 2016;54:2391–4.
39. Halachev MR, Chan JZ, Constantinidou CI, Cumley N, Bradley C, Smith-Banks M, Oppenheim B, Pallen MJ. Genomic epidemiology of a protracted hospital outbreak caused by multidrug-resistant Acinetobacter baumannii in Birmingham, England. Genome Med. 2014;6:70.
40. Lewis T, Loman NJ, Bingle L, Jumaa P, Weinstock GM, Mortiboy D, Pallen MJ. High-throughput whole-genome sequencing to dissect the epidemiology of Acinetobacter baumannii isolates from a hospital outbreak. J Hosp Infect. 2010;75:37–41.

An observational case study of hospital associated infections in a critical care unit in Astana, Kazakhstan

Dmitriy Viderman[1,3], Yekaterina Khamzina[1], Zhannur Kaligozhin[2], Makhira Khudaibergenova[2], Agzam Zhumadilov[2], Byron Crape[1] and Azliyati Azizan[1*]

Abstract

Background: Hospital Associated infections (HAI) are very common in Intensive Care Units (ICU) and are usually associated with use of invasive devices in the patients. This study was conducted to determine the prevalence and etiological agents of HAI in a Surgical ICU in Kazakhstan, and to assess the impact of these infections on ICU stay and mortality.

Objective: To assess the rate of device-associated infections and causative HAI etiological agents in an ICU at the National Research Center for Oncology and Transplantation (NRCOT) in Astana, Kazakhstan.

Methods: This retrospective, observational study was conducted in a 12-bed ICU at the NRCOT, Astana, Kazakhstan. We enrolled all patients who were admitted to the ICU from January, 2014 through November 2015, aged 18 to 90 years of age who developed an HAI.

Results: The most common type of HAI was surgical site infection (SSI), followed by ventilator-associated pneumonia (VAP), catheter-related blood stream infection (BSI) and catheter-associated urinary tract infection (UTI). The most common HAI was SSI with *Pseudomonas aeruginosa* as the most common etiological agent. The second most common HAI was VAP also with *P. aeruginosa* followed by BSI which was also associated with *P. aeruginosa* (in 2014) and *Enterococcus faecalis*, and *Klebsiella pneumoniae* (in 2015) as the most common etiological agents causing these infections.

Conclusion: We found that HAI among our study population were predominantly caused by gram-negative pathogens, including *P. aeruginosa*, *K. pneumoniae*, and *E. coli.* To our knowledge, this is the only study that describes ICU-related HAI situation from a country within the Central Asian region. Many developing countries such as Kazakhstan lack surveillance systems which could effectively decrease incidence of HAIs and healthcare costs for their treatment. The epidemiological data on HAI in Kazakhstan currently is underrepresented and poorly reported in the literature. Based on this and previous studies, we propose that the most important interventions to prevent HAI at the NRCOT and similar Healthcare Institutions in Kazakhstan are active surveillance, regular infection control audits, rational and effective antibacterial therapy, and general hygiene measures.

Keywords: Intensive care unit (ICU), Hospital associated infections (HAI), Surgical site infections (SSI), Ventilator associated pneumonia (VAP), Blood stream infections (BSI), Urinary tract infections (UTI)

* Correspondence: azliyati.azizan@nu.edu.kz
[1]Nazarbayev University School of Medicine (NUSOM), 5/1 Kerey and Zhanibek Khans Street, Astana, Kazakhstan010000
Full list of author information is available at the end of the article

Background

HAI influence the quality of health care and are a major source of adverse outcomes during health care delivery [1, 2]. HAI greatly increase morbidity and mortality of patients and healthcare costs [3]. The burden of HAI in developing countries is significant, whereby the incidence can be up to 15% of total hospitalized patients, and up to 50% among ICU patients [4]. HAI are challenging to treat because the etiological agents frequently develop multidrug, extensively drug and pandrug-resistance [5]. HAI have a big economic impact on healthcare by extending ICU stay, hospital stay, and increasing the need for invasive procedures. The most common HAI are primary bloodstream infections (BSI), ventilator-associated pneumonia (VAP), urinary tract infections (UTI) and surgical site infections (SSI), with SSI being the most prevalent in some studies [2, 6]. Prevention programs for HAI which could result in positive cost-benefit ratios typically originate with laboratory data from the clinical microbiology laboratory; this provides information regarding the causative pathogenic organisms causing the HAI [6].

The incidence of HAI in ICUs is about 2 to 5 times higher than those in general inpatient departments due to many associated risk factors [1, 7]. Furthermore, antimicrobial resistance rates in ICU are much greater than in general departments [7]. In order to reduce incidence of HAI, surveillance analysis is an essential step to identify problems and implement interventions [8]. National surveillance data form the basis for prevention and control of HAI in developed countries such as the USA and Australia, but this is rarely available in many developing countries, including Kazakhstan [9]. A recent systematic meta-analysis of the burden of HAI in Southeast Asia found that the most common HAI pathogens were mostly gram-negative bacilli, and were predominantly *Pseudomonas aeruginosa*, *Klebsiella* species and *Acinetobacter baumannii*; these findings are similar to those reported for many other developing countries [9]. According to the National Healthcare Safety Network (NHSN) report in 2013, ICU-related central-line associated BSI continued to decrease, whereas urinary catheter-associated tract infection rates increased in the majority of ICU types [10]. Several studies conducted in developing countries similar to ours, reported their findings in the literature; one study from Kuwait reported that their VAP rate was 4.0 per 1000 mechanical ventilator days, the central line–associated BSI rate was 3.5 per 1000 central line days, and the catheter-associated urinary tract infection (CAUTI) rate was 3.3 per 1000 urinary catheter days [11]. Another study from Ecuador showed that device associated HAIs rates in their ICUs were higher than the United States CDC/NSHN rates and similar to International Nosocomial Infection Control Consortium (INICC) international rates [12].

In an effort to evaluate the local HAI situation in Kazakhstan, we conducted an observational case study to assess incidence of the different types of HAI over a period of two years in 2014 and 2015. Our goal was to investigate if the patterns regarding type of HAI cases and the etiological agents were consistent from year to year, therefore we performed an analysis and comparison of data from at least two years. The data from the study was retrospectively analyzed in our effort to identify the causative HAI bacterial pathogens. We aimed to assemble and analyze epidemiological data associated with four different types of device associated HAI in an ICU at the National Research Center for Oncology and Transplantation (NRCOT) in Astana, Kazakhstan. The information summarized here will form the basis for a much larger surveillance study that could guide decisions regarding appropriate and potentially more efficacious use of prophylactic control within the ICU. This study could also guide the establishment of a national surveillance program to control and prevent HAI in hospitals in Kazakhstan and worldwide.

Methods

This retrospective, observational study was conducted from January 2014 through January 2016 in a 12 bed ICU at the National Research Center for Oncology and Transplantation (NRCOT), which is a 280-bed hospital in Astana, Kazakhstan. We undertook this pilot study comparing HAI cases and causative agents over a two year period to assess the current local infection control practices. We hope to understand from this study if intervention in the future would be appropriate to improve upon the current HAI scenario. The main change between 2014 and 2015 was access to better diagnostic capabilities within the hospital laboratory, though there are future plans to implement an improved HAI prevention program. This was considered by us to be a "retrospective" study because data analysis on the most part was done after these were collected (even though the staff collected the data during the patients' ICU visit). A standard screening protocol for HAI was used [13]. We tested all patients who spent more than 48 h in the ICU (whereby, all patients with less than 48 h stay in the ICU were excluded from this study). Samples for microbiological culture and analysis were obtained from patients who presented with HAI symptoms. Blood count, blood biochemistry, and blood coagulation tests were performed on all suspected patients who were at high risk of developing HAI following guidelines provided by the Healthcare Infection Control Practices Advisory Committee [14]. Clinical Pharmacologist and Hospital Infection Specialists visited the ICU every day. Chest radiography, deep tracheal aspirate, bronchoalveolar lavage (BAL) or mini-broncho-alveolar lavage (mini-BAL) were taken for pathogen identification if VAP was suspected. Blood samples, removed intravascular catheters, urine, urinary and wound catheters were also cultured for microbiological analysis if BSI, UTI or SSI were suspected. Samples were cultured using standard microbiological methods; isolated bacteria were identified by standard microbiological methods and tested for antibiotic susceptibility using Kirby-Bauer disk-diffusion technique according to Clinical and Laboratory Standards Institute (CLCI) specifications [15, 16].

Study ethics

Ethical clearance for this study was obtained from the Ethics committee of the Institutional Review Board of Nazarbayev University. The study was exempt from being classified as human subject research as no personal information related to any of the patients was made available to the Investigators at any time before, during or after the study.

Study population and microbiological culture and analysis

The patients admitted to the NRCOT ICU were from different surgical departments, which included the department of general, oncology, transplant, vascular, orthopedic, and gynecology surgeries. The patients with a diagnosis of HAI received treatment according to the hospital's standard protocol of management of HAI. Samples were taken from all patients admitted to the ICU aged 18 to 90 years of age who developed HAI based on clinical, laboratory and instrumental findings throughout the study duration. For microbiological culture and sensitivity testing, lower respiratory tract secretion, blood and urine samples were taken for diagnosis of VAP, catheter-related BSI, and catheter-associated UTI. Blood culture diagnostics was done for all samples from patients with suspected catheter-related blood stream infections. Data relevant to the diagnosis of HAI were taken by the hospital staff, but only microbiological data regarding etiological agents related to device associated HAI were provided for analysis in this study.

Statistical analysis

The rates of development of each type of HAI (BSI, VAP, UTI and SSI) as well as the total rate per 1000 cases were calculated. Relative risk for these groups was assessed using StataMP 13.0 software, and statistically significant cutoff was determined at a p-value of < 0.05, and highly statistically significant cutoff at a p-value of < 0.001. Prevalence of certain isolated strains of bacteria that caused hospital-acquired infections for each year was determined in percent and compared between the years 2014 and 2015 using Chi-square analysis in StataMP 13.0 software. Statistically significant level was determined at a p-value < 0.05; and highly statistically significant level at a p-value of < 0.001.

Results

General overview of ICU patients and the proportions with HAI

A total number of 1257 patients were admitted to the ICU from January 2014 to January 2016 of which, 56.6% (711 patients) were admitted in 2014 compared to the remaining 43.4% (546 patients) in 2015. The mean number of ICU stay was 18 days (with a range of 1–330 days) in 2014, while in 2015 the mean ICU stay was 36 days (with a range of 12–62 days); these variations are also a reflection of some changes in perioperative care that took place in between these two time periods. The change we mention here that led to increased mean number of ICU stay in 2015 compared to 2014 was due to the change in patient population. In 2014, the patient population consisted of patients who were transferred to the ICU after emergency surgeries (which were more than 85% of all transfers to ICU) such as patients who underwent appendectomy, cholecystectomy, hernia repair surgeries, etc. In 2015, the ICU patient population consisted of patients who were transferred to the ICU after oncological surgery (50%) and transplant surgery (30%). The period of ICU stay of patients after emergency surgery was generally shorter than the patients who were moved to the ICU after oncological or transplant surgery. Overall, the patients' general health conditions were better for the patients in 2014.

During the study period, 249 out of 1257 patients admitted to the ICU developed HAI; the p-value for the development of HAI between 2014 and 2015 was 0.000127 which is highly statistically significant. A total of 114 microbiological cultures were obtained and identified from patients suspected to have had HAI in 2014 compared to 135 cultures isolated in 2015 (with a p-value of 0.6582 which is not significant).

Device associated infections

The HAIs were classified into four categories: BSI, VAP, UTI and SSI. As evident from the Table 1, in 2014, SSI constituted the highest percentages of all HAIs followed by VAP, BSI and UTI. When compared to 2014, similar profile of device associated HAIs were observed for 2015, whereby SSI was again the most prominent category that caused HAI, followed by VAP. However in 2015, the percent of observed BSI was equal to the percent of UTI as the least frequent types of HAI.

Table 1 Types of Hospital Associated infections in percent for each year

Type of infection	Percent in 2014 (total number)	Percent in 2015 (total number)
BSI	24.6% (28)	18.5% (25)
VAP	25.4% (29)	29.6% (40)
UTI	19.3% (22)	18.5% (25)
SSI	30.7% (35)	33.3% (45)
Total	100% (114)	100% (135)

BSI: Catheter-associated Blood Stream Infections, *VAP*: Ventilator-associated Pneumonia, *UTI*: Catheter-associated Urinary Tract Infections, *SSI*: Surgical Site Infections

Variation in types of infections

Analysis of HAI categories (BSI, VAP, UTI, and SSI) in 2014 compared to 2015 was conducted and revealed significant variation between certain types of HAI (Fig. 1). Specifically, rates of VAP and SSI were found to be statistically different (p-value < 0.05) between the two years of the study period. Rates of VAP infections were higher in 2015 than in 2014. Similar results were obtained for SSI, whereby the rate of infection was again higher in 2015 (p-value < 0.05). On the other hand, no difference in rates of BSI and UTI was observed. The total rate of all types of infections was found to be significantly higher in 2015 when compared to the total infection rate in 2014 (p-value < 0.05). Data was available for the VAP incidence which was determined to be 8.4 per 1000 ventilator days while the incidence of catheter-related blood stream infections was 18 per 1000 line days.

Microbiological etiology of HAI

A total number of 249 microbial pathogens were isolated and identified in 2014 and 2015, and the percent distribution of these etiological agents is represented in Fig. 2a and b. The highest percent in 2014 corresponded to *Pseudomonas aeruginosa* at 23.68%, which was slightly reduced in 2015 to 13.33%. *Klebsiella pneumoniae, Escherichia coli, Staphylococcus aureus, Staphylococcus epidermidis,* and *Acinetobacter baumannii* were isolated and identified from many HAI cases for both 2014 and 2015. Unique and relatively widespread isolate for 2014 was *Enterobacter aerogenes*, representing 17.54% of the cases. Bacterial strains that had an incidence of less than 5% were combined into the subgroup 'Others'. In 2014 *Streptococcus viridans, Citrobacter* spp., *Enterococcus faecium, Achromobacter* spp., *Staphylococcus saprophyticus, Candida albicans and Serratia* spp. were included in this subgroup. In 2015 however, in addition to the above-mentioned *Citrobacter* spp., *S. saprophyticus* and *C. albicans,* unique pathogens such as *Staphylococcus haemolyticus*, *Enterococcus cloacae*, *Candida tropicalis*, *Burkholderia cepacia*, *Streptococcus mitis* and *Stenotrophomonas maltophilia* were isolated. When comparison analysis was conducted, highly significant difference between two years (p-value < 0.001) was identified. Even though many strains were similar for both years, case-wise analysis revealed important differences that should be taken into account. The types of pathogen described originated from cultures isolated from the different HAI categories as shown in Fig. 3a (VAP), Fig.3b (BSI), Fig. 3c (UTI), and Fig. 3d (SSI), and represented as percent (%) of total number of organisms isolated. We found that

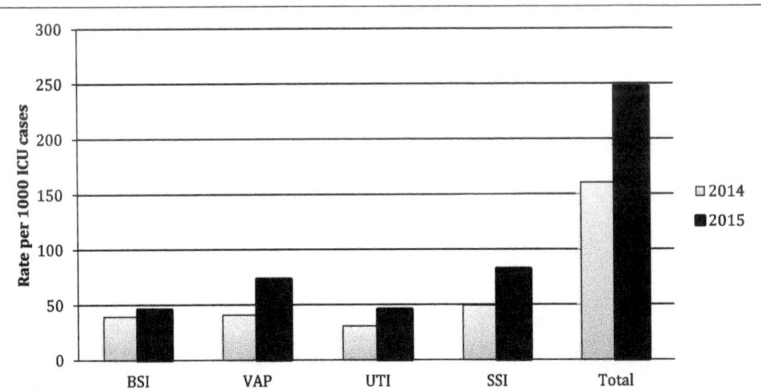

RR p-value 95%CI	1.18 0.4384	1.78 0.0024* (1.23-2.58)	1.48 0.0835 (0.949-2.32)	1.67 0.0032*	1.54 <0.0001**

Fig. 1 Samples for microbiological culture and analysis were obtained from patients who presented with HAI symptoms. Blood samples, removed intravascular catheters, urine, urinary and wound catheters were also cultured for microbiological analysis if BSI, UTI or SSI were suspected. Comparison of rates of case-specific infections between 2014 and 2015 were performed. Statistically significant level was determined at a p-value < 0.05; and highly statistically significant level at a p-value of < 0.001. Statistically significant difference is noted for VAP, SSI and combined total between years 2014 and 2015 (statistical significance: *p-value< 0.05; **p-value< 0.001)

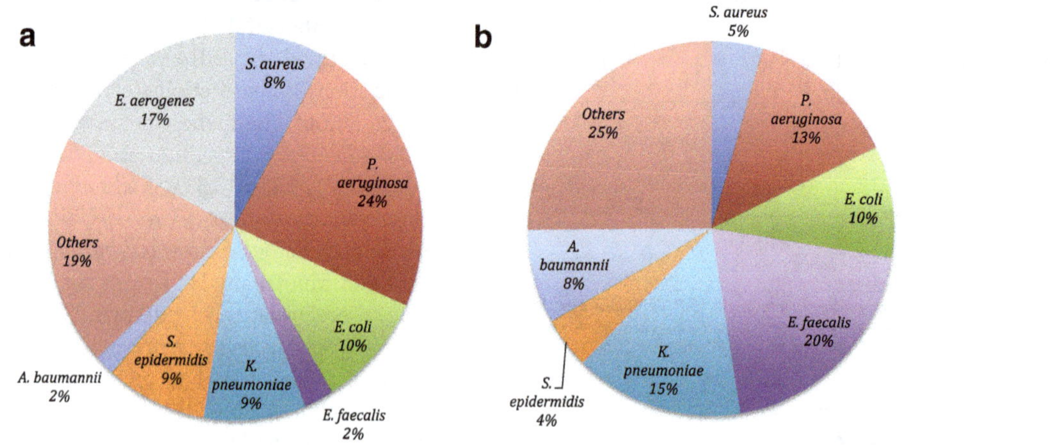

Fig. 2 Samples for bacterial culture and analysis were obtained from patients who presented with HAI symptoms. Samples were cultured using standard microbiological methods; isolated bacteria were identified by standard microbiological methods according to Clinical and Laboratory Standards Institute (CLCI) specifications [12, 13]. For comparison, Chi-square test was conducted with a *p*-value < 0.001**. The subgroup 'Others' includes rare strains of bacteria (with incidence of < 5%), which were different for each year (comparing 2014 and 2015).

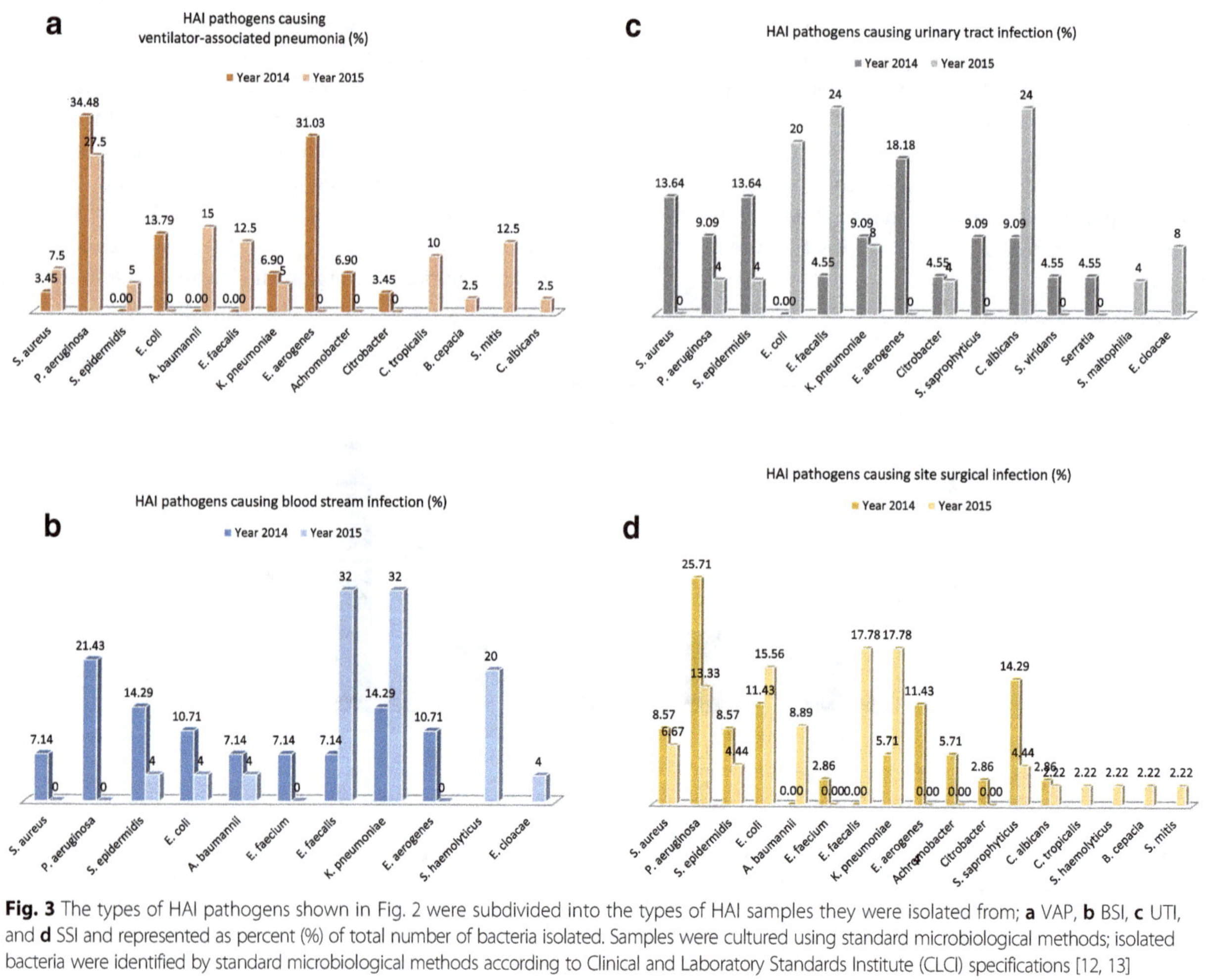

Fig. 3 The types of HAI pathogens shown in Fig. 2 were subdivided into the types of HAI samples they were isolated from; **a** VAP, **b** BSI, **c** UTI, and **d** SSI and represented as percent (%) of total number of bacteria isolated. Samples were cultured using standard microbiological methods; isolated bacteria were identified by standard microbiological methods according to Clinical and Laboratory Standards Institute (CLCI) specifications [12, 13]

HAI were predominantly caused by gram-negative bacterial pathogens, particularly *P. aeruginosa* and *K. pneumoniae*. These strains were most frequently associated with all the HAI types particularly SSI and BSI (as the first two most common types of HAI pathogens isolated) though there are some variations between the two years with these two pathogens as well as other types of bacterial pathogens that predominated, such as *Staphylococcus epidermidis, E. faecalis* and *Acinetobacter baumannii*. From our study, *P. aeruginosa* was recognized as a causal agent of the most serious HAI in the ICU. This organism was also causing the majority of VAP and BSIs in two consecutive years. SSI analogously was mainly caused by gram-negative bacteria, of which *P. aeruginosa* prevailed in 2014, while *K. pneumoniae* predominated in 2015.

Discussion

In this study, we have shown that healthcare-associated infections constitute a major healthcare burden in Kazakhstan, which is a rapidly developing nation. Kazakhstan is one of the five Central Asian countries (which also include Kyrgyzstan, Tajikistan, Turkmenistan and Uzbekistan) that achieved independence in 1991 after the collapse of the Soviet Union [17, 18]. At independence, these Central Asian Post-Soviet (CAPS) countries were faced with many problems; progress to build stronger economies varies between countries. Collapse of the Soviet Union led Kazakhstan as well as the other CAPS countries to economic recession. During the Soviet Union era, there were no wide informational, medical and pharmaceutical exchanges with other countries. On the other hand, the dissolution of the Soviet Union mobilized these countries to democracy which initiated important exchanges of products and knowledge with the other countries. Greater successes have been noted for Kazakhstan, Turkmenistan and Uzbekistan, which are the CAPS countries with the richest natural resources [17]. The healthcare systems of these CAPS countries have also gone through many decades of profound revolutions, whereby the rate and quality of progress of the healthcare sectors vary between these countries [19]. Since independence, the CAPS countries have steadily been receiving more attention at the international arena, especially due to the economic and geographical significance of the region. Over the last two decades, Kazakhstan has made significant progress in economy as well as healthcare sector, although there is still much room for improvement.

To our knowledge, this is the only study to be reported in an international journal describing ICU-related HAI situation from the Central Asian region. In our study, HAI represents a significant healthcare problem with ICU related HAI incidence being about 2 to 5 times higher than the incidence in other in-hospital departments [7]. In our study, patients frequently had the following universal host-related risk factors predisposing to HAI which included advanced age, severity of disease, hyperglycemia, neutropenia, immunosuppressive therapy, cancer diagnosis, and malnutrition. Majority of the patients had at least three of these risk factors. The most common type of HAI in our study was SSI whereby the rate increased significantly (p-value < 0.05) when comparing the year 2014 to 2015 (Table 1 and Fig. 1). Between both years, no intervention was introduced in terms of recommendations to improve upon infection control practices which may have been one of the reason there were no observed decrease in device-associated HAI rates. This high incidence of HAI associated with SSI was due to the fact that the Astana NRCOT is a multidisciplinary hospital focusing on multiple types of surgeries. In most cases, patients also had poor nutritional and altered immune status due to devastating diseases, which were either cancer, kidney and liver failure, diabetes, and coexisting infections at the remote body site. Multiple studies stated that the above mentioned medical conditions predispose patients to the development of SSI [20, 21]. Medical procedures in the hospital were typically prolonged, and patients were prone to intraoperative hypothermia, increasing the risk for SSI [22]. In our setting, colorectal surgery was the most frequently performed surgery, which is recognized as a risk factor for SSI worldwide [23].

From our study, VAP was identified as the second most common type of HAI. For patients on mechanical ventilation however, VAP was the leading type of infection, which is consistent with reports from multiple other studies [24, 25]. Majority of the patients who developed VAP had COPD, advanced age, H_2-antagonists and antibiotics use, and Multiple Organ System Failure [26]. Similar to the SSI associated HAI described above, the rates of VAP also increased significantly when comparing 2014 to 2015 (Table 1 and Fig. 1); this may have also been due to absence of intervention that was implemented to reduce the number of VAP cases in the studied ICU. The third most common type of HAI identified in our study was BSI. Almost all patients who developed BSI had the following risk factors; central vein catheterization, malnutrition and surgery, and infection with highly antibiotic resistant pathogens. These findings are supported by evidence from other studies, which report BSI to occur in 5% of all ICU patients [26, 27].

We found that HAI were predominantly caused by gram-negative pathogens, including *P. aeruginosa*, *K. pneumoniae*, and *E. coli*. These strains were most frequently associated with VAP, SSI, BSI and UTI. From our study, *P. aeruginosa* was recognized as a causal agent of the most serious HAI in the ICU [28]. This organism was also causing the majority of VAP and BSI in two consecutive years [9]. SSI analogously was mainly caused by gram-negative bacteria, of which *P. aeruginosa* prevailed in 2014, while *K. pneumoniae* predominated in 2015. Another interesting finding was with regards to the differences between the length of ICU patient stay, the patient population type, rate of HAI as well as the types of pathogens isolated in 2014 when compared to 2015. Since the period of ICU stay of patients after emergency surgeries was much shorter than after oncological or transplant surgeries, the overall period of ICU stay was longer in 2015. Furthermore, ICU patients' general condition was better among patients in 2014. Our results showed that the rate of HAIs was increased and the distribution of pathogen also changed in 2015 compared to 2014. We propose that the difference between patient populations in the ICU partially explained the reason for increased number and rates of HAI in 2015 (Table 1 and Fig. 1), as well as the differences in the types of HAI pathogens that were isolated when these pathogen types were compared between the two years of study. With regards to increased HAI rate, both the oncological and transplant patient populations were immunocompromised due to the surgical procedures, and these patients also received immunosuppressant drugs; this led to further decrease in their immune status. Plus, these patients stayed longer in the ICU thereby had higher risk of acquiring ICU-related HAIs. Interestingly, more HAI pathogens that are more commonly associated with multidrug resistance belonging to the "ESKAPE" pathogen group were identified in 2015. This included *P. aeruginosa, E. faecalis, K. pneumoniae and A. baumannii* (Fig. 2); this is not a surprising finding given that these pathogens are associated with many HAI infections within the last few decades [29].

There are limitations to this study, which include the fact that data collected did not include patients' age, sex, and other demographic variables, which might have contributed towards generation of more precise and valuable conclusions. For future studies, the design could include collection of these and other relevant information that would enhance the quality of data and conclusions that can be derived from the study. In this study, some organisms identified were usually not considered common causative agents (such as *Candida, Enterococcus faecalis, Staphylococcus epidermidis* and *Streptococcus mitis* for VAP as in Fig. 3a, and *S. epidermidis* and *S. viridans* for UTI as shown in Fig. 3c). Such unexpected findings further support our conclusion that there is an urgent and definitive need to improve upon HAI prevention practices which include incorporation of surveillance protocols that meet international standards that can more accurately detect and identify the correct etiological agent (which includes incorporation of quality control measures and established Standard operating procedure) in Kazakhstan and other developing countries within the region. These findings indicate that the surveillance protocols mentioned in the method section were not fully implemented during the study period, which is a major limitation of this study. Therefore the findings from this study demonstrates the need to improve training of infection control personnel regarding the use of and implementation of more stringent practices that meet the international HAI infection control and surveillance guidelines.

HAI is a critical problem for health-care providers worldwide, which should receive appropriate attention for further management. The integrated HAI control program was introduced more than 3 decades ago for the first time, being able to reduce both incidence of infections and related healthcare costs [30]. Unfortunately, many developing countries such as Kazakhstan lack surveillance systems which could effectively decrease incidence of HAIs and healthcare costs for their treatment. Currently, the international guidelines on prevention, diagnosis and treatment of HAI are not actively practiced, and access to newer antibacterial agents is not readily available in Kazakhstan. Within Kazakhstan, there are National and Regional Medical Centers (hospitals). There are no published epidemiological data on HAI from the Regional Medical Centers, therefore, the epidemiological characteristics of HAI from these Centers are unknown. If we compare the National Medical Centers with Regional hospitals, there is an unequal supply of medical equipment and uneven qualification of medical doctors and staff in the latter. For example, several National Medical Centers have internationally educated doctors and staff as well as equipment resembling those that can be found in the best World Class Medical Centers. These medical Centers can be effective in monitoring, diagnosing, treating and preventing the HAI, whereas many Regional (and rural) hospitals do not even follow any guidelines on diagnosis, treatment and preventions of HAIs. The National Medical Centers frequently receive severely ill patients with multiple undiagnosed multi- and pandrug resistant HAI from the Regional Medical Centers.

We propose that the most important recommended measures to prevent HAI at the NRCOT and similar Healthcare Institutions are rational antibacterial therapy, regular infection control audits, and general hygiene measures. Numerous studies in developing countries have shown that the International Nosocomial Infection Control Consortium (INICC) multidimensional infection control strategy with practice bundles can decrease the rate of HAI. Rosenthal et al. found that implementation of a multidimensional infection control strategy can significantly reduce the central line-associated BSI rates in the PICUs of developing countries [31]. In another study, Tao et al. demonstrated that a multidimensional infection control intervention for VAP contributed to a significant cumulative reduction in the VAP rate in their ICUs [32].

This is a first surveillance study on HAI at the NRCOT since its foundation eight years ago. An active surveillance system monitoring incidence and prevalence of HAI as preventative measures is necessary, and this study represents a first step towards this goal.

Conclusions

We conclude that HAI is one of the major problems in healthcare provision in Kazakhstan. SSI, VAP and BSI are the predominant types of HAI. Gram-negative bacteria such as *P. aeruginosa*, *K. pneumoniae* and *E. coli* are the most common causative agents of HAI. The most important risk factors are advanced age, severity of disease, hyperglycemia, neutropenia, immunosuppressive therapy, cancer diagnosis, and malnutrition. For more precise determination of its causality, an ongoing HAI surveillance program is needed to decrease HAI incidence and prevalence at the NRCOT and other healthcare institutions throughout the country. Kazakhstan has made significant effort and progress since independence to establish a healthcare system that is already an improvement over the centralized Semashko health system model inherited from the Soviet Union at independence [19]. One of the ways to continue on the positive trajectory of change for an improved healthcare system is implementation of an efficient active surveillance system for HAI that should be implemented nationwide. The system should include an organized and controlled data collection performed by trained personnel. The data collected should include not only infection-related data, but also patient-related data such as risk factors and history of present illness (such as history of HAI, diagnostic tests, surgeries and invasive methods, as well as the antimicrobial drugs used). A system of monthly HAI analysis and report should also be implemented. Such proactive surveillance system coupled with efficient infection control programs would be highly beneficial to control and reduce the rates of HAI within all Regional and National Medical Centers throughout Kazakhstan.

Acknowledgements
The Authors would like to acknowledge the staff for their contributions including sample retrieval, blinding and randomizing, as well as providing information on sample types available prior to randomizing. The Authors also would like to thank Reviewers for their valuable comments.

Funding
Nazarbayev University School of Medicine.

Author's contribution
DV, AA and YK participated in the study design. ZK and DV participated in the data collection. YK and BC performed the advanced statistical analyses and prepared the associated Figures and Table. YK, DV and AA wrote the manuscript. YK provided technical assistance related to manuscript development. DV and AA conceived of the study, reviewed the data, provided feedback for Figures and Table, and edited the manuscript. AZ and MK provided the technical support to data collection. All authors reviewed and approved the final version of manuscript.

Competing interests
The authors declare that they have no competing interests.

Author details
[1]Nazarbayev University School of Medicine (NUSOM), 5/1 Kerey and Zhanibek Khans Street, Astana, Kazakhstan010000. [2]National Research Center for Oncology and Transplantation, Astana, Kazakhstan. [3]National Research Neurosurgery Center, Astana, Kazakhstan.

References
1. WHO. The burden of health care-associated infection worldwide. 2016. Available at http://www.who.int/gpsc/country_work/burden_hcai/en/. Accessed 22 Apr 2018.
2. Horan TC, Gaynes R. Surveillance of nosocomial infections. In: Mayhall CG, editor. Hospital epidemiology and infection control. Philadelphia: Lippincott Williams & Wilkins; 1999. p. 1285–318.
3. Klevens RM, Edwards JR, Richards CL, et al. Estimating health care-associated infections and deaths in U.S. hospitals, 2002. Public Health Rep. 2007;122(2):160–6.
4. Vincent J. International Study of the Prevalence and Outcomes of Infection in Intensive Care Units. JAMA. 2009;302(21):2323.
5. Magiorakos A, Srinivasan A, Carey R, Carmeli Y, Falagas M, Giske C, et al. Multidrug-resistant, extensively drug-resistant and pandrug-resistant bacteria: an international expert proposal for interim standard definitions for acquired resistance. Clin Microbiol Infect. 2012;18(3):268–81.
6. Arefian H, Vogel M, Kwetkat A, Hartmann M. Economic evaluation of interventions for prevention of hospital acquired infections: a systematic review. PLoS One. 2016;11(1):e0146381.
7. Aly N, Al-Mousa H, Al Asar E. Nosocomial infections in a medical-surgical intensive care unit. Med Princ Pract. 2016;17(5):373–7. https://doi.org/10.1159/000141500
8. Choi J, Kwak Y, Yoo H, Lee S, Kim H, Han S, et al. Trends in the incidence rate of device-associated infections in intensive care units after the establishment of the Korean nosocomial infections surveillance system. J Hosp Infect. 2016;91(1):28–34. https://doi.org/10.1016/j.jhin.2015.06.002
9. Ling M, Apisarnthanarak A, Madriaga G. The burden of healthcare-associated infections in Southeast Asia: a systematic literature review and meta-analysis. Clin Infect Dis. 2016;60(11):1690–9. https://doi.org/10.1093/cid/civ095
10. Dudeck MA, Edwards JR, Allen-Bridson K, Gross C, Malpiedi PJ, Peterson KD, Sievert DM. National Healthcare Safety Network report, data summary for 2013, device-associated module. Am J Infect Control. 2015; 43(3):206–21.
11. Al-Mousa HH, Omar AA, Rosenthal VD, Salama MF, Aly NY, Noweir MED, George SM. Device-associated infection rates, bacterial resistance, length of stay, and mortality in Kuwait: international nosocomial infection consortium findings. Am J Infect Control. 2016;44(4):444–9.
12. Yepez ES, Bovera MM, Rosenthal VD, Flores HAG, Pazmiño L, Valencia F, Delgado V. Device-associated infection rates, mortality, length of stay and bacterial resistance in intensive care units in Ecuador: international nosocomial infection control Consortium's findings. World J Biol Chem. 2017;8(1):95.
13. Siegel J, Rhinehart E, Jackson M, Chiarello L. 2007 guideline for isolation precautions: preventing transmission of infectious agents in health care settings. Am J Infect Control. 2016;35(10):S65 S164. https://doi.org/10.1016/j.ajic.2007.10.007
14. CDC – HICPAC: 2016 Available at http://www.cdc.gov/hicpac/index.html. Accessed 22 Apr 2018.
15. Standards for microbiology investigations - GOV.UK: 2016. Available at https://www.gov.uk/government/collections/standards-for-microbiology-investigations-smi. Accessed 22 Apr 2018.

16. Clinical & Laboratory Standards Institute: CLSI Guidelines: 2016. Available at http://clsi.org/. Accessed 22 Apr 2018.
17. Central Asia after the breakup of the Soviet Union. Jeffrey Hays. Last updated April 2016. http://factsanddetails.com/central-asia/Central_Asian_Topics/sub8_8d/entry-4521.html. Accessed 22 Apr 2018.
18. Central Asia since 1991: The experience of the new independent states. Richard Pomfret. Research programme on: Market Access, Capacity Building and Competitiveness. Working Paper No. 212. OECD Development Centre, 29 July 2003.
19. Ulikpan A, Mirzoev T, Jimenez E, Malik A, Hill PS. Glob Health Action. 2014;7: 24978. https://doi.org/10.3402/gha.v7.24978.
20. Wick E, Vogel J, Church J, Remzi F, Fazio V. Surgical site infections in a "high outlier" institution. Dis Colon rectum. 2009;52(3):374–9.
21. Pedroso-Fernandez Y, Aguirre-Jaime A, Ramos M, Hernández M, Cuervo M, Bravo A, et al. Prediction of SSI after colorectal surgery. Am J Infect Control. 2016;44(4):450–4.
22. Seamon M, Wobb J, Gaughan J, Kulp H, Kamel I, Dempsey D. The effects of intraoperative hypothermia on surgical site infection. Ann Surg. 2012;255(4): 789–95. https://doi.org/10.1097/SLA.0b013e31824b7e35.
23. Kohut A, Liu J, Stein D, Sensenig R, Poggio J. Patient-specific risk factors are predictive for postoperative adverse events in colorectal surgery: an American College of Surgeons National Surgical Quality Improvement Program–based analysis. Am J Surg. 2015;209(2):219–29. https://doi.org/10.1016/j.amjsurg.2014.08.02.
24. Hunter J. Ventilator associated pneumonia. BMJ. 2012;344:e3325. https://doi.org/10.1136/bmj.e3325.
25. Afshari A, Pagani L, Harbarth S. Year in review 2011: critical care - infection. Crit Care. 2012;16(6):242. https://doi.org/10.1186/cc11421.
26. Elatrous S, Boujdaris R, Merghili S, Ouanes L, Boussarsar M, Nouira S, et al. Incidence and risk factors of VAP: a one-year prospective survey. Clin Intensive Care. 1996;7(6):276–81. https://doi.org/10.3109/tcic.7.6.276.281.
27. Vincent J, Rello J, Marshall J, Silva E, Anzueto A, Martin CD, et al. International study of the prevalence and outcomes of infection in ICU. JAMA. 2009;302(21):2323. https://doi.org/10.1001/jama.2009.1754.
28. Neuhauser M, Weinstein R, Rydman R, Danziger L, Karam G, Quinn J. Antibiotic resistance among gram-negative bacilli in US intensive care units. JAMA. 2003;289(7):885.
29. Santajit S, Indrawattana N. Mechanisms of antimicrobial resistance in ESKAPE pathogens. Biomed Res Int. 2016;2016:8. Article ID 2475067. https://doi.org/10.1155/2016/2475067.
30. Higuera F, Rosenthal V, Duarte P, Ruiz J, Franco G, Safdar N. The effect of process control on the incidence of central venous catheter–associated bloodstream infections and mortality in intensive care units in Mexico. Crit Care Med. 2005;33(9):2022–7.
31. Rosenthal VD, Ramachandran B, Villamil-Gomez W, Armas-Ruiz A, Navoa-Ng JA, Matta-Cortes L, Menco A. Impact of a multidimensional infection control strategy on central line-associated bloodstream infection rates in pediatric intensive care units of five developing countries: findings of the international nosocomial infection control consortium (INICC). Infection. 2012;40(4):415–23.
32. Tao L, Hu B, Rosenthal VD, Zhang Y, Gao X, He L. Impact of a multidimensional approach on ventilator-associated pneumonia rates in a hospital of shanghai: findings of the international nosocomial infection control consortium. J Crit Care. 2012;27(5):440–6.

Antimicrobial susceptibility among gram-positive and gram-negative blood-borne pathogens collected between 2012-2016 as part of the Tigecycline Evaluation and Surveillance Trial

Zhijie Zhang[1], Meng Chen[2], Ying Yu[3], Sisi Pan[3] and Yong Liu[1*]

Abstract

Background: Antimicrobial activity of tigecycline and comparator agents was assessed*in vitro*against 27857 isolates source from blood samples collected between 2012 and 2016 as part of the Tigecycline Evaluation and Surveillance Trial (TEST).

Methods: The broth microdilution methods was used to determine minimum inhibitory concentrations (MIC) of blood-borne isolates according to guildlines of the Clinical and Laboratory Standards Institute (CLSI). Antimicrobial susceptibility breakpoints from CLSI guidelines were used as standards to determine susceptibility against comparator agents, whereas tigecycline breakpoints were provided by the US Food and Drug Administration (FDA).

Results: More than 91% Enterobacteriaceae isolates, belonging to *Escherichia coli*, *Klebsiella pneumoniae*, *Enterobacter cloacae*and*Serratia marcescens*, were susceptible to amikacin, meropenem, and tigecycline. Meropenem resistance was observed in 8% of*K.pneumoniae* isolates worldwide. Extended-spectrum β-lactamase (ESBL) was produced in 15.9 and 20.9%*E.coli* and *K.pneumoniae*isolates, respectively. MIC_{90} of tigecycline against *Acinetobacter baumannii* was 2 μg/ml. The highest proportion of susceptible *A.baumannii*isolates was 70.8% for minocycline. Among *P.aeruginose* isolates worldwide, 71.1–94.9% were susceptible to six antibiotics. Almost all *Staphylococcus aureus*isolates were susceptible to linezolid(100%), vancomycin(100%), and tigecycline (99.9%). The proportion of methicillin-resistant *S.aureus* (MRSA) was 33.0% among *S.aureus*isolates worldwide; it was highest in Asia with 46.6%, followed by North America and Latin America with 37.7 and 34.2%, respectively. Vancomycin-resistant (VR) isolates represented 1.4% of*Enterococcus faecalis* (VR.*E.faecalis*) and 27.6% of *Enterococcus faecium*(VR.*E. faecium*). Highest percentages of VR.*E.faecium*were found in North America and Latin America, with 61.6 and 58.1% of the isolates, respectively. Production of penicillin-resistant *Streptococcus pneumoniae*(PRSP) represented 9.0% of *S. pneumoniae* isolates worldwide; the PRSP proportion was 25.8% in Asia, 13.0% in Africa, and 11.8% in Latin America.

Conclusions: In our study, tigecycline was the only antibiotic that was active against over 90% of all major blood-borne pathogens. A global comparison revealed that antimicrobial resistance was higher in Africa, Asia and Latin America than in Europe and North America.

Keywords: Antimicrobial drug resistance, Blood, Surveillance, tigecycline, Gram-positive bacteria, Gram-negative bacteria

* Correspondence: liuy@sj-hospital.org
[1]Shengjing Hospital of China Medical University, Shenyang, China
Full list of author information is available at the end of the article

Background

Bloodstream infections, acquired in clinics are major cause of mortality in severe disease patients. More attention has been recently paied to bloodstream infections because of the severe effects on health, longer hospital stays, expensive hospitalization costs, and an increase in mortality. In 2013, the incidence of severe sepsis in the United States was approximately 300 cases per 100,000 people associated with a mortality of 20–30% and an expenditure of about $14 billion/year [1].

Importantly, the mortality of bacteremia is directly correlated to the first adequate anti-infectious therapy. In a study on patients of intensive care units (ICU) in Japan,the initiation of an appropriate empirical antimicrobial treatment was associated with a lower 60-day mortality than that of an inappropriate therapy [2]. The selection of an empirical antimicrobial drug therapy should be based on clinical and epidemiological data. Hence, it is important for the clinical treatment of infections to have the information derived from epidemiological data, which differ in scope and focus, i.e., data collected from around the world, different regions,countries, provinces, and hospitals.

The Tigecycline Evaluation and Surveillance Trial (T.E.S.T.), which was initiated in 2004, is a global surveillance study focused on monitoring antimicrobial resistance worldwide. In this study, we report on the antimicrobial susceptibility of Gram-positive bacteria and Gram-negative bacteria isolated from blood specimen collected from around the world between 2012 and 2016.

Methods

Isolate collection

Each participating center was required to contribute at least 135 Gram-negative and 65 Gram-positive isolates per study year (Species and number of isolates: *Klebsiella* spp.,25; *Escherichia coli*, 25;*Enterobacter* spp., 25; *Pseudomonas aeruginosa*, 20; *Acinetobacter* spp., 15;*Haemophilus influenzae*, 15; and *Serratia* spp., 10; *Staphylococcus aureus*, 25; *Enterococcus* spp.,15;*Streptococcus pneumoniae*,15; and *Streptococcus agalactiae*,10). Isolates were collected from patients with an infectious disease and identified as the causative agent according to laboratory criteria. One isolate per patient was accepted. All body sites were acceptable for sample collection but the use of urine was limited to not more than 25% of all samples. Stored or duplicate isolates were not acceptable.

Antimicrobial susceptibility testing

Participating centers determined the minimum inhibitory concentrations(MICs) with the broth microdilution assay [3] using MicroScan® panels (Dade MicroScan Inc.,-West Sacramento,CA,USA) according to the manufacturer's instructions. To determine the susceptibility to antimicrobial agents, breakpoints from the Clinical and Laboratory Standards Institute (CLSI) guidelines [4] were used as interpretative standards except for the tigecycline breakpoints, which were obtained from the US Food and Drug Administration(FDA) [5]. The penicillin oral breakpoints (susceptible, ≤0.06 mg/L; resistant,≥2 mg/L) were used for *S. pneumoniae*.Breakpoint were not available for tigecycline against *Acinetobacter baumannii*. Methicillin-resistant *S.aureus*(MRSA) and extended-spectrum β-lactamase(ESBL)-producing *E.coli* and *Klebsiella spp.* were identified by the centers according to the CLSI guidelines [4].

The antimicrobials used in this study were listed in Tables 3 and 4. There were an additional four antimicrobials (azithromycin, clarithromycin, erythromycin and clindamycin) included in the panel for testing *S.pneumoniae.*

Quality control

The reference laboratory, International Health Management Associates(IHMA, Schaumburg, IL, USA), was responsible for the coordination of isolate collection, transport, and backup, as well as the administration of a database. Approximately 10–15% of the isolates were randomly selected each year by IHMA to verify isolate identity and MICs.

Results

Isolate collection

Between 2012 and 2016, 27,857 isolates, including 17,237 Gram-negative (61.9%) and 10,620(38.1%) Gram-positive isolates, were recovered from globally collected blood samples. The major Gram-negative bacteria were *E. Coli*(n = 5352;19.2%), *K.pneumoniae* (n = 3154;11.3%),*E. cloacae*(n = 1824;6.6%), *P .aeruginosa*(n = 1739;6.2%), *S.marcescens* (n = 1024;3.7%) and *A.baumannii* (n=749;2.7%). *S.aureus* (n = 3324;11.9%), *S.pneumoniae* (n = 1983;7.1%), *E.feacalis* (n = 1527;5.5%), *E.faecium* (n = 1000;3.6%) and *S.agalactiae* (n = 982;3.5%), were the dominating Gram-positive bacteria.

Europe and North America were the regions with the most participating centers and, therefore,contributed more isolates than the other regions. There were 132 and 54 participating centers collecting 17,456(62.7%) and 6785(24.3%) isolates in Europe and North America,respectively (Table 1). From all patients, 71.5% of the subjects were from non-ICUs and, 70.1% received in-patient treatment. The proportion of subjects of 61-80 years of age was 49.1% (Table 2).

Antimicrobial susceptibilities of isolates

Enterobacteriaceae

Four species of Enterobacteriaceae were isolated from blood-specimens, *E.coli, K.pneumoniae, E.cloacae,* and*S.marcescens*; most of these isolates (99,91,95, and 96%, respectively)were

Table 1 Participating centers and collected isolate per world region

Region[a]	Number of Centers	Percent of centers (%)	Number of isolates	Percent of isolates (%)
Africa	8	3.4	375	1.4
Asia	29	12.1	1989	7.1
Europe	132	55.2	17,456	62.7
North America	54	22.6	6785	24.3
LatinAmerica	16	6.7	1252	4.5
Total	239	100	27,857	100

[a]Africa:= Egypt, Morocco, South Africa, Tunisia; Asia: =China, Kuwait, Hong Kong, India, Japan, Jordan, Saudi Arabia, South Korea, Malaysia, Pakistan, Philippines, Singapore, Taiwan, Thailand, Vietnam; Europe:=Austria, Belgium, Croatia, Czech Republic, Denmark, Finland, France, Germany, Greece, Hungary, Ireland, Italy, Lithuania, Latvia, Netherlands, Poland, Portugal, Romania, Serbia, Spain, Sweden, Switzerland, United Kingdom; Latin America: = Argentina, Brazil, Chile, Colombia, Mexico, Panama, Guatemala,Venezuela; North American: =Canada, United States

susceptible to amikacin, meropenem, and tigecycline. The most meropenem-resistant isolates were found in*K.pneumoniae,* with 8% of resistant isolates globally. A lower proportion of resistant isolates was found in *E.cloacae, S.marcescens,* and *E.coli,* with only 1.6,1.6, and 0.4% of the isolates, respectively. There were large differences in the occurrence of meropenem-resistant*K.pneumoniae*, which was highest in Africa (15.4%), followed by Europe, Asia, and Latin America (12.1,10.5, and 8.4%, respectively), and lowest in North America (2%) (Table 3, Fig. 1).

Susceptibility to cephalosporins(ceftriaxone,ceftazidime, and cefepime) was found in 78.4–86.3%, 69.4–73.6%, 61.6–78.4%, and 84.3–95.1% of isolates of*E.coli, K.pneumoniae, E.cloacae,* and *S.marcescens*, respectively. The most cephalosporin-susceptible organism was *S.marcescens,*whereas *K.pneumoniae* and *E.cloacae*were less susceptible. In the four species of Enterobacteriaceae, *E.coli, K.pneumoniae, E.cloacae,* and *S.marcescens*, susceptibility to piperacillin/tazobactam(pip/taz) and amoxicillin/clavulanic acid(amoxy/clav) was found in 94.1%/72.1, 81.7%/69.2, 77.2%/3.2, and 94.2%/3.0% of the isolates, respectively. The in vitro activity of pip/taz was lower against *K. pneumoniae* and *E. cloacae* than *E. coli* and *S .marcescens.* The activity of amoxy/clav against *E. coli* and *K. pneumoniae* was weak as compared to that of pip/taz, and it had almost no effect on *E. cloacae* and *S. marcescens* (Table 3).

Minocycline was more active against the four Enterobacteriaceae with a similar susceptibility in 87.0, 81.7, 86.2, and 91.7% of the isolates of *E. coli, K .pneumoniae, E .cloacae,*and *S. marcescens,*respectively. The activity of levofloxacin was lowest against *E. coli*(65.2%) and highest against *S. marcescens*(95.2%) (Table 3).

Table 2 Distribution of patients according to location and age

Demographic parameter	Number of patients	Percent of patients(%)
Patient location		
ICU[a]	5419	19.5
non-ICU	19,907	71.5
Unknown	2531	9.1
In-patient	19,520	70.1
Out-patient	5806	20.8
Unknown	2531	9.1
Patient age		
0–20 years	2627	9.4
21–40 years	2471	8.9
41–60 years	6507	23.4
61–80 years	10,901	39.1
≥ 81 years	4674	16.8
Unknown	677	2.4
Total	27,857	100

[a]*ICU*= intensive care unit

ESBL production was found in 15.9% of *E. coli* and 20.9% of *K. pneumoniae* isolates. Africa had the highest proportion of ESBL-producers, with 40.4%(19/47) and 55.8%(29/52) of *E. coli* and *K. pneumoniae* isolates, respectively, followed by Latin America(23.0%,43/187), Asia(22.7%,90/396), Europe(17.2%,555/3235), and North America(9.8%,145/1487) in *E. coli,*as well as Latin America(37.4%,62/166), Europe (26.2%,462/1761), Asia (16.3%,45/276), and North America(6.8%,61/899) in *K. pneumoniae* (Fig. 1).

Susceptibility to amikacin, meropenem, and tigecycline was found in more than 98.4% of ESBL-producing *E. coli* isolates, as well as in 95.8,84.8 and 90.4% of ESBL-producing *K.pneumoniae* isolates, respectively. Over than 86% of ESBL-producing *E. coli* isolates were susceptible to pip/taz and minocycline,but only 59.6–70.3% of ESBL-producing *K. pneumoniae.* Susceptibility to other antibiotics was observed in less than 50% of Enterobacteriaceae isolates (Table 3).

A. baumannii and P. aeruginosa

Antibiotics exhibited a very poor activity against *A. baumannii.* The most active antibiotic was minocycline; 70.8% of *A. baumannii* isolates were susceptible. Susceptibility to meropenem was found in 31.2% of the isolates. The MIC_{90} of tigecycline was 2 μg/ml (Table 3).

Table 3 Antimicrobial susceptibility among Gram negative isolates including ESBL-producing strains from blood specimens collected between 2012 and 2016

	Africa	Asia	Europe	North America	Latin America	Global				Global			
	S%	S%	S%	S%	S%	MIC_{90}(mg/L)	MIC range(mg/L)	S%	R%	MIC_{90}(mg/L)	MIC range(mg/L)	S%	R%
	E.coli					*E.coli*, all isolates				*E.coli* ESBL isolates			
	N = 47	*N* = 396	*N* = 3235	*N* = 1487	*N* = 187	N = 5352				*N* = 852			
Amikacin	97.9	97.7	99.5	99.9	98.9	4	0.5–128	99.4	0.2	8	0.5–64	98.4	0.2
Amoxy/clav	48.9	72.0	70.1	78.1	64.7	32	0.25–64	72.1	10.1	32	0.5–64	48.6	14.4
Ampicillin	12.8	18.4	32.8	43.4	26.2	64	0.5–64	34.3	65.0	64	1–64	0.6	99.4
Cefepime	57.5	59.6	82.0	88.8	73.8	16	0.5–64	81.8	13.1	64	0.5–64	13.9	64.7
Ceftazidime	63.8	70.0	86.5	91.6	79.1	8	1–32	86.3	9.4	32	1–32	35.3	42.7
Ceftriaxone	48.9	49.8	78.8	87.4	67.4	64	0.06–64	78.4	21.0	64	0.06–64	0.9	97.8
Levofloxacin	51.1	48.0	64.9	71.6	58.8	16	0.008–16	65.2	31.9	16	0.008–16	16.3	78.9
Meropenem	95.7	98.2	99.9	99.7	97.3	0.06	0.06–32	99.6	0.4	0.12	0.06–16	99.5	0.4
Minocycline	74.5	83.3	85.9	91.3	81.8	8	0.5–32	87.0	7.4	8	0.5–32	86.0	7.3
Pip/taz	80.9	95.0	92.7	97.4	94.4	8	0.06–256	94.1	3.2	16	0.06–256	91.2	4.5
Tigecycline	100	100	99.9	99.9	100	0.25	0.008–16	99.9	0.04	0.5	0.008–2	100	0.0
	K.pneumoniae					*K.pneumoniae*, all isolates				*K.pneumoniae* ESBL isolates			
	N = 52	*N* = 276	*N* = 1761	*N* = 899	*N* = 166	N = 3154				*N* = 659			
Amikacin	84.6	90.2	96.7	99.4	96.4	8	0.5–128	96.7	1.8	16	0.5–128	95.8	2.7
Amoxy/clav	25.0	66.7	60.8	90.9	59.0	64	0.12–64	69.2	18.8	64	2–64	19.6	40.2
Ampicillin	1.8	2.2	2.6	6.2	1.2	64	0.5–64	3.5	85.1	64	16–64	0	99.9
Cefepime	34.6	66.7	65.0	93.3	57.2	64	0.5–64	72.3	23.4	64	0.5–64	8.4	78.0
Ceftazidime	34.6	69.2	67.0	91.2	68.7	32	1–32	73.6	21.7	32	1–32	18.1	65.0
Ceftriaxone	21.2	62.7	62.5	90.6	54.2	64	0.06–64	69.4	29.8	64	0.06–64	1.8	97.3
Levofloxacin	57.7	76.5	70.8	91.4	80.7	16	0.008–16	77.5	18.7	16	0.03–16	40.5	47.7
Meropenem	84.6	89.5	87.9	98.0	91.6	1	0.06–32	91.1	8.0	8	0.06–32	84.8	11.7
Minocycline	71.2	83.3	78.6	87.5	83.7	16	0.5–32	81.7	11.5	16	0.5–32	70.3	18.2
Pip/taz	55.8	80.8	76.7	94.1	77.1	256	0.06–256	81.7	15.0	256	0.5–256	59.6	29.1
Tigecycline	96.2	93.1	94.4	95.6	97.6	2	0.008–16	94.8	0.7	2	0.008–16	90.4	1.2
	S.marcescens												
	N = 29	*N* = 88	*N* = 591	*N* = 224	*N* = 92	N = 1024							
Amikacin	100.0	96.6	99.0	100.0	85.9	4	0.5–128	97.9	0.9				
Amoxy/clav	0.0	8.0	3.1	1.3	3.3	64	0.5–64	3.0	92.4				
Ampicillin	0.0	6.8	6.3	4.0	4.4	64	0.5–64	5.5	87.3				
Cefepime	89.7	85.2	96.6	98.7	80.4	1	0.5–64	94.4	3.8				

Table 3 Antimicrobial susceptibility among Gram negative isolates including ESBL-producing strains from blood specimens collected between 2012 and 2016 *(Continued)*

	Africa	Asia	Europe	North America	Latin America	Global				Global			
	S%	S%	S%	S%	S%	MIC_{90}(mg/L)	MIC range(mg/L)	S%	R%	MIC_{90}(mg/L)	MIC range(mg/L)	S%	R%
Ceftazidime	96.6	88.6	96.1	98.2	87.0	2	1–32	95.1	3.8				
Ceftriaxone	89.7	79.6	85.3	88.0	71.7	4	0.06–64	84.3	11.8				
Levofloxacin	100.0	94.3	95.8	96.0	89.1	1	0.008–16	95.2	2.9				
Meropenem	96.6	95.5	99.0	99.1	93.5	0.25	0.06–32	98.1	1.6				
Minocycline	100.0	88.6	90.4	94.2	88.0	4	0.5–32	91.9	2.3				
Pip/taz	100.0	89.8	94.1	97.3	90.2	8	0.06–256	94.2	2.4				
Tigecycline	96.6	95.5	97.0	97.8	93.5	2	0.03–16	96.7	0.3				
	E.cloacae												
	N = 47	*N* = 157	*N* = 1084	*N* = 404	*N* = 132	N = 1824							
Amikacin	95.7	96.8	99.0	100.0	97.0	4	0.5–128	98.8	0.9				
Amoxy/clav	2.1	1.9	3.7	3.0	1.5	64	0.12–64	3.2	95.4				
Ampicillin	4.3	3.2	6.8	4.5	4.6	64	0.5–64	5.8	89.5				
Cefepime	51.1	76.4	77.2	86.9	74.2	16	0.5–64	78.4	12.0				
Ceftazidime	51.1	63.1	65.0	74.5	65.9	32	1–32	66.7	29.6				
Ceftriaxone	40.4	59.2	59.7	70.5	60.6	64	0.06–64	61.6	36.2				
Levofloxacin	91.5	87.9	85.8	94.6	86.4	4	0.008–16	88.1	9.8				
Meropenem	100.0	94.3	97.2	99.5	97.7	0.25	0.06–32	97.6	1.6				
Minocycline	85.1	84.1	86.0	86.9	88.6	8	0.5–32	86.2	8.2				
Pip/taz	78.7	75.2	76.3	81.7	79.6	128	0.06–256	77.7	11.5				
Tigecycline	95.7	96.8	95.4	95.5	97.0	2	0.008–16	95.7	0.8				
	P.aeruginosa												
	N = 29	*N* = 150	*N* = 1081	*N* = 387	*N* = 95	N = 1739							
Amikacin	96.6	95.3	94.3	97.9	88.4	8	0.5–128	94.9	2.7				
Cefepime	65.5	76.0	75.5	86.3	85.3	16	0.5–64	78.4	9.1				
Ceftazidime	79.3	77.3	78.8	88.9	82.1	32	1–32	81.1	11.4				
Levofloxacin	86.2	82.7	72.4	76.5	75.8	16	0.015–16	74.6	19.8				
Meropenem	75.9	69.3	69.6	75.7	69.5	16	0.06–32	71.1	22.0				
Pip/taz	82.8	78.0	78.3	86.8	85.3	64	0.12–256	80.7	7.9				
	A.baumannii												
	N = 32	*N* = 123	*N* = 424	*N* = 118	N = 52	*N* = 749							
Amikacin	31.3	43.1	37.0	74.6	28.9	128	0.5–128	43.1	49.1				
Cefepime	12.5	27.6	24.1	54.2	15.4	64	0.5–64	28.3	65.7				

Table 3 Antimicrobial susceptibility among Gram negative isolates including ESBL-producing strains from blood specimens collected between 2012 and 2016 *(Continued)*

	Africa	Asia	Europe	North America	Latin America	Global				Global			
	S%	S%	S%	S%	S%	MIC_{90}(mg/L)	MIC range(mg/L)	S%	R%	MIC_{90}(mg/L)	MIC range(mg/L)	S%	R%
Ceftazidime	15.6	35.0	27.1	50.0	23.1	32	1–32	31.2	64.2				
Ceftriaxone	9.4	22.8	16.0	31.4	11.5	64	0.06–64	19.0	67.0				
Levofloxacin	21.9	30.9	23.6	51.7	15.4	16	0.008–16	28.6	61.7				
Meropenem	25.0	26.8	26.9	60.2	15.4	32	0.06–32	31.2	66.8				
Minocycline	81.3	73.2	61.8	89.0	90.4	8	0.5–32	70.8	8.8				
Pip/taz	12.5	26.0	24.5	52.5	13.5	256	0.06–256	27.9	68.2				
Tigecycline						2	0.008–4						

Abbreviations: *S%* percentage of susceptible isolates, *R%* percentage of resistant isolates, *MIC* minimum inhibitory concentration, *Amoxy/clav* Amoxicillin/clavulanic acid, *Pip/taz* Piperacillin/tazobactam

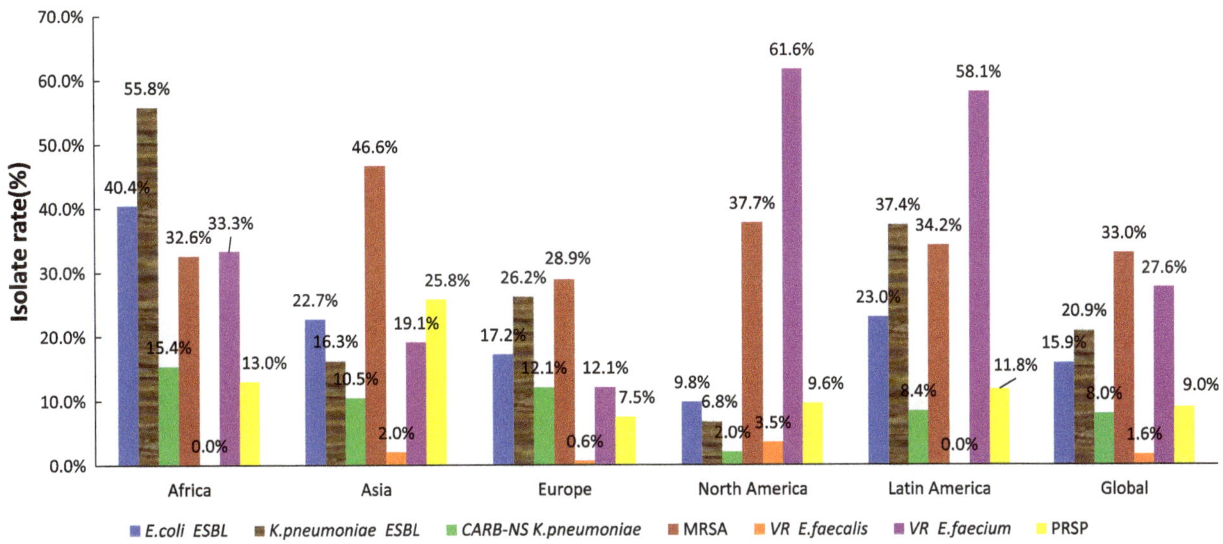

Fig. 1 Distribution of multi-drug resistant (MDR) bacteria among isolates from blood specimen collected in various international regions. Percent on every column indicates percentage of resistant isolates in each region for each organism. ESBL, extended-spectrum β-lactamase; CARB-NS, cabapanem non-susceptibility; MRSA, methicillin-resistant *S. aureus*; VR, vancomycin resistant; PRSP, Penicillin-resistant *S. pneumoniae*

Amikacin was the most active antibiotic in *P. aeruginose,* i.e., 94.9% susceptible isolates. Susceptibility to ceftazidime and pip/taz was found in over 80% of the isolates. Susceptibility to other antibiotics was confirmed for over 70% of the isolates (Table 3).

S. aureus

Almost all *S. aureus* isolates were susceptible to linezolid(100%), vancomycin(100%), and tigecycline(99.9%). The isolates were also highly susceptible to minocycline (98.8%). The lowest susceptibility in *S. aureus* was observed for penicillin; only14.7% of susceptible isolates (Table 4). Moreover, the proportion of MRSA was 33.0% globally; it was highest in Asia with 46.6%, followed by North America(37.7%) and Latin America (34.2%), whereas the MRSA percentage was lower in Africa(32.6%) and Europe(28.9%) (Fig. 1).

E. faecalis and E. faecium

In this study, *E. faecalis was* susceptible to five (penicillin, ampicillin, tigecycline, linezolid, and vancomycin) out of seven antibiotics at a rate of ≥98%. The susceptibility of *E. faecium* was 99.4 and 99.5% to tigecycline and linezolid, respectively, but only 12.9 and 11.9% to penicillin and ampicillin, respectively. The susceptibility of *E. faecium* to vancomycin was 71.6, and 70.7% of *E. faecalis* and 10.6% of *E .faecium* isolates were susceptible to levofloxacin. Further, 36.3% of *E. faecalis* and 65.6% of *E.faecium* isolates were susceptible to minocycline (Table 4).

The isolate rates of vancomycin-resistant *E. faecalis*(VR *E. faecalis*) and *E. faecium*(VR *E. faecium*) were 1.4 and 27.6%, respectively. Most VR E. *faecium* isolates were collected in North America and Latin America with isolate rate of 61.6 and 58.1%, respectively (Fig. 1). Tigecycline and linezolid were active against 98.9% of VR E. *faecium*.

S. pneumoniae

No linezolid- or vancomycin-resistant isolates were found in our study. Over than 97% susceptibility was observed for tigecycline, levofloxacin, ceftriaxone, and amoxy/clav. Susceptibility to clindamycin was 84.7%, which was higher than that to macrolides, including erythromycin,clarithromycin and azithromycin with similar susceptibility(72.7–74.0%). Meropenem and minocycline were active in 87.8 and 77.5% of the isolates, respectively (Table 4).

The lowest susceptibility among all antibiotics was observed for penicillin with 68.3% of susceptible isolates. The global rate for penicillin-resistant *S. pneumoniae* (PRSP) isolates was 9.0% in globally; regionly, it was 25.8% in Asia,13.0% in Africa,11.8% in Latin America, 9.6% in North America and 7.5% in Europe (Fig. 1).The activity of many antibiotics decreased in PRSP. The rate of isolates susceptible to macrolides decreased to 28.7–30.5% and clindamycin, meropenem, and minocycline were reduced to 53.5, 3.4 and 46.1%, respectively. However, 100% susceptibility was observed for linezolid, vancomycin, tigecycline, and levofloxacin (Table 4).

S. agalactiae

The proportion of antimicrobial-susceptible*S. agalactiae* isolates was higher than 97%, except for minocycline

Table 4 Antimicrobial susceptibility among Gram-positive isolates including multi-drug resistance(MDR) strains from blood specimens collected between 2012 and 2016

	Africa	Asia	Europe	North America	Latin America	Global				Global			
	S%	S%	S%	S%	S%	MIC_{90}(mg/L)	MIC range(mg/L)	S%	R%	MIC_{90}(mg/L)	MIC range(mg/L)	S%	R%
	S.aureus				*S.aureus*, all isolates					MRSA			
	N = 43	*N* = 298	*N* = 2008	*N* = 814	*N* = 161	N = 3324				*N* = 1096			
Levofloxacin	65.1	57.4	69.3	67.3	77.0	16	0.06–64	68.1	30.2	64	0.06–64	21.9	75.6
Linezolid	100.0	100.0	100.0	100.0	100.0	2	0.5–4	100.0	0.0	2	0.5–4	100.0	0.0
Minocycline	83.7	97.3	99.5	98.3	100.0	0.25	0.25–16	98.8	0.1	0.5	0.25–16	97.5	0.1
Penicillin	2.3	6.0	15.9	16.6	8.1	16	0.06–16	14.7	85.4	16	0.12–16	0.1	99.9
Tigecycline	100	99.7	100.0	100.0	100.0	0.12	0.008–1	99.9	0.0	0.25	0.015–1	99.9	0.0
Vancomycin	100.0	100.0	100.0	100.0	100.0	1	0.12–2	100.0	0.0	1	0.12–2	100.0	0.0
	E.faecalis				*E.faecalis*, all isolates					VR *E.faecalis*			
	N = 26	*N* = 99	*N* = 910	*N* = 406	*N* = 86	*N* = 1527				N = 22			
Ampicillin	100.0	96.0	98.9	99.8	96.5	1	0.06–32	98.8	1.2	32	0.5–32	86.4	13.6
Levofloxacin	69.2	70.7	68.6	73.4	81.4	64	0.06–64	70.7	28.5	64	0.5–64	13.6	86.4
Linezolid	100.0	97.0	100.0	100.0	97.7	2	0.5–8	99.7	0.1	2	0.5–2	100.0	0.0
Minocycline	30.8	35.4	36.8	35.2	38.4	8	0.25–16	36.3	6.3	8	0.25–8	27.3	0.0
Penicillin	100.0	95.0	98.8	99.8	96.5	4	0.06–16	98.7	1.3	16	2–16	86.4	13.6
Tigecycline	100.0	100.0	99.9	100.0	100.0	0.12	0.008–0.5	100.0	0.0	0.12	0.03–0.12	100.0	0.0
Vancomycin	96.2	98.0	99.0	96.6	98.8	2	0.12–64	98.2	1.4	64	32–64	0.0	100.0
	E.faecium				*E.faecium*, all isolates					VR *E.faecium*			
	N = 9	N = 89	*N* = 603	*N* = 268	N = 31	N = 1000				N = 276			
Ampicillin	11.1	12.4	11.1	14.2	6.5	32	0.06–32	11.9	88.1	32	4–32	0.7	99.3
Levofloxacin	22.2	9.0	9.8	12.3	12.9	64	0.06–64	10.6	87.0	64	8–64	0.0	100.0
Linezolid	100.0	100.0	99.7	98.8	100.0	2	0.5–8	99.5	0.2	2	0.5–8	98.9	0.4
Minocycline	88.9	47.2	70.2	59.0	80.7	8	0.25–16	65.6	6.2	8	0.25–16	58.7	6.2
Penicillin	11.1	14.6	13.1	12.7	6.5	16	0.06–16	12.9	87.1	16	4–16	1.5	98.6
Tigecycline	100.0	100.0	99.5	98.9	100.0	0.12	0.008–1	99.4	0.0	0.12	0.008–1	98.9	0.0
Vancomycin	66.7	78.7	87.1	38.1	41.9	64	0.12–64	71.6	27.6	64	32–64	0.0	100.0
	S.pneumoniae				*S.pneumoniae*, all isolates					PR *S.pneumoniae*			
	N = 23	*N* = 66	*N* = 1248	*N* = 553	*N* = 93	N = 1983				*N* = 178			
Amoxy/clav	91.3	95.5	98.0	96.2	93.6	1	0.03–16	97.1	1.1	8	0.03–16	68.5	11.8
Azithromycin	69.6	38.1	81.1	63.0	44.6	64	0.03–512	72.7	26.0	128	0.03–512	28.7	69.0
Ceftriaxone	100.0	94.0	98.7	99.0	98.9	0.5	0.03–8	98.6	0.1	2	0.03–8	86.0	1.1
Clarithromycin	69.6	39.7	80.9	63.0	69.6	128	0.015–128	73.9	26.0	128	0.015–128	30.5	69.0

Table 4 Antimicrobial susceptibility among Gram-positive isolates including multi-drug resistance(MDR) strains from blood specimens collected between 2012 and 2016 *(Continued)*

	Africa	Asia	Europe	North America	Latin America	Global				Global			
	S%	S%	S%	S%	S%	MIC_{90}(mg/L)	MIC range(mg/L)	S%	R%	MIC_{90}(mg/L)	MIC range(mg/L)	S%	R%
Clindamycin	78.3	61.9	85.3	87.4	79.4	128	0.015–128	84.7	14.8	128	0.015–128	53.5	45.4
Erythromycin	69.6	39.7	80.8	63.6	69.6	64	0.015–128	74.0	25.8	128	0.015–128	29.9	69.0
Levofloxacin	100.0	98.5	99.6	99.6	98.9	1	0.06–16	99.6	0.4	1	0.12–16	99.4	0.6
Linezolid	100.0	100.0	100.0	100.0	100.0	1	0.5–2	100.0	0.0	1	0.5–2	100.0	0.0
Meropenem	81.0	60.6	89.7	87.0	86.0	0.5	0.12–8	87.8	7.1	1	0.12–8	3.4	70.8
Minocycline	73.9	37.9	77.5	83.7	69.9	4	0.25–16	77.5	16.8	8	0.25–16	46.1	45.0
Penicillin	69.6	34.9	70.4	69.8	55.9	1	0.06–16	68.3	9.0	4	2–16	0.0	100.0
Tigecycline	100.0	98.5	99.8	99.5	100.0	0.03	0.008–4	99.7	0.0	0.03	0.008–0.12	100.0	0.0
Vancomycin	100.0	100.0	100.0	100.0	100.0	0.5	0.12–1	100.0	0.0	0.5	0.12–1	100.0	0.0
	S.agalactiae												
	N = 8	*N* = 64	*N* = 505	*N* = 373	N = 32	N = 982							
Ampicillin	100.0	100.0	100.0	100.0	100.0	0.12	0.06–0.25	100.0	0.0				
Ceftriaxone	100.0	100.0	100.0	100.0	100.0	0.12	0.03–0.5	100.0	0.0				
Levofloxacin	100.0	95.3	98.2	96.5	87.5	1	0.06–64	97.1	2.7				
Linezolid	100.0	100.0	100.0	100.0	100.0	1	0.5–2	100.0	0.0				
Meropenem	100.0	100.0	100.0	100.0	100.0	0.12	0.12–0.5	100.0	0.0				
Minocycline	12.5	20.3	17.8	22.0	50.0	16	0.25–16	20.6	62.7				
Penicillin	100.0	100.0	100.0	100.0	100.0	0.12	0.06–0.12	100.0	0.0				
Tigecycline	100.0	96.9	99.8	100.0	100.0	0.06	0.008–4	99.7	0.0				
Vancomycin	100.0	100.0	100.0	100.0	100.0	0.5	0.12–1	100.0	0.0				

Abbreviations: *S%* percentage of susceptible isolates, *R%* percentage of resistant isolates, *MIC* minimum inhibitory concentration, *Amoxy/clav* Amoxicillin/clavulanic acid

with 20.6% of susceptible isolates. A susceptibility of 100% was found for penicillin, ampicillin, linezolid, meropenem, and vancomycin (Table 4).

Variations insusceptibility between the major world regions

Antibiotics with a global susceptibility rate of less than 90% were selected and the ones with the lowest susceptibility rate in two regions were marked. The occurrence of each region due to the marked antibiotics reflected the situation of antimicrobial resistance in this region (Table 5). Africa was the region with the most occurrences of marked antibiotics, 38 times and at the proportion of 34.2%, followed by Latin America (27,24.3%) and Asia(26,23.4%). The proportion was less than 12% for Europe and North America.

Discussion

Bacteria isolated from blood are typically the causative agents for a circulatory system infection or a local infection(e.g., the special respiratory system) [6], and they often indicate poor prognosis [7]. Therefore, bacteria isolated from blood are important for physicians and studies on pathogenic bacteria and their resistance to antibiotics have a great practical significance and a high clinical value.

Bacterial species isolated from blood specimens in our study were common pathogens of community-acquired and hospital-acquired bloodstream infection [8, 9]. The patients were mostly from non-ICU departments and had the highest proportion in elderly patients 61–80 years of age. A surveillance program performed for 18 years by a large hospital of Malawi in Africa pathogens from bloodstream infections [8] found that the organisms causing differed with the age. Except for children below 4 years of age, bacterial infections were likely to be caused by *Salmonella typhimurium*, *Salmonella enteritidis*,*S. pneumoniae,* and yeast in adults of less than 60 years old of age. Morbidity in bloodstream infections caused by Enterobacteriaceae(such as *E. coli* or *K. pneumoniae)* and *S. aureus* increased with the age and occurred most frequently in elderly people ≥60 years old of age. In this investigation,the proportion of Enterobacteriaceae and *S. aureus* was 52.7% and the trend of the occurrence of the infection increased with age; these observations are in agreement with the findings in the study from Africa.

The high activities determined for amikacin, meropenem, and tigecycline against Enterobacteriaceae from blood samples in our study indicated that these antibiotics can be used as the first choice in the empirical treatment of clinical bloodstram infections caused by Enterobacteriaceae.

Low in vitro activity was observed for cephalosporin and pip/taz against *K. pneumonia.* ESBL production was higher in *K. pneumoniae* than in *E. coli* (20.9% vs. 15.9%). Meropenem resistance found globally in 8% of *K. pneumoniae,* far exceeds that in other Enterobacteriaceae. These results indicated that the lower activity of cephalosporins and pip/taz against *K. pneumoniae* is related to the production of ESBL and carbapenemases.

ESBL was the main reason for *E. coli* and *K. pneumoniae* resistance against the third and fourth generation of cephalosporins because of the hydrolytic activity [10]. Production of ESBL monitored by many large disease surveillance organizations. In this study, the production of ESBL in *E. coli* and *K. pneumoniae* were 22.7%/16.3%, 23.0%/37.4% and 9.8%/6.8% in Asia, Latin America, and North America, respectively. The data from the 2011–2014 SENTRY surveillance, ESBL in *E. coli* and *K. pneumoniae* in Asia-Pacific [11], Latin America [12], and the USA [13] were 60%/47%,37.7%/57.3%, and 11.1%/20.4%, respectively, which was higher than the

Table 5 Occurrence of every regions with low susceptibility to antibiotics in major blood-borne pathogens (%)

bacterial	number of antibiotics[a] × 2	Africa	Asia	Europe	North America	Latin America
E. coli	14	7 (50.0)	4 (28.6)	0 (0.0)	0 (0.0)	3 (14.3)
K .pneumoniae	16	8 (50.0)	0 (0.0)	3 (18.8)	0 (0.0)	5 (31.3)
S. marcescens	6	2 (33.1)	1 (16.7)	0 (0.0)	2 (33.3)	1 (16.7)
E. cloacae	16	5 (31.3)	6 (37.5)	2 (12.5)	0 (0.0)	3 (18.8)
P. aeruginosa	10	1 (10.0)	3 (30.0)	4 (40.0)	0 (0.0)	2 (20.0)
A. baumannii	16	7 (43.8)	1 (6.3)	1 (6.3)	0 (0.0)	7 (43.8)
S. aureus	4	2 (50.0)	2 (50.0)	0 (0.0)	0 (0.0)	0 (0.0)
E. faecalis	4	2 (50.0)	0 (25.0)	1 (25.0)	1 (25.0)	0 (0.0)
E. faecium	11[b]	2[b](18.2)	2 (18.2)	2[b](18.2)	2 (18.2)	3 (27.3)
S. pneumoniae	14	2 (14.3)	7 (50.0)	0 (0.0)	2 (14.3)	3 (21.4)
Total	111	38 (34.2)	26 (23.4)	13 (11.7)	7 (6.3)	27 (24.3)

[a] There were antibiotics with a global susceptibility of less than 90%

[b] Same susceptibility in Africa and Europe of ampicillin to *E. faecium*

data in our study. In a meta- analysis from West Africa [14], ESBL in *E. coli* and *K. pneumoniae* were11.9 and 24.2%, respectively, which was less than 40.4 and 55.8% in our study. In a report of the TEST study between 2004 and 2013 [15], ESBL of *E. coli* and *K. pneumoniae* were 14.0 and 20.4% globally, similar to 15.9 and 20.9%, respectively, in our study. Different procedures implemented by different organizations involved in various surveillance programs lead to disparities in surveillance data specific for each region. It is critical to organize very active surveillance stations and collect accurate data to assess the true status of antimicrobial resistance in a local area.

Carbapenemases cause carbapenem resistance in Enterobacteriaceae [16]. *K. pneumoniae* carbapenemases(KPC) and metallo-β-lactamases(MBL)are common epidemic carbapenemases. KPC is reportedly prevalent in Latin-America, Europe and the Middle-East and the MBL is also prevalent in Europe and Asia [16]. No article has mentioned an increase of carbapenemases in Africa, but we found the highest rate of non-susceptibility to carbapenem(15.4%) in Africa. The number of participating centers and the collected strains were minimal in Africa(8 centers; 47*E. coli* and 52 *K. pneumoniae* isolates) as compared to other regions. There is a high probability that specific data by a single center can lead to a resistance rate increase that is not representative for the entire continent. Another reason was that we could not acquire correct information is the rarity of reports from Africa. To enhance the surveillance of bacterial resistance in developing regions is imperative for future infectious disease management. Non-susceptibility of meropenem against *K. pneumoniae* was 8.4 and 10.5% in Latin America and Asia, respectively, in our study, which is similar to the results of SENTRY [11, 12]. However, there is a large difference between our data for North America(2.0%) and the SENTRY data for this region (10.8%) [13].

Similar results were obtained on the susceptibility of cephalosporins and pip/taz to *E. cloacae* comparing our results to the SENTRY report [12]; 61.6–78.4% of cephalosporin-susceptible *E. cloacae* indicated the prudent use of cephalosporins in *E. cloacae* bacteremia. The results of our antimicrobial susceptible tests should be used as a reference. For *S. marcescens* bacteremia, there are several antibiotics available for empirical antibiotic treatment.

High in vitro activity was observed for minocycline against Enterobacteriaceae, but it was lower against ESBL-producing *K. pneumoniae.* Poor levofloxacin susceptibility exists in *E. coli* and *K. pneumoniae* (65.2 and 77.5%, respectively), which is worse in ESBL-producing *E. coli* and *K. pneumoniae*(16.3 and 40.5%, respectively),- but better in *E. cloacae* and *S. marcescens*(88.1 and 95.2%, respectively). Thus, levofloxacin could be used to treat bacteremia caused by *E. cloacae* or *S. marcescens,* but not in bacteremia caused by *E. coli* or *K. pneumoniae.*

Susceptibility to carbapenem in *A.baumannii* has also been closely monitored. Consistency has been demonstrated by a 31.2% of susceptibility in this investigation and less than 30% from SENTRY [12] and SMART [17] in Latin America. The clinical effect of carbapenem against *A. baumannii* is very limited because the epidemic caused by the global emergence of multi-drug resistant(MDR) isolates. The separation rate of MDR *A. baumannii* between 2004 and 2014 was calculated by Anna et al. [18]. The result was 44.3% globally and up to 60–70% in Latin America, Middle-East, and Africa. Strong resistance is challenging for clinical disease management. The emergence of MDR *A. baumannii* in bloodstream infections significantly increased the mortality in patients [19]. Only minocycline has a better activity against *A. baumannii* in our study(70.8% susceptible isolates), which was similar to that in the SENTRY report (79.1%) [20]. The meta-analysis by Lashinskyet al. [21] on several clinical investigations found that the treatment success rate of minocycline single and combination on *A. baumannii* was 78.2%,verifying the recommendation to use minocycline treatment for an infection caused by *A. baumannii.*

The susceptibility for six antibiotics by *P. aeruginosa* were 71.1–94.9% globally, and 66.7–91.7% and 54.4–75.4% in Asia and Latin America, respectively, which was higher than TEST result (63.9–90.2%) of 2004–2013 [15] for all specimen globally collected, and the SENTRY result for Asia-Pacific(66.7–91.7%) [11] and Latin America(54.4–75.4%) [22] in 2011. *P. aeruginose* isolated from blood may be more susceptible to common antibiotics than the specimens collected from other body sites.

Best in vitro activity was found for linezolid, vancomycin, tigecycline and minocycline against *S. aureus.* Very poor penicillin-susceptibility was observed for *S. aureus,* only 14.7%, which was in accordance with several other investigations [15, 23]. The rate of 33.0% MRSA isolates in globally of our study agreed with 40.2% in the TEST report for 2004–2013 [15]. The isolate rates of MRSA in Asia-Pacific [11], Latin America [12], and the USA [13] were 37,44.7, and 53.1% in the SENTRY surveillance report. In a comparison with our study, the rate for the USA was higher than that for North America(37.7%), whereas the Asia-Pacific rate was lower than the Asia rate (46.6%). A meta- analysis on *S. aureus* in Africa summarized by Matthew [24] found <50% separation of MRSA, which is a smaller difference to our study. Further, 21.2% isolation of MRSA by the EARS-Net surveillance network in Europe is close to 28.9% in our study.

In our investigation, the susceptibility to primary drugs was significantly lower in *E. faecium* than in *E. faecalis*,except for linezolid, tigecycline and minocycline. High resistance levels are a complication during infection treatment. Resistance to vancomycin was significantly higher in *E. faecium* (27.6%) than in *E. faecalis*(1.4%). In VR E. *faecium,* it increased to 61.6 and 58.1% in North America and Latin America, respectively, which is in accordance with the result for the USA (74.7%)[13] and Latin America(50.3%) [12] in the SENTRY surveillance report.

The global occurrence rate of PRSP was 9.0%, and 25.8,13.0,11.8,7.5, and 9.6% in Asia, Africa, Latin America, Europe, and North America, respectively, which was lower than the TEST data from 2009 to 2012(14.4% globally; and 33.1,32.3,15.1,10.1, and 16.3% in the respective regions) [25]. The difference may be linked to the source specimens used for recovering the isolates. Isolates from blood may be more susceptible than these from other body sites. The same situation may apply to other antibiotics. Susceptilbility to macrolides, clindamycin, meropenem and minocycline was 47.5–47.9, 70.2, 83.4, and 51.7%, respectively, in the TEST study from 2009 to 2012 [25], which was significantly less than these in our study. The resistance is higher against many antibiotics in PRSP as compared to that in *S. pneumoniae,* which has been verified by other investigations [26]. The highest activity was determined for linezolid, vancomycin, tigecycline, and levofloxacin irrespective of the resistance against penicillin.

Many research groups investigated and monitored the emergence of macrolide resistance in *S.agalactiae.* A resistance level of even less than 20% is serious for *S.agalactiae,* which is still susceptible to almost all antibiotics [27, 28]. It is very unfortunate that we did not detect the activity of macrolides in our study. *S. agalactiae* is fully susceptible to penicillin, which is critical for decolonization management in pregnant women and infections in other patients. However, the resistance to penicillin is emerging. In a study on *S.agalactiae* isolates from 2012 by Crespo et al. [28], 2% of penicillin-resistant *S. agalactiae* were detected. The mechanism of penicillin resistance in *S.agalactiae* is related to changes in penicillin-binding proteins(PBPs) [29], based on an investigation of resistant strains isolated from cattle.

Tigecycline has the highest in vitro activity against bacteria recovered from blood. Susceptibility to tigecycline in Gram-positive bacteria, including MRSA, VR E. *faecalis,* and PRSP, was above 99.4, except for VR E. *faecium* (98.9%). In Gram-negative bacteria, the susceptibility was high in *E. coli,* and more than 95% in *S. marcescens* and *E. cloacae,* but lower in *K. pneumoniae*(94.8%) and ESBL-producing *K. pneumoniae*(90.4%). Tigecycline was the only antibiotic with over 90% susceptibility in all major pathogens(except for *P.aeruginosa* because of its natural resistance) isolated from blood. High susceptibility values and the difference in various organisms were similar in the SENTRY report from 2016 [30], indicating the reliability of our results and the stability in the efficacy of tigecycline.

The data in Table 5 show that Africa, Asia and Latin America have a serious problem with antimicrobial resistance. There is a higher probability for the people in these regions that they have acquired an antibiotic-resistant organism if they fall ill with a bloodstream infection. Both difficult clinical management and high mortality increase the hardship. Hence, it is imperative to implement rational usage guidelines for antibacterial agents to reduce the occurrence and control the spread of antimicrobial-resistant bacteria globally and especially in the developing countries.

Conclusion

In our study, tigecycline was the only antibiotic associated with susceptibility in over 90% of all major pathogen isolates collected from blood specimens. In the comparison that included all world regions, the occurrence of antimicrobial-resistant bacteria was higher in Africa, Asia and Latin America than in Europe and North America. Therefore, reinforcement of the surveillance is important in all regions,but it is very critical in developing countries.

Abbreviations

CARB-NS: Cabapanem non-susceptibility; CLSI: Clinical and Laboratory Standards Institute; ESBL: Extended-spectrum β-lactamase; FDA: US Food and Drug Administration; ICU: Intensive care unit; IHMA: International Health Management Associates; KPC: *K. pneumonia* carbapenemases; MBL: Metallo-β-lactamases; MDR: Multi-drugs resistance; MIC: Minimum inhibitory concentration; MRSA: Methicillin-resistance *S. aureus*; PBP: Penicillin-binding protein; PRSP: Penicillin-resistance *S.pneumoniae*; TEST: Tigecycline Evaluation and Surveillance Trail; VR: Vancomycin resistant

Acknowledgements

The authors would like to acknowledge and thank all T.E.S.T investigators and laboratories for their participation in the study, as well as the staff at IHMA for the coordination of T.E.S.T. and at Pfizer for the involvement in study design and the decision to submit this article for publication.

Funding

This study was sponsored by Pfizer, Inc., providing funds for designing the study, performing the tests and managing the data.

Authors' contributions

ZZ and MC participated in data collection and interpretation. ZZ wrote the manuscript. YL and PS reviewed the manuscript. YY was involved in the data interpretation and drafting the manuscript. All authors read and approved the final manuscript.

30. Pfaller MA, Huband MD, Streit J, Flamm RK, Sader HS. Surveillance of tigecycline activity tested against clinical isolates from a global (North America, Europe, Latin America and Asia-Pacific) collection (2016). Int J Antimicrob Agents. 2018;51:848–53.

Consent for publication

Not applicable.

Competing interests

ZZ, MC and YL declare no competing interests. YY and PS are employees of Pfizer, Inc.

Author details

[1]Shengjing Hospital of China Medical University, Shenyang, China. [2]Affiliated Hospital of Hebei University, Baoding, China. [3]Pfizer Investment Co.,Ltd, Shanghai, China.

References

1. Mayr FB, Yende S, Angus DC. Epidemiology of severe sepsis. Virulence. 2014; 5:4–11.
2. Yamaga S, Shime N. Association between appropriate empiric antimicrobial therapy and mortality from bloodstream infections in the intensive care unit. J Infect Chemother. 2018;24:267–71.
3. Clinical and Laboratory Standards Institute (CLSI). Methods for dilution antimicrobial susceptibility tests for bacteria that grow aerobically; approved standards – Tenth edition.CLSI Document M07-A10. Wayne, PA.CLSI; 2015.
4. Clinical and Laboratory Standards Institute (CLSI). Performance standards for antimicrobial susceptibility testing – Twenty-fifth informational supplement. CLSI Document M100-S25. Wayne, PA.CLSI; 2015.
5. Pfizer Inc. (Wyeth Pharmaceuticals). Tygacil® product insert. [Philadelphia, PA]. http://labeling.pfizer.com/showlabeling.aspx?id=491&pagename= tygacil_fly. 2016.
6. Ruiz-Giardin JM, Jimenez BC, Martin RM, Ortiz J, Condori Arenas MH, Sanmartin JV, et al. Clinical diagnostic accuracy of suspected sources of bacteremia and its effect on mortality. Eur J Intern Med. 2013;24:541–5.
7. Skovgaard M, Schønheyder HC, Benfield T, Nielsen RB, Knudsen JD, Bangsborg J, et al. Impact of positive chest X-ray findings and blood cultures on adverse outcomes following hospitalized pneumococcal lower respiratory tract infection: a population-based cohort study. BMC Infect Dis. 2013;13:197.
8. Musicha P, Cornick JE, Bar-Zeev N, French N, Masesa C, Denis B, et al. Trends in antimicrobial resistance in bloodstream infection isolates at a large urban hospital in Malawi (1998–2016): a surveillance study. Lancet Infect Dis. 2017; 17:1042–52.
9. De Angelis G, Fiori B, Menchinelli G, D'Inzeo T, Liotti FM, Morandotti GA, et al. Incidence and antimicrobial resistance trends in bloodstream infections caused by ESKAPE and *Escherichia coli* at a large teaching hospital in Rome, a 9-year analysis (2007-2015). Eur J Clin Microbiol infect dis. 2018. https://doi.org/10.1007/s10096-018-3292-9 [Epub ahead of print].
10. Sanders CC, Sanders WE. β-Lactama resistance in gram-negative bacteria: global trends and clinical impact. Clin Infect Dis. 1992;15:824–39.
11. Mendes RE, Mendoza M, Banga SK, Castanheira M, Bell JM, Turnidge JD, et al. Regional Resistance Surveillance Program Results for 12 Asia-Pacific Nations (2011). Antimicrob Agents Chemother. 2013;57:5721–6.
12. Sader HS, Castanheira M, Farrell DJ, Flamm RK, Mendes RE, Jones RN. Tigecycline antimicrobial activity tested against clinical bacteria from Latin American medical centers: results from SENTRY antimicrobial surveillance program (2011–2014). Int J Antimicrob Agents. 2016;48:144–50.
13. Helio SS, David JF, Robert KF, Ronald NJ. Variation in potency and Spectrum of Tigecycline activity against bacterial strains from U.S. medical centers since its approval for clinical use (2006 to 2012). Antimicrob Agents Chemother. 2014;58:2274–80.
14. Kerlly JB, Céline L, Nathan F, Ronatd JB, Richard AM. Antimicrobial resistance in West Africa:a systematic review and meta-analysis. Int J Antimicrob. 2017; 50:629–39.
15. Hoban DJ, Reinert RR, Bouchillon SK, Dowzicky MJ. Global in vitro activity of tigecycline and comparator agents:Tigecycline evaluation and surveillance trial 2004-2013. Ann Clin Microbiol Antimicrob. 2015;14:27.
16. van Duin D, Doi Y. The global epidemiology of carbapenemase-producing Enterobacteriaceae. Virulence. 2017;8:460–9.
17. Karlowsky JA, Hoban DJ, Hackel MA, Lob SH, Sahm DF. Resistance among gram-negative ESKAPE pathogens isolated from hospitalized patients with intra-abdominal and urinary tract infections in Latin American countries: SMART 2013-2015. Braz J Infect Dis. 2017;21:343–8.
18. Giammanco A, Calà C, Fasciana T, Dowzicky MJ. Global assessment of the activity of tigecycline against multidrug-resistant Gram-negative pathogens between 2004 and 2014 as part of the Tigecycline Evaluation and Surveillance Trial. mSphere. 2017;2:e00310–6. https://doi.org/10.1128/mSphere.00310-16.
19. Sirijatuphat R, Sripanidkulchai K, Boonyasiri A, Rattanaumpawan P, Supapueng O, Kiratisin P, et al. Implementation of global antimicrobial resistance surveillance system (GLASS) in patients with bacteremia. PLoS ONE. 2018;13:e0190132.
20. Castanheira M, Mendes RE, Jones RN. Update on Acinetobacter species: mechanisms of antimicrobial resistance and contemporary in vitro activity of minocycline and other treatment options. Clin Infect Dis. 2014;59Suppl 6: 367–373.
21. Lashinsky JN, Henig O, Pogue JM, Kaye KS. Minocycline for the treatment of Multidrug and extensively drug-Resistant *A. baumannii*: a review. Infect Dis Ther. 2017;6:199–211.
22. Jones RN, Blanco MG, Gales AC, Gallegos B, ALL C, MDV M, et al. Susceptibility rates in Latin American Nations:Report from a Regional Resistance Surveillance Program. Brazi J Infec Dis. 2013;17:672–81.
23. Bielicki JA, Lundin R, Sharland M. ARPEC project. Antibiotic resistance prevalence in routine bloodstream isolates from Children's hospitals varies substantially from adult surveillance data in Europe. Pediatr Infect Dis J. 2015;34:734–41.
24. Falagas ME, Karageorgopoulos DE, Leptidis J. KorbilaIP.MRSA in Africa: Filling the Global Map of Antimicrobial Resistance. PLoS ONE. 2013;8: e68024.
25. Viktorija T, Michael JD. Regional and global antimicrobial susceptibility among isolates of *Streptococcus pneumoniae* and *Haemophilus influenzae* collected as part of the Tigecycline Evaluation and Surveillance Trial (T.E.S.T.) from 2009 to 2012 and comparison with previous years of T.E.S.T. (2004–2008). Ann Clin Microbiol Antimicrob. 2014;13:52.
26. Kim SH, Song JH, Chung DR, Thamlikitkul V, Yang Y, Wang H, et al. Changing trends in antimicrobial resistance and serotypes of *Streptococcus pneumoniae* isolates in Asian countries: an Asian network for surveillance of resistant pathogens (ANSORP) study. Antimicrob Agents Chemother. 2012; 56:1418–26.
27. Numanović F, Smajlović J, Gegić M, Delibegović Z, Bektaš S, Halilović E, et al. Presence and resistance of *Streptococcus agalactiae* in vaginal specimens of pregnant and adult non-pregnant women and association with other aerobic bacteria. Med Glas (Zenica). 2017;14:98–105.
28. Crespo-Ortiz Mdel P, Castañeda-Ramirez CR, Recalde-Bolaños M, Vélez-Londoño JD. Emerging trends in invasive and noninvasive isolates of *Streptococcus agalactiae* in a Latin American hospital: a 17-year study. BMC Infect Dis. 2014;14:428.
29. Hu Y, Kan Y, Zhang Z, Lu Z, Li Y, Leng C, et al. New mutations of penicillin-binding proteins in *Streptococcus agalactiae* isolates from cattle with decreased susceptibility to penicillin. Microb Drug Resist. 2018. https://doi.org/10.1089/mdr.2017.0223 . [Epub ahead of print].

26

Prevalence and molecular characterization of *Staphylococcus aureus* from human stool samples

A. E. Kates[1], D. Thapaliya[2], T. C. Smith[2] and M. L. Chorazy[3*]

Abstract

Background: To determine the prevalence of intestinal *S. aureus* colonization of patients at a large teaching hospital and determine the molecular characteristics of the identified strains. The second objective of this research was to determine risk factors associated with *S. aureus* intestinal colonization.

Methods: A cross-sectional study of 781 specimens from inpatients and outpatients at the University of Iowa Hospitals and Clinics Clinical Microbiology Laboratory was conducted. *S. aureus* was identified using traditional culture methodologies. Methicillin-resistance was determined via PCR of the *mecA* gene. PVL PCR, *spa* typing, and antimicrobial sensitivity testing were also done. A nested case-control study was done on a subset of patients with all colonized patients defined as cases and non-colonized controls. Medical record abstractions were done to identify risk factors for intestinal colonization in the nested study.

Results: Out of 625 patients included in the final study, 58 were positive for *S. aureus* (9.3%). One isolate was positive for the PVL gene. A high number of isolates were resistant to multiple antibiotics including oxacillin (43.1%), erythromycin (51.7%), and levofloxacin (41.4%). All isolates were susceptible to vancomycin, daptomycin, linezolid, and quinupristin-dalfopristin. In the nested study, having a disease or condition of the gastrointestinal tract significantly increased the odds of intestinal colonization (OR: 1.96, 95% CI: 1.04–3.7; aOR: 13.9, 95% CI: 1.67–115.7). No other variables were significantly associated with increased odds of colonization.

Conclusions: *S. aureus* was identified from the stool of patients at the University of Iowa Hospitals and Clinics, with a large number of those isolates being resistant to antibiotics and may serve a reservoir for subsequent infections as well as asymptomatic transmission.

Keywords: Methicillin-resistant *Staphylococcus aureus*, Hospitals, Antibiotic resistance, Intestinal carriage

Background

Staphylococcus aureus is a commensal bacterium and important cause of healthcare-associated infections [1]. Nasal carriage is considered to be the most important site of *S. aureus* colonization [2] and is the best-studied [3]. However, other extra-nasal body sites, including the gastrointestinal tract, are known to harbor *S. aureus* [4–6]. Recent studies have found *S. aureus* in the intestines of healthy humans [7, 8] as well as the intestines of hospitalized patients [9].

S. aureus, an in particular methicillin-resistant *S. aureus* (MRSA) intestinal colonization, may be more common than previously thought and has been shown to be clinically important [10, 11]. Rectal carriers have been found to be at increased risk of developing *S. aureus* infections [10] and gastrointestinal carriage of MRSA has been associated with nosocomial antibiotic-associated diarrhea [11]. Screening for gastrointestinal carriage has been shown to identify colonized patients who would have been otherwise missed [12]. *S. aureus* gastrointestinal carriage may be an overlooked reservoir, contributing to hospital infection and transmission.

The objectives of this study were to determine the prevalence of *S. aureus* and MRSA in human stool

* Correspondence: margaret-chorazy@uiowa.edu
[3]Department of Epidemiology, College of Public Health, University of Iowa, Iowa City, IA, USA
Full list of author information is available at the end of the article

samples at a large university hospital, to characterize the identified isolates by molecular methods, and to assess potential risk factors for intestinal carriage. We hypothesized *S. aureus* and MRSA prevalence in stool will be similar to what has been reported previously in the literature [3]. Furthermore, we hypothesized having a gastrointestinal condition would increase the risk of intestinal *S. aureus* carriage.

Methods

Population and design

We conducted a cross-sectional study of 781 stool specimens retrieved from the University of Iowa Hospitals and Clinics (UIHC) Clinical Microbiology Laboratory between September 2010 and March 2011. UIHC is Iowa's only comprehensive academic medical center, consisting of 811 beds. Though patients are primarily drawn from eastern Iowa, the hospital serves the entire state and into the region beyond (including parts of Illinois, Wisconsin, Minnesota). The specimens were provided from a bank of existing biologic specimens originally collected for the purpose of patient clinical care as part of standard clinical practice. Samples remaining after completion of diagnostics that would have otherwise been disposed by the Clinical Microbiology Laboratory were collected by the researchers and stored at − 80 °C for further analysis. This convenience sample included both inpatients and outpatients from Iowa, Northern Missouri, and Western Illinois. A nested case-control study was conducted using electronic patient medical records to assess potential risk factors for *S. aureus* intestinal carriage. All patients positive for intestinal *S. aureus* carriage were included in the nested study and considered cases. Two controls were chosen for every case based on admission date and time of stool sample collection within ± 24 h. Only one stool sample per patient was included. If more than one stool sample per patient was included in the biobank, only the first stool provided by the patient was included in this analysis.

Ethics, consent, and approval

The University of Iowa Institutional Review Board approved all study protocols.

Identification and characterization of *S. aureus*

50 μL of stool was plated onto Baird-Parker Agar and CHROMagar MRSA media (Becton Dickinson and Company, Sparks, Maryland, USA) and incubated for 48 h at 35 °C. Presumptive positive colonies were streaked onto Columbia CNA with 5% sheep blood (Becton Dickinson and Company, Sparks, Maryland, USA), and incubated for 24 h at 35 °C. All isolates were tested for *S. aureus* using the catalase, coagulase, and Pastorex Staph Plus rapid latex agglutination (Bio-Rad, Redmond, Washington, USA) tests. Any patient who was culture positive for *S. aureus* and/or MRSA in the stool was considered intestinally colonized.

All *S. aureus* isolates were tested for antimicrobial susceptibility using broth dilution as described by the Clinical and Laboratory Standards Institute [13]. Isolates were tested for susceptibility to oxacillin, tetracycline, erythromycin, clindamycin, trimethoprim-sulfamethoxazole, gentamycin, levofloxacin, vancomycin, daptomycin, quinupristin/dalfopristin, linezolid, and rifampin.

Whole, genomic DNA was extracted using the Wizard Genomic DNA purification kit (Promega Corporation, Madison, Wisconsin, USA) adapted for *S. aureus*. Presence of the *mecA* [14] and PVL [15] genes were determined through end-point PCR. *spa* typing was carried out using the primers and methodologies described by Ridom Bioinformatics and sequences were interpreted utilizing the Ridom StaphType software (Ridom GmbH, Würzburg, Germany). For phenotypically MRSA isolates negative for the *mecA* gene, the presence of the *mecC* gene was determined [16]. All molecular procedures were carried out using known positive and negative controls, including USA300 (*mecA*, PVL) and LGA251 (*mecC*).

Medical record abstraction

Medical record abstractions were done on all *S. aureus* and MRSA-positive patients (cases) and two culture-negative patients (controls). Controls were chosen based on date of admission and time of sample collection relative to cases. Demographic information (gender, age, and race/ethnicity), reason for specimen collection, hospital admission and discharge dates, ICU admission and discharge dates, death date, co-infections, recent antimicrobial use, recent anti-motility medication use, history of gastrointestinal disorders, and history of immunosuppressive conditions were abstracted from the electronic medical record.

Statistical analysis

Statistical analyses were performed using SAS, version 9.3 (SAS Institute, Cary, NC). There were 781 banked samples available to the investigators from the UIHC. Two controls for each case was decide upon because it has been shown more than two controls per case does not greatly increase the statistical power of the analysis [17]. Logistic regression was performed to assess risk factors for intestinal colonization. The primary exposure of interest, having a disorder of the gastrointestinal tract, was modeled as dichotomous (yes/no). Backwards selection was used to determine which variables to include into the model ($p > 0.2$ threshold to stay in the model).

Interaction terms were assessed between all covariates. If the term was significantly associated with *S. aureus* infections, it was included into the final model and the Akaike information criterion (AIC) was assessed. If the model including the interaction term increased the AIC by more than three over the model without the term, the interaction term was not included in the final model. Odds ratios and 95% Confidence Intervals were calculated and a significance level of $p = .05$ was used.

Results

Of the 781 samples retrieved from the UIHC Clinical Microbiology Laboratory, six samples were excluded due to the tubes breaking during the freezing process. An additional 148 samples were excluded due to patients providing more than one stool sample and six additional samples were excluded due to medical records that were not able to be located, leaving 621 patients included in the study (Fig. 1). Demographic and clinical characteristics of the 621 patients included in the study are described in Table 1. The average age for all patients was 51.6 years (stan. Dev.: 19 years, range: 0 to 94 years). A majority of patients were female (320, 51.5%) and Caucasian (560, 90.2%). A majority were inpatients (487, 78.4%) with 20.1% (126/625) being outpatients, and 1.3% (8/625) being housed outpatients. The average length of stay for inpatients as defined as the entire time they were admitted for the stay when their stool samples was collected was 15.8 days (stan. Dev.: 28.6 days). There were no significant differences between carriers and non-carriers for any variables listed in Table 1.

Of the 621 samples, 58 (58/621, 9.3%) were positive for *S. aureus*, 26 of which (26/621, 4.2%) were MRSA via the presence of the *mecA* gene, with an MRSA prevalence of 44.8% (26/58). One isolate was positive for PVL. Thirty unique *spa* types were identified, with t002 being the most prevalent at 66.7% ($n = 20$) followed by t012 and t1635 both at 10% ($n = 3$). The BURP analysis resulted in one major cluster with the hospital-associated strain t002 as the founder. The *spa* cc-002 grouping accounted for 24 strains (42% of all strains) and four *spa* types (13% of all *spa* types). Two *spa* types (three isolates) were excluded as they had less than 5 repeat sequences present in the *spa* gene.

Antimicrobial susceptibility testing was performed on all isolates positive for *S. aureus* (Fig. 2). Resistance was observed for most antibiotics tested. The highest prevalence of resistance was to erythromycin at 51.7% ($n = 37$) followed by oxacillin at 43.1% ($n = 25$) and levofloxacin at 41.4% ($n = 24$). Resistance to clindamycin was observed at 22.4% ($n = 16$). No isolates were resistant to vancomycin, daptomycin, or quinupristin/dalfopristin. Resistance to all other antimicrobials was low (Fig. 3). Twenty-six (44.8%) isolates met the definition for multi-drug resistance (MDR) with having acquired non-susceptibility to at least one agent in three or more antimicrobial categories [18]. Of the MDR isolates, one isolate was resistant to at least one agent in six antimicrobial categories and one isolate was resistant to ≥1 agent in five categories. Twelve isolates were resistant to ≥1 agent in four categories and 9 isolates were resistant to ≥1 agent in 3 categories. Three isolates met the definition of MDR by being MRSA. Twenty-two of the 58 isolates (37.9%) were susceptible to all antibiotics tested. Six isolates (10.3%) were resistant to only one antimicrobial and two were resistant to two antimicrobials (3.4%). Two isolates were phenotypically resistant to oxacillin according to the AST (both isolates had a minimum inhibitory concentration

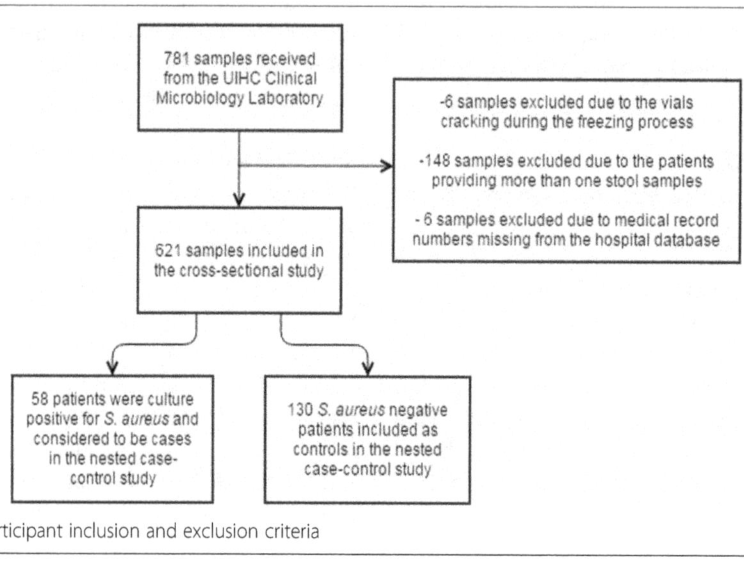

Fig. 1 Flow chart of the participant inclusion and exclusion criteria

Table 1 Patient demographic data by *S. aureus* intestinal colonization status

	Carriers $n = 58$	Non-carriers $n = 567$	*P*	Total $n = 621$
Age (Mean years ± Std. dev.)	51.2 (±20.4)	51.6 (±18.9)	0.897	51.6 (±19.0)
Sex				
Male	24 (41.4%)	277 (49.2%)		301 (48.5%)
Female	34 (58.6%)	286 (50.8%)	0.256	320 (51.5%)
Race/ Ethnicity				
Caucasian	52 (89.7%)	508 (90.2%)		560 (90.2%)
African American	2 (3.5%)	24 (4.3%)		26 (4.2%)
Hispanic or Latino	3 (5.2%)	8 (1.4%)		11 (1.8%)
Other[a]	1 (1.7%)	24 (4.2%)	0.486	25 (4.0%)
Visit Type				
Inpatient	44 (75.9%)	443 (78.7%)		487 (78.4%)
Outpatient	13 (22.4%)	113 (20.1%)		126 (20.3%)
Housed outpatient[b]	1 (1.7%)	7 (1.2%)	0.865	8 (1.3%)
Length of Stay (Mean days ± Std. dev.)	21.7 (±51.7)	15.2 (± 25.1)	0.992	15.8 (± 28.6)

[a]Other includes American Indian or Alaskan Natives, Asian, Native Hawaiian or Pacific Islander, as well as individuals who declined to provide a race or ethnicity

[b]Housed outpatient refers to patients being held for observation

[MIC] of ≥4 μg/mL); however, both isolates were negative for the presence of the *mecA* and *mecC* genes.

Medical record abstractions were completed on 189 patients (58 cases and 131 controls). A majority of cases were Caucasian ($n = 168$, 88.9%) and slightly over half were male ($n = 98$, 51.8%). In the univariate analysis, most covariates were not significantly associated with *S. aureus* intestinal colonization. We observed a borderline significant association with sex with females having increased odds of intestinal colonization, though the confidence interval included 1.0 (OR: 1.84, 95% CI: 0.98–3.44). Having a history of a gastrointestinal condition, the primary predictor, was significant in the unadjusted, univariate model with those having any disorder of the gastrointestinal tract having increased odds of intestinal colonization (OR: 1.96, 95% CI: 1.04–3.7). The most prevalent disorder of the GI tract was gastroesophageal reflux disease (GERD) at 31 of the 189 patients (16.4%) of the total population analyzed for the nested study. The second most prevalent condition was lower GI bleed ($n = 16$, 7.4%) followed by Crohn's disease ($n = 13$, 6.9%) and any inflammatory disorder of the intestines including inflammatory bowel disorder ($n = 13$, 6.9%). No other covariates were significantly associated with intestinal colonization in the univariate analyses (Table 2).

The final adjusted model included having a disorder of the gastrointestinal tract, age, sex, laxative usage, anti-motility agent usage, having a *S. aureus* infection, whether the patient died, ICU length of stay, and the reason for specimen collection. An interaction between having a gastrointestinal disorder and age was forced

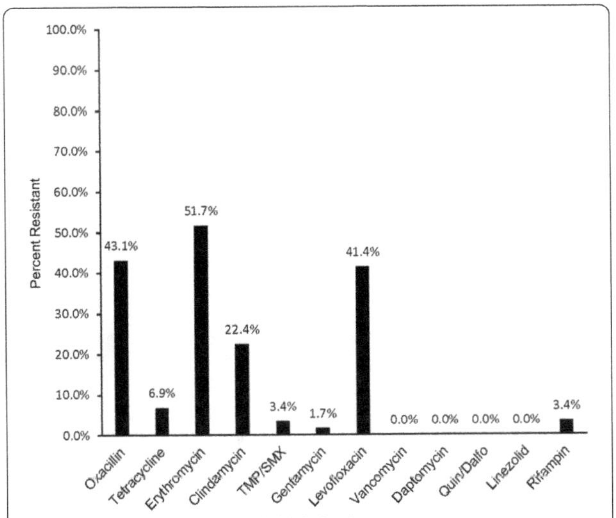

Fig. 2 Antibiotic susceptibility testing using minimum inhibitory concentrations ($n = 58$)

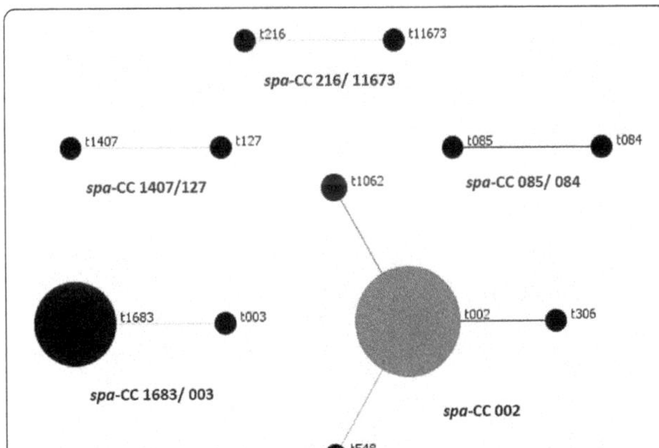

Singletons: 20 strains (35% of all isolates) and 16 *spa* types (53% of all *spa* types). t008, t012, t019, t126, t166, t209, t272, t277, t333, t630, t1635, t3446, t3682, t3719, t4947, t11674

Excluded *spa* types: 3 strains (5% of all isolates) and 2 *spa* types (7% of all *spa* types) t026, t3022

Fig. 3 Based Upon Repeat Pattern Analysis of all positive *S. aureus* isolates ($n = 58$). Based Upon Repeat Pattern (BURP) analysis was used to group all 58 *S. aureus* isolates into cluster complexes. Cost distances of ≤4 were used to define clusters and *spa* types with 5 or fewer repeats were excluded from the analysis

Table 2 Associations between potential risk factors and *S. aureus* intestinal colonization

Risk Factor	Cases (N = 58)	Controls (*N* = 131)	Unadjusted OR (95% CI)	Adjusted OR (95% CI)
Age				
0–29 years	9	13	Ref	Ref
30–49 years	14	34	0.58 (0.020–1.65)	2.94 (0.43–19.88)
50–69 years	28	60	0.67 (0.026–1.77)	5.02 (0.81–30.9)
Over 70 years	7	23	0.44 (0.13–1.5)	1.42 (0.15–13.6)
Sex				
Male	24	74	Ref	Ref
Female	33	58	1.84 (0.98–3.44)	1.93 (0.94–3.96)
Race/ Ethnicity				
Caucasian	53	115	Ref	
African American	2	5	0.9 (0.17–4.8)	
Hispanic/ Latino	3	2	3.35 (0.54–20.63)	
Other	1	8	0.28 (0.03–2.29)	
S. aureus Infection[a]				
No	53	121	Ref	Ref
Yes	5	10	1.14 (0.37–3.50)	0.83 (0.19–3.54)
Other Coinfections				
No Coinfections	26	46	Ref	
One	21	60	0.62 (0.34–1.23)	
Two	4	18	0.49 (0.16–1.48)	
Three or more	7	7	0.67 (0.19–2.34)	
Collection Reason				
Abdominal pain	5	13	Ref	Ref
Clostridium difficile	23	37	1.61 (0.51–5.13)	1.87 (0.49–7.11)
Diarrhea	11	72	0.67 (0.21–2.14)	0.59 (0.15–2.25)
Other	19	9	2.25 (0.63–8.03)	2.74 (0.64–11.7)
Deceased[b]				
No	44	83	Ref	Ref
Yes-within 30 days	3	11	0.71 (0.18–2.8)	0.74 (0.13–4.67)
Yes- after 30 days	14	26	0.4 (0.16–0.98)	0.29 (0.1–0.86)
Undeterminable	4	7	1.08 (0.3–3.9)	0.71 (0.17–2.96)
Gastrointestinal Disease				
No	21	69	Ref	Ref
Yes	37	62	1.96 (1.04–3.7)	13.9 (1.67–115.7)
Immunocompromised				
No	15	34	Ref	
Yes	43	97	1.01 (0.47–2.04)	
ICU Stay				
No	47	98	Ref	
Yes	11	33	0.69 (0.32–1.5)	
ICU Unit				
No ICU stay	47	98	Ref	
MICU	5	21	0.5 (0.18–1.4)	

Table 2 Associations between potential risk factors and *S. aureus* intestinal colonization *(Continued)*

Risk Factor	Cases (N = 58)	Controls (*N* = 131)	Unadjusted OR (95% CI)	Adjusted OR (95% CI)
SICU	2	6	0.7 (0.14–3.58)	
Other	4	6	1.4 (0.4–5.2)	
ICU Length of Stay				
0 days	47	99	Ref	Ref
1 to 4 days	1	14	0.15 (0.02–1.18)	0.15 (0.02–1.36)
Greater than 4 days	10	18	1.18 (0.5–2.73)	1.38 (0.46–4.15)
Total Length of Stay				
0 days	12	23	Ref	
1 to 10 days	23	59	0.75 (0.32–1.75)	
11 to 29 days	10	26	0.74 (0.27–2.02)	
Greater than 30 days	13	23	1.08 (0.41–2.87)	
Antibiotics used				
No	26	40	Ref	
Yes	32	91	0.54 (0.29–1.02)	
Laxatives used				
No	43	100	Ref	Ref
Yes	15	31	1.13 (0.56–2.3)	1.94 (0.8–4.6)
Anti-motility agent used				
No	57	122	Ref	Ref
Yes	1	9	0.238 (0.03–1.92)	0.16 (0.02–1.53)

[a]*S. aureus* infections are defined as clinical infections extracted from the patients medical record
[b]Mortality is not considered a risk factor colonization. For this variable, *S. aureus* colonization is a risk factor for mortality

into the model as the interaction term was verging on significance ($p = 0.058$) and did not increase the AIC by more than 3. In the final model, having a disorder of the GI tract was significantly associated with increased odds of being intestinally colonized with *S. aureus*, though the confidence interval is very wide (OR: 13.9, 95% CI: 1.67–115.7). No other covariates included in the final model were significantly associated with intestinal *S. aureus* colonization (Table 2).

Discussion

We identified *S. aureus* in the intestines of patients at UIHC and report an intestinal colonization rate of 9.3%. During the 1950's, *S. aureus* intestinal colonization was studied in greater detail than seen in the current literature [19]. Studies from this time report carriage prevalence ranges between 8% and 30% [3, 20, 21]. While researchers have known of the relationship between intestinal *S. aureus* carriage and antibiotic-associated diarrhea, as well as the increased risk of other *S. aureus* infections, intestinal carriage has been studied far less than carriage at other anatomical sites, particularly the nares. Recent studies of *S. aureus* intestinal carriage have detected intestinal carriage rates ranging from 10% [22] to as high as 37% [10]. It has been estimated the average rate of intestinal colonization in hospitalized patients is roughly 20% [3], though the number of studies included in reaching this estimate is small and the populations vary greatly. Our observed prevalence of 9.3% is lower than the estimated average and lower than most studies have reported to date. This may be due to the fact the population screened for this study included patients from many departments across a large teaching hospital as well as outpatients seen in the emergency department. Use of frozen instead of fresh stools may also have reduced our recovery rate.

Many of the studies in recent years have focused on MRSA carriage and have reported MRSA intestinal carriage rates frequently ranging from 5% [22, 23] to 10% [24] with some studies finding a MRSA prevalence as high as 22% in high-risk populations [25]. The observed prevalence of MRSA reported here is 4.2%, which is lower than others have reported. Of the *S. aureus* isolates identified, 44.8% met the definition for MDR-SA. Two of these isolates were phenotypically resistant to oxacillin; however, they were not positive for either resistance gene – *mecA* or *mecC* –tested for.

We found one isolate to be positive for the PVL gene [26]. As PVL genes are mainly associated with community- associated *S. aureus*, it is not surprising we found such a low prevalence in clinical cohort. *Spa* type t002 was the most frequently identified *spa* type accounting for 66.7% of all identified *spa* types. This *spa* type is most frequently associated with hospital strains and typically belongs to the pulsed-field type USA100 [27]. *Spa* type t012, the second most prevalent *spa* type observed in this study (10% of all *spa* types) is frequently found in community settings and may be associated with younger age [28].

Prevalence of intestinal carriage is dependent on the method of specimen collection employed. Varying rates of colonization are seen by method and anatomical site used to define "gastrointestinal." The two main methods used to collect specimens are swabs and stool samples. Swabs collected from the rectum, anus, perineum, and the groin or inguinal region are typically accepted as representing intestinal carriage of *S. aureus* in addition to stool specimens [3]. Several studies have assessed which method and region provide the most consistent rate of colonization, but these studies are few and do not provide a consensus. Rectal swabbing has been shown to yield more *S. aureus* than stool cultures [29]. This may explain why our study reports a lower prevalence compared to many of the studies cited above which used rectal or perineal swabbing.

Intestinal colonization may be an important reservoir for the dissemination of *S. aureus* in the health care setting. Intestinal colonization is known to lead to increased risk of infection [30–32], though the mechanism is not clear. It has been hypothesized intestinal colonization increases colonization or contamination of the skin which in turn increases contamination of the patient's environment. Environmental contamination then increases both the risk of infection as well as the potential for nosocomial transmission [31]. While we were unable to investigate colonization of other body sites in this study, *S. aureus* intestinal colonization has been associated with an increased risk of skin colonization [10]. Nasal and intestinal carriage are also frequently observed in the same patient; however, intestinal colonization alone does increase the detection sensitivity [3, 22, 23, 33–35]. In a meta-analysis by McKinnell et al., it was found rectal screening increased yield by 20%, with rectal screening having the greatest impact in hospitals with a low MRSA prevalence (23% increase) [35].

To assess potential risk factors for intestinal colonization, we performed a nested case-control study. We hypothesized having a disease or condition of the gastrointestinal tract would put patients at increased risk of *S. aureus* intestinal colonization. In the univariate analysis we found gastrointestinal conditions did significantly increase the odds of being colonized with *S. aureus* (OR: 1.96, 95% CI: 1.04–3.7) and this association remained significant after adjusting for the other variables included in the final model (OR: 13.9, 95% CI: 1.67–115.7), though the 95% confidence interval was very wide due to a small sample size. No other variables abstracted from the medical record were significantly associated with an increased risk of intestinal colonization in either the univariate or adjusted models. Other studies have reported several potential risk factors for intestinal *S. aureus* colonization. It has been shown that a stay in an extended care facility or nursing home can significantly increase the risk of intestinal colonization [36]; however, we were unable to assess nursing home stays in the present study. Studies have also reported length of stay [37], a recent history of antimicrobial usage [37–39], a history of MRSA infection [38], and dependence on healthcare workers to perform activities of daily living [37] all significantly increasing the risk of intestinal *S. aureus* carriage. While we were not able to assess activities of daily living in the medical record, we did not detect a significant association with LOS, antibiotic usage, or the history of MRSA infections and colonization in our population. This may be due to the inclusion of a single hospital in this study, smaller sample size, and the reliance on medical record data.

Our study has several limitations. The first is the specimens analyzed were not collected for research purposes, but for routine medical care and as such we were only able to address intestinal colonization in a cross-sectional study and were unable to determine the duration of colonization in these patients. Future studies are needed to determine colonization duration, as well as the rates of persistent versus intermittent carriage. Furthermore, we were unable to determine if the *S. aureus* strain the patient was colonized with was the same strain causing an *S. aureus* infection, or otherwise present in other locations of the patient's body or environment. This study was conducted in a single hospital in Iowa with a predominantly white population which may limit the generalizability of the study findings. However, UIHC is a large teaching hospital with a catchment area including several surrounding mid-western states. *S aureus* was identified from the stool of patients at the UIHC. Lastly, the samples used for this study were collected as part of routine clinical care and as such, all participants had some degree of gastrointestinal symptoms. A history of gastrointestinal conditions increased the risk of intestinal *S. aureus* carriage. Many of those isolates are resistant to antibiotics and may serve as a reservoir for subsequent infections and transmission events.

Conclusions

S. aureus colonization was found in 9.3% of tested stool samples. Having a disease or condition of the gastrointestinal tract significantly increased the odds of intestinal colonization. A diverse array of molecular types were isolated, and antibiotic resistance was common, including methicillin resistance and multi-drug resistant strains.

Abbreviations

AIC: Akaike information criterion; BURP: Based Upon Repeat Pattern.; GERD: Gastroesophageal reflux disease; LOS: Length of stay; MDR: Multi-drug resistant; MIC: Minimum inhibitory concentration; MRSA: Methicillin-resistant *Staphylococcus aureus*; UIHC: University of Iowa Hospitals and Clinics

Acknowledgements

The authors would like to thank the Clinical Microbiology Laboratory and the University of Iowa Hospitals and Clinics and Dr. Bradley Ford for their assistance with medical record abstraction. Thanks to Yesenia C. Romero-Herazo for retrieving the specimens.

Funding

No funding was received.

Authors' contributions

Conception and design of the study: AK, MC, TS. Acquisition of data: AK, MC. Molecular characterization: AK, DT. Analysis and interpretation of data: AK, DT. Drafting and revising of the manuscript: all authors. Final approval of the manuscript: all authors.

Consent for publication

Not applicable.

Competing interests

The authors declare that they have no competing interests.

Author details

[1]Division of Infectious Disease, Department of Medicine, School of Medicine and Public Health, University of Wisconsin-Madison, Madison, WI, USA. [2]Department of Biostatistics, Epidemiology and Environmental Health Services, College of Public Health, Kent State University, Kent, OH, USA. [3]Department of Epidemiology, College of Public Health, University of Iowa, Iowa City, IA, USA.

References

1. Wertheim HF, Melles DC, Vos MC, van Leeuwen W, van Belkum A, Verbrugh HA, Nouwen JL. The role of nasal carriage in Staphylococcus aureus infections. Lancet Infect Dis. 2005;5(12):751–62.
2. Williams RE. Healthy carriage of Staphylococcus aureus: its prevalence and importance. Bacteriol Rev. 1963;27:56–71.
3. Acton DS, Plat-Sinnige MJ, van Wamel W, de Groot N, van Belkum A. Intestinal carriage of Staphylococcus aureus: how does its frequency compare with that of nasal carriage and what is its clinical impact? Eur J Clin Microbiol Infect Dis. 2009;28(2):115–27.
4. Wertheim HF, Verveer J, Boelens HA, van Belkum A, Verbrugh HA, Vos MC. Effect of mupirocin treatment on nasal, pharyngeal, and perineal carriage of Staphylococcus aureus in healthy adults. Antimicrob Agents Chemother. 2005;49(4):1465–7.
5. Ridley M. Perineal carriage of Staph. Aureus. Br Med J. 1959;1(5117):270–3.
6. Rimland D, Roberson B. Gastrointestinal carriage of methicillin-resistant Staphylococcus aureus. J Clin Microbiol. 1986;24(1):137–8.
7. Benito D, Lozano C, Gomez-Sanz E, Zarazaga M, Torres C. Detection of methicillin-susceptible Staphylococcus aureus ST398 and ST133 strains in gut microbiota of healthy humans in Spain. Microb Ecol. 2013;66(1):105–11.
8. Gurnee EA, Ndao IM, McGhee JE, Warner BB, Tarr PI, Fritz SA, Burnham CA. Fecal carriage of methicillin-resistant Staphylococcus aureus and vancomycin-resistant enterococcus in healthy children. Antimicrob Agents Chemother. 2014;58(2):1261–2.
9. Nakao A, Ito T, Han X, Lu YJ, Hisata K, Tsujiwaki A, Matsunaga N, Komatsu M, Hiramatsu K, Shimizu T. Intestinal carriage of methicillin-resistant Staphylococcus aureus in nasal MRSA carriers hospitalized in the neonatal intensive care unit. Antimicrob Resist Infect Control. 2014;3:14.
10. Bhalla A, Aron DC, Donskey CJ. Staphylococcus aureus intestinal colonization is associated with increased frequency of S. Aureus on skin of hospitalized patients. BMC Infect Dis. 2007;7:105.
11. Boyce JM, Havill NL. Nosocomial antibiotic-associated diarrhea associated with enterotoxin-producing strains of methicillin-resistant Staphylococcus aureus. Am J Gastroenterol. 2005;100(8):1828–34.
12. Nishikawa M, Tanaka T, Nakashima K, Senda K, Shibasaki M, Miura H, Tamakoshi A, Ohta T, Yagi T. Screening for methicillin-resistant Staphylococcus aureus (MRSA) carriage on admission to a geriatric hospital. Arch Gerontol Geriatr. 2009;49(2):242–5.
13. CLSI. Performance standards for antimicrobial susceptibility testing: twenty-second informational supplement, vol. In: 32: Clinical & Laboratory Standards Institute; 2012.
14. Bosgelmez-Tinaz G, Ulusoy S, Aridogan B, Coskun-Ari F. Evaluation of different methods to detect oxacillin resistance in *Staphylococcus aureus* and their clinical laboratory utility. Eur J Clin Microbiol Infect Dis. 2006;25(6):410–2.
15. Lina G, Piemont Y, Godail-Gamot F, Bes M, Peter MO, Gauduchon V, Vandenesch F, Etienne J. Involvement of Panton-valentine leukocidin-producing *Staphylococcus aureus* in primary skin infections and pneumonia. Clin Infect Dis. 1999;29(5):1128–32.
16. Garcia-Alvarez L, Holden MT, Lindsay H, Webb CR, Brown DF, Curran MD, Walpole E, Brooks K, Pickard DJ, Teale C, et al. Meticillin-resistant Staphylococcus aureus with a novel mecA homologue in human and bovine populations in the UK and Denmark: a descriptive study. Lancet Infect Dis. 2011;11(8):595–603.
17. Lewallen S, Courtright P. Epidemiology in practice: case-control studies. Community Eye Health. 1998;11(28):57–8.
18. Magiorakos AP, Srinivasan A, Carey RB, Carmeli Y, Falagas ME, Giske CG, Harbarth S, Hindler JF, Kahlmeter G, Olsson-Liljequist B, et al. Multidrug-resistant, extensively drug-resistant and pandrug-resistant bacteria: an international expert proposal for interim standard definitions for acquired resistance. Clin. Microbiol. Infect. 2012;18(3):268–81.
19. Altemeier WA, Hummel RP, Hummel RP, Hill EO. Staphylococcal enterocolitis following antibiotic therapy. Ann Surg. 1963;157:847–58.
20. Greendyke RM, Constantine HP, Magruder GB, Dean DC, Gardner JH, Morgan HR. Staphylococci on a medical ward, with special reference to fecal carriers. Am J Clin Pathol. 1958;30(4):318–22.
21. Grun L. Studies on intestinal staphylococci. Arch Hyg Bakteriol. 1958;142(1):3–7.
22. Cavalcanti SM, Franca ER, Cabral C, Vilela MA, Montenegro F, Menezes D, Medeiros AC. Prevalence of Staphylococcus aureus introduced into intensive care units of a university hospital. Braz J Infect Dis. 2005;9(1):56–63.
23. Eveillard M, de Lassence A, Lancien E, Barnaud G, Ricard JD, Joly-Guillou ML. Evaluation of a strategy of screening multiple anatomical sites for methicillin-resistant Staphylococcus aureus at admission to a teaching hospital. Infect Control Hosp Epidemiol off j Soc Hosp Epidemiol Am. 2006;27(2):181–4.
24. Roghmann MC, Gorman PH, Wallin MT, Kreisel K, Shurland S, Johnson JA. Staphylococcus aureus colonization in community-dwelling people with spinal cord dysfunction. Arch Phys Med Rehabil. 2007;88(8):979–83.
25. Grmek-Kosnik I, Ihan A, Dermota U, Rems M, Kosnik M, Jorn Kolmos H. Evaluation of separate vs pooled swab cultures, different media, broth enrichment and anatomical sites of screening for the detection of methicillin-resistant Staphylococcus aureus from clinical specimens. J hosp infect. 2005;61(2):155–61.
26. Vandenesch F, Naimi T, Enright MC, Lina G, Nimmo GR, Heffernan H, Liassine N, Bes M, Greenland T, Reverdy ME, et al. Community-acquired methicillin-resistant Staphylococcus aureus carrying Panton-valentine leukocidin genes: worldwide emergence. Emerg Infect Dis. 2003;9(8):978–84.
27. McDougal LK, Steward CD, Killgore GE, Chaitram JM, McAllister SK, Tenover FC. Pulsed-field gel electrophoresis typing of oxacillin-resistant Staphylococcus aureus isolates from the United States: establishing a national database. J Clin Microbiol. 2003;41(11):5113–20.
28. Sangvik M, Olsen RS, Olsen K, Simonsen GS, Furberg AS, Sollid JU. Age- and gender-associated Staphylococcus aureus spa types found among nasal carriers in a general population: the Tromso staph and skin study. J Clin Microbiol. 2011;49(12):4213–8.

29. Crossley K, Solliday J. Comparison of rectal swabs and stool cultures for the detection of gastrointestinal carriage of Staphylococcus aureus. J Clin Microbiol. 1980;11(4):433–4.
30. Tulloch LG, Alder VG, Gillespie WA. Treatment of chronic furunculosis. Br Med J. 1960;2(5195):354–6.
31. Squier C, Rihs JD, Risa KJ, Sagnimeni A, Wagener MM, Stout J, Muder RR, Singh N. Staphylococcus aureus rectal carriage and its association with infections in patients in a surgical intensive care unit and a liver transplant unit. Infect control hosp epidemiol off j Soc Hosp Epidemiol Am. 2002;23(9):495–501.
32. Solberg CO. A study of carriers of Staphylococcus aureus with special regard to quantitative bacterial estimations. Acta Medica Scand Suppl. 1965;436:1–96.
33. Mody L, Kauffman CA, Donabedian S, Zervos MJ, Bradley SF. Epidemiology of Staphylococcus aureus colonization in nursing home residents. Clin infect dis off publ Infect Dis Soc Am. 2008;46(9):1368–73.
34. Simor AE, Ofner-Agostini M, Paton S, McGeer A, Loeb M, Bryce E, Mulvey M. Clinical and epidemiologic features of methicillin-resistant Staphylococcus aureus in elderly hospitalized patients. Infect control hosp epidemiol off j Soc Hosp Epidemiol Am. 2005;26(10):838–41.
35. McKinnell JA, Huang SS, Eells SJ, Cui E, Miller LG. Quantifying the impact of extranasal testing of body sites for methicillin-resistant Staphylococcus aureus colonization at the time of hospital or intensive care unit admission. Infect control hosp epidemiol off j Soc Hosp Epidemiol Am. 2013;34(2):161–70.
36. Lee DC, Barlas D, Ryan JG, Ward MF, Sama AE, Farber BF. Methicillin-resistant Staphylococcus aureus and vancomycin-resistant enterococci: prevalence and predictors of colonization in patients presenting to the emergency department from nursing homes. J Am Geriatr Soc. 2002;50(8):1463–5.
37. Trick WE, Weinstein RA, DeMarais PL, Kuehnert MJ, Tomaska W, Nathan C, Rice TW, McAllister SK, Carson LA, Jarvis WR. Colonization of skilled-care facility residents with antimicrobial-resistant pathogens. J Am Geriatr Soc. 2001;49(3):270–6.
38. Hogardt M, Proba P, Mischler D, Cuny C, Kempf VA, Heudorf U. Current prevalence of multidrug-resistant organisms in long-term care facilities in the Rhine-main district, Germany, 2013. Euro Surveill. 2015;20(26).
39. Papadimitriou-Olivgeris M, Spiliopoulou I, Christofidou M, Logothetis D, Manolopoulou P, Dodou V, Fligou F, Marangos M, Anastassiou ED. Co-colonization by multidrug-resistant bacteria in two Greek intensive care units. Euro j clin microb infect dis off publ Euro Soc Clin Microbiol. 2015; 34(10):1947–55.

High prevalence of ESBL-Producing *E. coli* in private and shared latrines in an informal urban settlement in Dar es Salaam, Tanzania

Stefan Erb[1*†], Lauren D'Mello-Guyett[2,3†], Hamisi M. Malebo[4], Robert M. Njee[4,5], Fatuma Matwewe[3], Jeroen Ensink[2^], Vladimira Hinic[6], Andreas Widmer[1] and Reno Frei[1,6]

Abstract

Background: Data about the burden of extended-spectrum beta-lactamase (ESBL)-producing microorganisms in Africa are limited. Our study aimed to estimate the prevalence of human faecal ESBL carriage in the community of an informal urban settlement in Dar es Salaam (Tanzania, East Africa) by using environmental contamination of household latrines with ESBL as a surrogate marker.

Methods: Within the context of a large survey in February 2014 assessing 636 randomly selected household latrines for faecal contamination by the detection of growth of *E. coli* and total faecal coliform bacteria, a randomly selected subset of the samples were screened for ESBL.

Results: Seventy latrines were screened for ESBL. An average of 11.4 persons (SD ±6.5) were sharing one latrine. Only three (4.3%) latrines had hand-washing facilities and 50 showed faeces on the floor. ESBL-producing *Enterobacteriaceae* were confirmed in 17 (24.3%) of the 70 latrine samples: 16 *E. coli* and 1 *Klebsiella pneumoniae*. Five ESBL *E. coli* strains were detected on door handles. The most prevalent ESBL type was CTX-M-1 group (76.5%). Pulsed-field gel electrophoresis typing of a subset of ESBL-producing *E. coli* isolates revealed both diverse singular types and a cluster of 3 identical isolates. There was no significant difference of the latrine and household characteristics between the group with ESBL ($n = 17$) and the group with non-ESBL *E. coli* ($n = 53$) ($p > 0.05$).

Conclusions: Almost a quarter of private and shared latrines in an informal urban settlement in Tanzania are contaminated with ESBL-producing microorganisms, suggesting a high prevalence of human ESBL faecal carriage in the community. Shared latrines may serve as a reservoir for transmission in urban community settings in Tanzania.

Keywords: Extended-spectrum beta-lactamase ESBL, Community, Carriage, Prevalence, Latrines, Sub-Saharan Africa

Background

Extended-spectrum beta-lactamase (ESBL)-producing gram-negative bacteria have become an emerging global health threat and have been associated with high mortality [1, 2]. Whereas ESBL infections were initially associated with nosocomial outbreaks, there is now increasing recognition of high rates of faecal carriage and the importance of community-acquired infections due to ESBL-producing *Escherichia coli* in industrialized countries [3, 4].

Data about the prevalence of ESBL-producing microorganisms in Africa are limited. A wide variation from 0.6% up to 77.8% has been reported in hospital-based surveys of clinical isolates [5–11]. There is little published data on the magnitude of the community carriage of ESBL in African countries like Tanzania.

Our study aimed to estimate the prevalence of human faecal ESBL carriage in the community in an urban setting in Tanzania, East Africa, by using environmental

* Correspondence: stefan.erb@usb.ch
†Equal contributors
^Deceased
[1]Division of Infectious Diseases and Hospital Epidemiology, University Hospital Basel, University of Basel, Basel, Switzerland
Full list of author information is available at the end of the article

contamination of household latrines with ESBL as a surrogate marker.

Methods

The study was performed in February 2014 in an urban study site in Keko Machungwa, part of the largest unplanned and under-serviced settlement in Temeke district, Dar es Salaam, Tanzania.

Within the context of a large survey assessing the improvement of sanitation facilities [12], 636 randomly selected household latrines were screened for the presence and concentration of faecal contamination (*E. coli* and total faecal coliform bacteria) [13]. Surface swipe swabs from high frequency contact points (10 cm^2) like door handle and footrest were taken and analysed using direct membrane filtration technique (Merck Millipore, Billerica, MA, USA) with commercial medium m-ColiBlue® (HACH, Loveland, CO, USA) [14]. In this survey, 492 latrines showed growth of *E. coli* or coliform bacteria either at the footrest, the door handle or both (unpublished data, Fig. 1).

From latrines with *E. coli* growth, samples were selected using a calculator based random number generator and further screened for ESBL-producing *Enterobacteriaceae* using the chromogenic selective culture medium chromID® ESBL (bioMérieux, Marcy-l'Étoile, France) according to the manufacturer's instructions. ESBL or carbapenemase production was confirmed with standard microbiological techniques following EUCAST guideline [15]. ESBL molecular types (specifically CTX-M-1 and CTX-M-9 groups) were determined by isothermal amplification (eazyplex® SuperBug CRE Assay [Amplex Biosystems, Gießen, Germany] for use on Genie® II platform [Optigene, Horsham, UK]). Antimicrobial susceptibility testing and interpretation was done using Vitek® 2 automated system (bioMérieux) or Etest® (bioMérieux) according to EUCAST clinical breakpoints (version 5.0, 2015; http://www.eucast.org/clinical_breakpoints). Molecular typing was performed by pulsed-field gel electrophoresis (PFGE) as described previously [16].

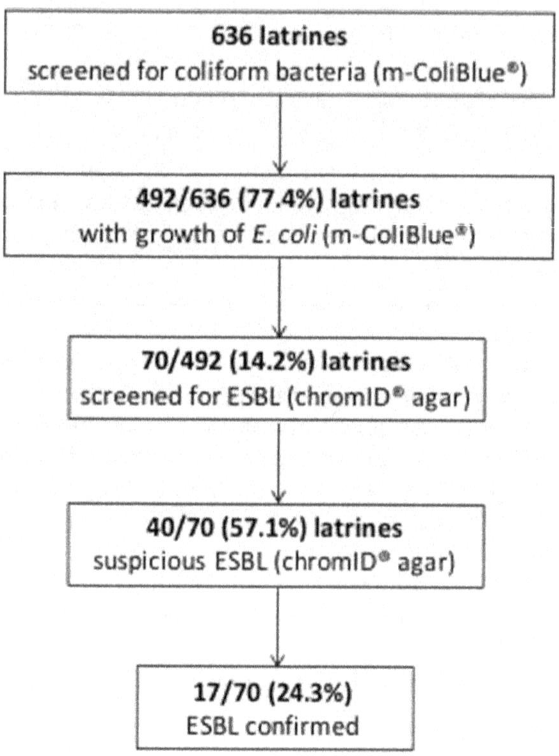

Fig. 1 ESBL screening algorithm. ESBL, extended-spectrum beta-lactamase-producing microorganisms

Table 1 Baseline characteristics of latrines screened for ESBL ($n = 70$)

Characteristics		
Screened latrines (*n*, %)	70	100%
Households sharing one latrine (*n*, %)		
1 houshold (private latrine)	24	34.3%
2 households	26	37.1%
3 households	13	18.6%
4–10 households	4	5.7%
10–23 households	3	4.3%
Persons sharing one latrine (mean, ±SD)	11.4	6.5
Household leader male (*n*, %)	23	32.9%
Household leader's educational level (*n*, %)		
none	5	7.1%
primary school	43	61.4%
secondary school	22	31.4%
Household leader's monthly income in US$ (mean, ±SD)	102.7	78.9
Latrines used by children <5 years (*n*, %)	58	82.9%
Latrines with stored bucket for anal cleaning (*n*, %)	26	37.1%
Handwashing facilities <1 m (n, %)	3	4.3%
Soap available in latrine (*n*, %)	6	8.6%
Age of latrines in years (mean, ±SD)	4.6	3.4
Latrine floor material (*n*, %)		
brick	60	85.7%
cement	10	14.3%
Cracked or broken slab (*n*, %)	54	77.1%
Condition of latrine (*n*, %)		
clean	20	28.6%
Dirty - faeces on the floor	50	71.4%
Lid available (*n*, %)	3	4.3%
Latrine separation (*n*,%)		
no door	6	8.6%
curtain	5	7.1%
wood door	59	84.3%
Flies in latrine (*n*, %)	40	57.1%
Animals in the compound (*n*, %)	14	20.0%

SD standard deviation

Table 2 Microbiological results of the screened latrines (n = 70)

ESBL-producing bacteria total (n, %)	17	24.3%
ESBL *E. coli*	16	
ESBL *K. pneumoniae*	1	
Screening sites positive (n, %)	17	
Footrests	12	70.6%
Door handles ± footrests	5	29.4%
Antibiotics resistant/intermediate[a] (n, %)		
Ampicillin	17	100%
Amoxicillin/Clavulanic acid	16	94.1%
Piperacillin/Tazobactam	4	23.5%
Cefoxitin	11	64.7%
Ceftazidime	16	94.1%
Ceftriaxone	17	100%
Cefepime	16	94.1%
Ertapenem	0	0%
Meropenem	0	0%
Ciprofloxacin	16	94.1%
Tobramycin	15	88.2%
Amikacin	6	35.3%
Trimethoprim/Sulfamethoxazole	14	82.4%
Nitrofurantoin	1	5.9%
Fosfomycin	0	0%
Colistin	0	0%
ESBL types (n, %)	17	
CTX-M-1 group	13	76.5%
CTX-M-9 group	1	5.9%
Other than CTX-M-1/9 group	3	17.6%

ESBL extended-spectrum beta-lactamase-producing microorganisms
[a]Interpretation according to EUCAST breakpoints version 5.0 (2015)

Data about household and latrine characteristics were collected by visual inspection and questionnaire.

Univariable analysis was performed by the chi-square test or Fisher's exact test, where appropriate, for categorical variables and two-tailed Student's t test for continuous variables. Two-tailed p-values of <0.05 were considered statistically significant.

The study was approved by the national ethics committee of the National Institute for Medical Research Tanzania (NIMR/HQ/R.8a/Vol.IX/1632).

Results

From the 492 latrines with growth of *E. coli*, 70 latrines were randomly selected for ESBL screening. All 70 latrines had either a cement, tile or brick floor and met the WHO/UNICEF Joint Monitoring Program for Water Supply and Sanitation definitions for improved latrines [12]. Only 3 (4.3%) latrines had hand-washing facilities and 50 showed faeces on the floor. An average of 11.4 persons (SD ±6.5) were sharing one latrine.

Twenty-four (34.3%) latrines were private (i.e. each of these latrines were used by only one household), the remaining latrines were shared by ≥2 households. The latrines were not accessible for the public but restricted to individuals living in the respective household (Table 1).

Forty samples showed ESBL suspected colonies on chromID® ESBL culture medium. ESBL-producing *Enterobacteriaceae* were finally confirmed in 17 (24.3%) of the 70 latrine samples: 16 *E. coli* and 1 *Klebsiella pneu-*

Table 3 Microbiological and household characteristics of the 17 detected ESBL microorganisms

No	Sample ID	ESBL organism	ESBL type	Amoxicillin/ Clavulanic acid	Piperacillin/ Tazobactam	Ceftriaxone	Meropenem	Amikacin	TMP/SMX	Nitrofurantoin	Ciprofloxacin	Fosfomycin	Colistin
1	91BH	*E. coli*	CTX-M-1	R	S	R	S	S	S	S	R	S	S
2	124CM	*E. coli*	CTX-M-1	R	R	R	S	S	R	S	R	S	S
3	107AH	*E. coli*	CTX-M-1	R	R	R	S	S	R	S	R	S	S
4	115AH	*E. coli*	CTX-M-1	R	R	R	S	S	R	S	R	S	S
5	106CH	*E. coli*	other	R	R	R	S	S	R	S	R	S	S
6	104DS	*E. coli*	other	R	S	R	S	S	R	S	R	S	S
7	102DS	*E. coli*	CTX-M-1	R	S	R	S	R	R	S	R	S	S
8	90S	*E. coli*	other	R	S	R	S	S	R	S	R	S	S
9	86BS	*E. coli*	CTX-M-1	R	S	R	S	S	R	S	R	S	S
10	84BS	*E. coli*	CTX-M-1	R	S	R	S	R	R	S	R	S	S
11	83BS	*E. coli*	CTX-M-1	R	S	R	S	R	R	S	R	S	S
12	97DS	*E. coli*	CTX-M-1	R	S	R	S	R	R	S	R	S	S
13	93AS	*E. coli*	CTX-M-1	R	S	R	S	R	R	S	R	S	S
14	70DS	*E. coli*	CTX-M-1	R	S	R	S	S	S	S	R	S	S
15	67BS	*E. coli*	CTX-M-9	R	S	R	S	S	R	S	R	S	S
16	94AS	*E. coli*	CTX-M-1	R	S	R	S	R	R	S	R	S	S
17	64BA	*K. pneumoniae*	CTX-M-1	S	S	R	S	S	S	R	S	S	S

Susceptibility testing according to EUCAST: *R* resistant or intermediate, *S* susceptible, *TMP/SMX* Trimethoprim/Sulfamethoxazole

Table 3 Microbiological and household characteristics of the 17 detected ESBL microorganisms *(Continued)*

No	Screening site	Age of latrine in years	Persons sharing 1 latrine	Children <5y using 1 latrine	Latrine floor material	Condition of the slab	Condition of the latrine	Lid available	Latrines with stored bucket for anal cleaning	Handwashing facilities	Soap available in latrine	Latrine separation	Flies in latrine	Animals in the compound
1	handle	6	14	3	brick	broken	clean	no	no	no	no	door	yes	yes
2	handle	2	6	1	brick	broken	dirty	no	yes	no	no	door	no	no
3	handle	3	2	0	cement	broken	dirty	no	yes	no	yes	door	yes	yes
4	handle	1	5	1	brick	broken	dirty	no	yes	no	no	door	no	no
5	handle	6	6	1	brick	broken	dirty	no	no	no	no	curtain	no	yes
6	floor	0.5	15	1	brick	no cracks	dirty	no	no	no	no	door	yes	no
7	floor	4	15	1	brick	broken	dirty	no	no	no	no	door	yes	no
8	floor	4	15	1	brick	broken	dirty	no	no	no	no	door	no	no
9	floor	0.5	5	1	cement	broken	dirty	yes	yes	yes	yes	door	no	no
10	floor	0.5	23	1	brick	broken	clean	no	no	no	no	door	yes	no
11	floor	0.5	12	2	brick	no cracks	clean	no	no	no	no	door	yes	no
12	floor	2	9	1	cement	broken	dirty	no	yes	no	no	door	no	yes
13	floor	0.5	10	1	brick	broken	dirty	no	yes	no	no	door	no	yes
14	floor	1	15	4	brick	broken	dirty	no	no	no	no	door	yes	no
15	floor	2	4	1	brick	broken	clean	no	no	no	no	no	yes	no
16	floor	9	7	0	cement	broken	dirty	yes	no	no	no	curtain	yes	no
17	floor	6	10	1	brick	no cracks	clean	no	no	no	no	door	yes	yes

moniae (Table 2). Five ESBL *E. coli* strains were detected on door handles. Antimicrobial resistance to ciprofloxacin and trimethoprim/sulfamethoxazole was detected in 94.1% and 82.4% of the ESBL isolates, respectively. No carbapenem resistance or indication for carbapenemase production was detected. The most prevalent ESBL type was CTX-M-1 group (76.5%) (Table 2). Microbiological and household/latrine characteristics of the 17 detected ESBL microorganisms are summarized in Table 3. PFGE typing of a subset of ESBL-producing *E. coli* isolates revealed both diverse singular types and a cluster of 3 identical isolates (Fig. 2). Ten isolates were nontypable by PFGE as observed in other studies [17].

There was no significant difference of the latrine and household characteristics between the group with ESBL (n = 17) and the group with non-ESBL *E. coli* (n = 53) ($p > 0.05$).

Discussion

In this study, we found that a quarter of the *E. coli* from contaminated latrines in an urban informal settlement in Dar es Salaam express ESBL, suggesting a high prevalence of human ESBL faecal carriage in the community, and that shared latrines may serve as a reservoir for transmission in urban areas of Tanzania.

In a recent meta-analysis, the median proportion of ESBL-producing *Enterobacteriaceae* in patients of Tanzanian healthcare facilities was 39% (range 14.2–75.9%) [11]. Only little is known about the ESBL burden in a community setting in Tanzania. Tellevik et al. reported an ESBL faecal carriage rate in healthy community children in Dar es Salaam of 11.6% [18]. An elderly survey from 2004 found ESBL in 16% of Enterobacteriaceae causing community-

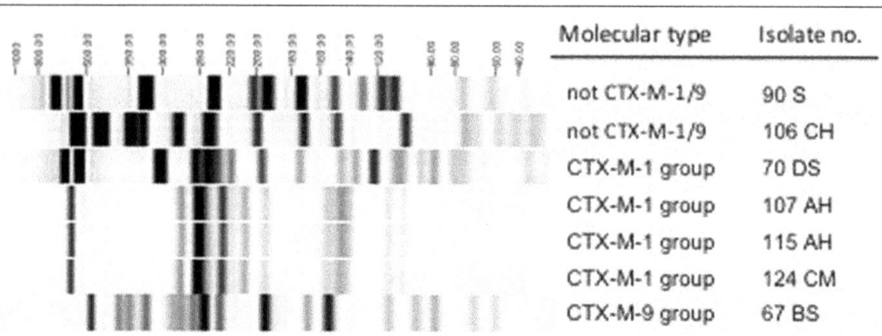

Fig. 2 PFGE of seven ESBL-producing *E. coli* isolates. PFGE, pulsed-field gel electrophoresis; ESBL, extended-spectrum beta-lactamase-producing microorganisms. PFGE shows a cluster of 3 isolates (107AH, 115AH, 124CM) with identical PFGE band pattern. Other isolates show different PFGE pattern

acquired urinary tract infections [19]. Studies from other African countries like Senegal, Niger and Madagascar have reported ESBL carriage rates in the community ranging as high as 10% to 31% [3]. In cases where they have been identified, CTX-M enzymes were predominantly of CTX-M-1 group as in our isolates.

Community-onset infections with ESBL-producing pathogens are now increasingly reported. Empirical and targeted antibiotic treatment of such infections is challenging particularly in resource-limited countries. ESBL producing gram-negative bacteria are by definition resistant to extended-spectrum cephalosporins and frequently carry additional resistance genes conferring reduced susceptibility to many other antibiotics like e.g. fluoroquinolones. In many cases the carbapenems remain the only choice for treatment of infections caused by these resistant bacteria. However, the access to antimicrobial agents active against ESBL is limited in many regions of East Africa, thus common infections with multidrug-resistant pathogens cannot be treated adequately.

Intestinal colonization with ESBL-producing microorganisms may last several weeks, months or even years and is a potential source for human-to-human transmission. Precarious hygienic conditions of latrines, which are commonly shared amongst different households and household members, and the presence of ESBL-producing microorganisms on door handles may enable further spread. The cluster of 3 identical *E. coli* strains from 3 different latrines detected by PFGE typing in our study points to the potential of ESBL transmission in the community.

Our study has limitations: 1) Due to ethical and logistical reasons rectal swabs were not feasible. However, environmental samples of the latrines may give a valuable estimate of the frequency and distribution of ESBL-producing microorganisms. In addition, there is a lower risk of selection bias in the community and the results provide information about potential transmission pathways of multidrug-resistant pathogens in the community, similar to a recent study from airport toilet door handles [20]. 2) Our study was restricted to one informal urban settlement in Dar es Salaam and might differ from other urban and rural settings in Tanzania and East Africa. 3) Due to financial constraints only 70 latrines could be screened for ESBL.

Conclusions

Our study provides evidence of a high prevalence of human ESBL faecal carriage in the community of a resource-limited country such as Tanzania. Further larger surveillance studies are needed in Africa to better describe the epidemiology of ESBL, to raise awareness of the need of strategies to prevent further dissemination, and to improve the access and responsible use of appropriate antimicrobial agents in the empirical treatment of infections caused by otherwise deadly multidrug-resistant microorganisms.

Acknowledgements
We thank Danica Nogarth, Elisabeth Schultheiss and Judith Shipili for performing the special microbiological analyses.

Funding
Division of Clinical Microbiology, University Hospital Basel, Switzerland. SHARE Research Consortium, London School of Hygiene and Tropical Medicine, UK.

Authors' contributions
All authors have seen and approved the manuscript and have significantly contributed to the work.

Consent for publication
Not applicable

Competing interests
The authors declare that they have no competing interests.

Author details
[1]Division of Infectious Diseases and Hospital Epidemiology, University Hospital Basel, University of Basel, Basel, Switzerland. [2]Environmental Health Group, Faculty of Infectious and Tropical Diseases, London School of Hygiene and Tropical Medicine, London, UK. [3]Maji Safi kwa Afya Bora Ifakara (MSABI), Morogoro, Tanzania. [4]National Institute for Medical Research, Dar es Salaam, Tanzania. [5]Ministry of Health, Community Development, Gender, Elderly and Children, Dar es Salaam, Tanzania. [6]Division of Clinical Microbiology, University Hospital Basel, University of Basel, Basel, Switzerland.

References

1. WHO. Antimicrobial resistance: Global report on surveillance. Geneva: World Health Organization; 2014.
2. Schwaber MJ, Carmeli Y. Mortality and delay in effective therapy associated with extended-spectrum b-lactamase production in Enterobacteriaceae bacteraemia: a systematic review and meta-analysis. J Antimicrob Chemother. 2007;60:913–20.
3. Woerther PL, Burdet C, Chachaty E, Andremont A. Trends in human fecal carriage of extended-spectrum beta-lactamases in the community: toward the globalization of CTX-M. Clin Microbiol Rev. 2013;26:744–58.
4. Ny S, Lofmark S, Borjesson S, et al. Community carriage of ESBL-producing 253 Escherichia coli is associated with strains of low pathogenicity: A Swedish 254 Nationwide Study. J Antimicrob Chemother. 2017;72(2):582–588.
5. Frank T, Arlet G, Gautier V, Talarmin A, Bercion R. Extended-spectrum beta-lactamase-producing Enterobacteriaceae, Central African Republic. Emerg Infect Dis. 2006;12:863–5.
6. Moyo SJ, Aboud S, Kasubi M, Lyamuya EF, Maselle SY. Antimicrobial resistance among producers and non-producers of extended spectrum beta-lactamases in urinary isolates at a tertiary hospital in Tanzania. BMC Res Notes. 2010;3:348.
7. Mshana SE, Matee M, Rweyemamu M. Antimicrobial resistance in human and animal pathogens in Zambia, Democratic Republic of Congo,

Mozambique and Tanzania: an urgent need of a sustainable surveillance system. Ann Clin Microbiol Antimicrob. 2013;12:28.
8. Tansarli GS, Poulikakos P, Kapaskelis A, Falagas ME. Proportion of extended-spectrum beta-lactamase (ESBL)-producing isolates among Enterobacteriaceae in Africa: evaluation of the evidence - systematic review. J Antimicrob Chemother. 2014;69:1177–84.
9. Sangare SA, Maiga AI, Guindo I, et al. Prevalence of extended-spectrum beta-lactamase-producing Enterobacteriaceae isolated from blood cultures in Africa. Med Mal Infect. 2015;45:374–82.
10. Storberg V. Esbl-producing Enterobacteriaceae in Africa - a non-systematic literature review of research published 2008–2012. Infect Ecol Epidemiol. 2014;4. https://doi.org/10.3402/iee.v4.20342. eCollection 2014.
11. Sonda T, Kumburu H, van Zwetselaar M, et al. Meta-analysis of proportion estimates of extended-spectrum-beta-lactamase-producing Enterobacteriaceae in East Africa hospitals. Antimicrob Resist Infect Control. 2016;5:18.
12. Bain RE, Gundry SW, Wright JA, Yang H, Pedley S, Bartram JK. Accounting for water quality in monitoring access to safe drinking-water as part of the millennium development goals: lessons from five countries. Bull World Health Organ. 2012;90:228–235A.
13. Exley JL, Liseka B, Cumming O, Ensink JH. The sanitation ladder, what constitutes an improved form of sanitation? Environ Sci Technol. 2015;49: 1086–94.
14. Rusin P, Orosz-Coughlin P, Gerba C. Reduction of faecal coliform, coliform and heterotrophic plate count bacteria in the household kitchen and bathroom by disinfection with hypochlorite cleaners. J Appl Microbiol 1998; 85: 819-828.
15. EUCAST. Eucast guideline for the detection of resistance mechanisms and specific resistances of clinical and/or epidemiological importance. Version 1. 0. European Committee on Antimicrobial Susceptibility Testing .2013. http://www.eucast.org/resistance_mechanisms/.
16. Pfaller M, Hollis R, Sader H, editors. Chromosomal restriction fragment analysis by pulsed-field gel electrophoresis. Washington, D.C.: American Society for Microbiology; 1992.
17. Oethinger M, Conrad S, Kaifel K, et al. Molecular epidemiology of fluoroquinolone-resistant Escherichia Coli bloodstream isolates from patients admitted to European cancer centers. Antimicrob Agents Chemother. 1996;40:387–92.
18. Tellevik MG, Blomberg B, Kommedal O, Maselle SY, Langeland N, Moyo SJ. High prevalence of faecal carriage of ESBL-producing Enterobacteriaceae among children in Dar es Salaam, Tanzania. PLoS One. 2016;11:e0168024.
19. Manyahi J, Moyo SJ, Tellevik MG, et al. Detection of CTX-M-15 beta-lactamases in Enterobacteriaceae causing hospital- and community-acquired urinary tract infections as early as 2004, in Dar es Salaam, Tanzania. BMC Infect Dis. 2017;17:282.
20. Schaumburg F, Kock R, Leendertz FH, Becker K. Airport door handles and the global spread of antimicrobial-resistant bacteria: a cross sectional study. Clin Microbiol Infect. 2016;22:1010–1.

Permissions

All chapters in this book were first published in AR&IC, by BioMed Central; hereby published with permission under the Creative Commons Attribution License or equivalent. Every chapter published in this book has been scrutinized by our experts. Their significance has been extensively debated. The topics covered herein carry significant findings which will fuel the growth of the discipline. They may even be implemented as practical applications or may be referred to as a beginning point for another development.

The contributors of this book come from diverse backgrounds, making this book a truly international effort. This book will bring forth new frontiers with its revolutionizing research information and detailed analysis of the nascent developments around the world.

We would like to thank all the contributing authors for lending their expertise to make the book truly unique. They have played a crucial role in the development of this book. Without their invaluable contributions this book wouldn't have been possible. They have made vital efforts to compile up to date information on the varied aspects of this subject to make this book a valuable addition to the collection of many professionals and students.

This book was conceptualized with the vision of imparting up-to-date information and advanced data in this field. To ensure the same, a matchless editorial board was set up. Every individual on the board went through rigorous rounds of assessment to prove their worth. After which they invested a large part of their time researching and compiling the most relevant data for our readers.

The editorial board has been involved in producing this book since its inception. They have spent rigorous hours researching and exploring the diverse topics which have resulted in the successful publishing of this book. They have passed on their knowledge of decades through this book. To expedite this challenging task, the publisher supported the team at every step. A small team of assistant editors was also appointed to further simplify the editing procedure and attain best results for the readers.

Apart from the editorial board, the designing team has also invested a significant amount of their time in understanding the subject and creating the most relevant covers. They scrutinized every image to scout for the most suitable representation of the subject and create an appropriate cover for the book.

The publishing team has been an ardent support to the editorial, designing and production team. Their endless efforts to recruit the best for this project, has resulted in the accomplishment of this book. They are a veteran in the field of academics and their pool of knowledge is as vast as their experience in printing. Their expertise and guidance has proved useful at every step. Their uncompromising quality standards have made this book an exceptional effort. Their encouragement from time to time has been an inspiration for everyone.

The publisher and the editorial board hope that this book will prove to be a valuable piece of knowledge for researchers, students, practitioners and scholars across the globe.

List of Contributors

Chao Liu
Department of Respiratory Medicine, Peking Union Medical College, Chinese Academy of Medical Sciences, China-Japan Friendship Hospital, Beijing, China

Jun Guo
Department of Respiratory Medicine, School of Clinical Medicine, Beijing Tsinghua Changgung Hospital, Tsinghua University, Beijing, China
Department of Geriatric Respiratory Medicine, Chinese PLA General Hospital, Beijing, China

Zhen Zhu, Mingze Cao, Xuzheng Zhou, Bing Li and Jiyu Zhang
Key Laboratory of New Animal Drug Project of Gansu Province, Key Laboratory of Veterinary Pharmaceutical Development of Ministry of Agriculture, Lanzhou Institute of Husbandry and Pharmaceutical Sciences of CAAS, Jiangouyan, Qilihe District, Lanzhou, People's Republic of China

Rafael Manuel Ortí-Lucas and Julio Muñoz-Miguel
Social Medicine and Public Health Department, Universidad Católica de Valencia San Vicente Mártir, C/ Espartero,7, Valencia 46007, Spain
Preventive Medicine Department, Hospital Clínico Universitario de Valencia, Valencia, Spain

Liang-an Chen
Department of Respiratory Medicine, Chinese PLA General Hospital, Fuxing Road No. 28, Beijing 100853, China

Yangyang Zhang
Department of Respiratory Medicine, Chinese PLA General Hospital, Fuxing Road No. 28, Beijing 100853, China
Department of Respiratory Medicine, Affiliated Hospital of Chengde Medical University, Nanyingzi Street No. 36, Chengde, Hebei Province 067000, China

Qing Zhang
Department of Respiratory Medicine, Affiliated Hospital of Chengde Medical University, Nanyingzi Street No. 36, Chengde, Hebei Province 067000, China

Mingmei Du
Department of Infection Management and Disease Control, Chinese PLA General Hospital, Beijing 100853, China

Yan Chang
Department of Respiratory Medicine, The General Hospital of the PLA Rocket Force, Xinjiekou Street No. 16, Beijing 100088, China

Maria-Lucia M. Lee, Victor Zecchin and Antonio S. Petrilli
Oncology Pediatric Institute (IOP-GRAACC), Escola Paulista de Medicina, Federal University of Sao Paulo (UNIFESP), Sao Paulo, Brazil

Fabianne Carlesse
Oncology Pediatric Institute (IOP-GRAACC), Escola Paulista de Medicina, Federal University of Sao Paulo (UNIFESP), Sao Paulo, Brazil
Department of Pediatrics, Escola Paulista de Medicina, Federal University of Sao Paulo (UNIFESP), Sao Paulo, Brazil

Anna-Paula C. Amaral
Department of Pediatrics, Escola Paulista de Medicina, Federal University of Sao Paulo (UNIFESP), Sao Paulo, Brazil

Sarah S. Gonçalves, Hemilio Xafranski and Arnaldo L. Colombo
Division of Infectious Diseases, Escola Paulista de Medicina, Federal University of Sao Paulo (UNIFESP), Rua Pedro de Toledo, 669 e 5° -andar, Sao Paulo CEP 04039-032, Brazil

Abdullah M. Al-Hatmi
Westerdijk Fungal Biodiversity Centre, Utrecht, The Netherlands
Center of Expertise in Mycology Radboudumc/ CWZ, Nijmegen, The Netherlands

Jacques F. Meis
Center of Expertise in Mycology Radboudumc/ CWZ, Nijmegen, The Netherlands
Department of Medical Microbiology and Infectious Diseases, Canisius Wilhelmina Hospital (CWZ), Nijmegen, The Netherlands

Ferry Hagen
Department of Medical Microbiology and Infectious Diseases, Canisius Wilhelmina Hospital (CWZ), Nijmegen, The Netherlands

Ido Orlin
The Faculty of Medicine in the Galilee, Bar-Ilan University, Galilee, Israel

Avi Onn
The Faculty of Medicine in the Galilee, Bar-Ilan University, Galilee, Israel
Pediatric Gastrointestinal Unit, Padeh Poriya Medical Center, Poriya, Tiberias, Israel

Daniel Glikman
The Faculty of Medicine in the Galilee, Bar-Ilan University, Galilee, Israel
Pediatric Infectious Diseases Service, Galilee Medical Center, Nahariya, Israel

Avi Peretz
The Faculty of Medicine in the Galilee, Bar-Ilan University, Galilee, Israel
Clinical Microbiology Laboratory, Padeh Poriya Medical Center, Poriya, Hanna Senesh 818/2, Tiberias, Israel

Assaf Rokney
National Staphylococcus aureus Reference Center, Central Laboratories, Israel Ministry of Health, Jerusalem, Israel

Xia Zheng, Jun Xu and Juan Hu
Intensive Care Unit, The First Affiliated Hospital, College of Medicine, Zhejiang University, 79 Qingchun Road, Hangzhou 310003, People's Republic of China

Jian-feng Wang
Department of Respiratory Diseases, The Affiliated Hospital of Hangzhou Normal University, Hangzhou, Zhejiang, No. 126 Wenzhou Road, Hangzhou 310009, People's Republic of China

Wang-lan Xu
Intensive Care Unit, Hospital of Zhejiang General Corps of Armed Police Forces, No. 16 Nanhu Road, Jiaxing, 314000 Zhejiang, People's Republic of China

Zhichang Zhao and Maobai Liu
Department of Pharmacy, Fujian Medical University Union Hospital, Fuzhou, Fujian 350001, China

Fangjun Lan and Bin Li
Department of Clinical Laboratory, Fujian Medical University Union Hospital, 29 Xinquan Rd, Fuzhou, Fujian 350001, People's Republic of China

Weiyuan Chen, Liya Huang and Qili Lin
Medical Technology and Engineering College, Fujian Medical University, Fuzhou 350004, Fujian, People's Republic of China

Bin Li, Fangjun Lan, Qingwen He and Yingping Cao
Department of Clinical Laboratory, Fujian Medical University Union Hospital, 29 Xinquan Rd, Fuzhou, Fujian 350001, People's Republic of China

Yanfang Lu
Department of Clinical Laboratory, Maternal and Children's Health Hospital of Fujian Province, Fuzhou, Fujian 350001, China

Chen Li
Department of Infectious Disease, Fujian Medical University Union Hospital, Fuzhou, Fujian 350001, China

E.A. Reuland, B.B. Wintermans, A. Koek and C.M.J.E. Vandenbroucke-Grauls
Medical Microbiology and Infection Control, VU University Medical Center, Amsterdam, The Netherlands

N. Alnaiemi
Medical Microbiology and Infection Control, VU University Medical Center, Amsterdam, The Netherlands
Laboratory for Medical Microbiology and Public Health, Hengelo, The Netherlands
Department of Microbiology, Faculty of Veterinary Medicine, Zagazig University, Zagazig, Egypt

H.M. Abdallah
Medical Microbiology and Infection Control, VU University Medical Center, Amsterdam, The Netherlands
Department of Microbiology, Faculty of Veterinary Medicine, Zagazig University, Zagazig, Egypt

A.M. Abdelwahab
Department of Microbiology, Faculty of Veterinary Medicine, Zagazig University, Zagazig, Egypt

A. Samy
National Laboratory for Veterinary Quality Control on Poultry Production, Animal Health Research Institute, Dokki, Giza, Egypt

K. W. Abdelsalam
Department of Virology, Faculty of Veterinary Medicine, Zagazig University, Zagazig, Egypt

Jörg Wüllenweber, Karsten Becker and Evgeny A. Idelevich
Institute of Medical Microbiology, University Hospital Münster, Domagkstr. 10, 48149 Münster, Germany

Robin Köck
Institute of Medical Microbiology, University Hospital Münster, Domagkstr. 10, 48149 Münster, Germany
Institute of Hospital Hygiene, University of Oldenburg, European Medical School Oldenburg-Groningen, Rahel-Straus-Str. 10, 26133 Oldenburg, Germany

Dagmar Horn
Pharmacy Department, University Hospital Münster, Albert-Schweitzer-Campus 1, 48149 Münster, Germany

Christian Lanckohr
Department for Anaesthesiology, Intensive Care Medicine and Pain Therapy, University Hospital Münster, Albert-Schweitzer-Campus 1, 48149 Münster, Germany

Stefanie Kampmeier, Mike H. Pillukat, Annelene Kossow and Alexander Mellmann
Institute of Hygiene, University Hospital Münster, Robert–Koch–Strasse 41, 48149 Münster, Germany

Evgeny A. Idelevich
Institute of Medical Microbiology, University Hospital Münster, Münster, Germany

Aleksandra Pettke
Institute of Medical Microbiology, University Hospital Münster, Münster, Germany
Science for Life Laboratory, Division of Translational Medicine and Chemical Biology, Department of Medical Biochemistry and Biophysics, Karolinska Institute, Stockholm, Sweden

Young Eun Ha, Cheol-In Kang and Kyong Ran Peck
Division of Infectious Diseases, Department of Internal Medicine, Samsung Medical Center, Sungkyunkwan University School of Medicine, 81 Irwon-ro, Gangnam-gu, Seoul 06351, Republic of Korea

Sun Young Cho
Division of Infectious Diseases, Department of Internal Medicine, Samsung Medical Center, Sungkyunkwan University School of Medicine, 81 Irwon-ro, Gangnam-gu, Seoul 06351, Republic of Korea
Center for Infection Prevention and Control, Samsung Medical Center, Seoul, South Korea

Doo Ryeon Chung
Division of Infectious Diseases, Department of Internal Medicine, Samsung Medical Center, Sungkyunkwan University School of Medicine, 81 Irwon-ro, Gangnam-gu, Seoul 06351, Republic of Korea
Center for Infection Prevention and Control, Samsung Medical Center, Seoul, South Korea
Asia Pacific Foundation for Infectious Diseases, Seoul, South Korea

Yu Ri Kang, So Hyun Kim and Jae-Hoon Song
Division of Infectious Diseases, Department of Internal Medicine, Samsung Medical Center, Sungkyunkwan University School of Medicine, 81 Irwon-ro, Gangnam-gu, Seoul 06351, Republic of Korea
Asia Pacific Foundation for Infectious Diseases, Seoul, South Korea

So Yeon Park
Division of Infectious Diseases, Department of Internal Medicine, Samsung Medical Center, Sungkyunkwan University School of Medicine, 81 Irwon-ro, Gangnam-gu, Seoul 06351, Republic of Korea
Division of Infectious Diseases, Kangdong Sacred Heart Hospital, Hallym University College of Medicine, Seoul, South Korea

Chhorvoin Om and Mary-Louise McLaws
School of Public Health and Community Medicine, UNSW Medicine, UNSW, Level 3 Samuels Building, Sydney 2052, NSW, Australia

Frances Daily and James C. McLaughlin
Diagnostic Microbiology Development Program, # 23 (First Floor), Street 310, BKK 1, Khan Chamcar Morn, Phnom Penh, Cambodia

Erika Vlieghe
Department of Clinical Sciences, Institute of Tropical Medicine, Nationalestraat 155, 2000 Antwerp, Belgium

Katrin Zurfluh, Magdalena Nüesch-Inderbinen and Roger Stephan
Institute for Food Safety and Hygiene, Vetsuisse Faculty University of Zurich, Winterthurerstrasse 272, 8057 Zurich, Switzerland

Jochen Klumpp
Institute of Food, Nutrition and Health, ETH Zurich, Schmelzbergstr. 7, 8092 Zurich, Switzerland

Laurent Poirel and Patrice Nordmann
Emerging Antibiotic Resistance, Medical and Molecular Microbiology Unit, Department of Medicine, University of Fribourg, Fribourg, Switzerland
National Reference Center for Emerging Antibiotic Resistance, University of Fribourg, Fribourg, Switzerland

Aina Gomila
Hospital Universitari de Bellvitge-IDIBELL, Barcelona, Spain
VINCat program, Catalonia, Spain

Josep M Badia
VINCat program, Catalonia, Spain
Hospital General de Granollers, Universitat Internacional de Catalunya, Barcelona, Spain

Francesc Aguilar
VINCat program, Catalonia, Spain
Consorci Sanitari de Terrassa, Barcelona, Spain

Robert Redwood
Division of Infectious Disease, Department of Medicine, University of Wisconsin-Madison School of Medicine and Public Health, 750 Highland Ave, Madison, Wisconsin 53705, USA

Mary Jo Knobloch and Nasia Safdar
Division of Infectious Disease, Department of Medicine, University of Wisconsin-Madison School of Medicine and Public Health, 750 Highland Ave, Madison, Wisconsin 53705, USA
William S. Middleton Memorial Veterans Hospital, 2500 Overlook Terrace, Madison, Wisconsin 53705, USA

Daniela C. Pellegrini
Department of Infectious Disease, University of Chicago Medical Center, 5841 S Maryland Ave, Chicago, Illinois 60637, USA

Matthew J. Ziegler
Division of Infectious Disease, Perelman School of Medicine, University of Pennsylvania, 3400 Civic Center Blvd, Philadelphia, Pennsylvania 19104, USA

Michael Pulia
BerbeeWalsh Department of Emergency Medicine, University of Wisconsin-Madison School of Medicine and Public Health, 800 University Bay Drive, Madison, Wisconsin 53705, USA

Andreas F. Wendel, Monika Malecki, Robin Otchwemah and Frauke Mattner
Institute of Hygiene, University Hospital I of Witten/Herdecke, Cologne Merheim Medical Centre, Cologne, Germany

Carlos J. Tellez-Castillo
Department of Clinical Microbiology, MVZ synlab Leverkusen GmbH, Köln-Merheim, Germany

Samir G. Sakka
Department of Anesthesiology and Operative Intensive Care Medicine, University of Witten/Herdecke, Cologne Merheim Medical Centre, Cologne, Germany

Baoguang Liu, Hua Wu, Yajun Zhai, Zhipei He, Huarun Sun, Tian Cai, Dandan He, Jianhua Liu, Yushan Pan, Li Yuan and Gongzheng Hu
College of Animal Husbandry and Veterinary Science, Henan Agricultural University, Zhengzhou 450002, China

Shanmei Wang
Medical Microbiology Laboratory, Henan Provincial People's Hospital, Zhengzhou 450002, China

Deborah H. L. Ng, Jia Jun Lee, Wei Xin Khong and Oon Tek Ng
Institute of Infectious Diseases and Epidemiology, Tan Tock Seng Hospital, 11 Jalan Tan Tock Seng, Singapore 304833, Singapore

Kalisvar Marimuthu and Brenda Ang
Institute of Infectious Diseases and Epidemiology, Tan Tock Seng Hospital, 11 Jalan Tan Tock Seng, Singapore 304833, Singapore
National University of Singapore, 21 Lower Kent Ridge Road, Singapore 119077, Singapore

Wei Zhang and Bee Fong Poh
Infection Control Unit, Tan Tock Seng Hospital, 11 Jalan Tan Tock Seng, Singapore 304833, Singapore

Pooja Rao, Maya Devi Rajinder Raj and Partha Pratim De
Department of Laboratory Medicine, Tan Tock Seng Hospital, 11 Jalan Tan Tock Seng, Singapore 304833, Singapore

Florian Salm
Institute for Infection Prevention and Hospital Epidemiology, Medical Center - University of Freiburg, Faculty of Medicine, Freiburg, Germany
Institute of Hygiene and Environmental Medicine, Charité - Universitätsmedizin, Berlin, Germany
National Reference Center for the Surveillance of Nosocomial Infections, Berlin, Germany

Frank Schwab, Michael Behnke, Christine Geffers and Petra Gastmeier
Institute of Hygiene and Environmental Medicine, Charité - Universitätsmedizin, Berlin, Germany
National Reference Center for the Surveillance of Nosocomial Infections, Berlin, Germany

Frank M. Brunkhorst
Center for Sepsis Control and Care, Jena University Hospital, Jena, Germany
Center for Clinical Studies, Jena University Hospital, Jena, Germany
Department of Anesthesiology and Intensive Care Medicine, Jena University Hospital, Jena, Germany

André Scherag
Center for Sepsis Control and Care, Jena University Hospital, Jena, Germany
Institute of Medical Statistics, Computer Sciences and Documentation, Jena University Hospital, Jena, Germany

Zhannur Kaligozhin, Makhira Khudaibergenova and Agzam Zhumadilov
National Research Center for Oncology and Transplantation, Astana, Kazakhstan

Rosimara Gonçalves Leite Vieira, Thaís da Silva Moraes, Larissa de Oliveira Silva, Thamires Chiquini Bianchi, Rodrigo Cassio Sola Veneziani, Sérgio Ricardo Ambrósio, Regina Helena Pires and Carlos Henrique Gomes Martins
Nucleus of Research in Sciences and Technology, Laboratory of Research in Applied Microbiology, University of Franca, Avenida Armando Salles de Oliveira, 201, Franca - São Paulo 14404-600, Brazil

Jairo Kenupp Bastos
School of Pharmaceutical Sciences of Ribeirão Preto, University of São Paulo, Avenida do Café, s/n, Ribeirão Preto - São Paulo 14040-903, Brazil

Chloe Bogaty
University of Manitoba, Winnipeg, MB, Canada

Laura Mataseje and Michael Mulvey
National Microbiology Laboratory, Winnipeg, MB, Canada

Andrew Gray
Northern Health, Prince George, BC, Canada

Brigitte Lefebvre and Simon Lévesque
Laboratoire de santé publique du Québec, Sainte-Anne-de-Bellevue, QC, Canada

Yves Longtin
McGill University, Montreal, QC, Canada

Yekaterina Khamzina, Byron Crape and Azliyati Azizan
Nazarbayev University School of Medicine (NUSOM), 5/1 Kerey and Zhanibek Khans Street, Astana, Kazakhstan010000

Dmitriy Viderman
Nazarbayev University School of Medicine (NUSOM), 5/1 Kerey and Zhanibek Khans Street, Astana, Kazakhstan010000
National Research Neurosurgery Center, Astana, Kazakhstan

Zhijie Zhang and Yong Liu
Shengjing Hospital of China Medical University, Shenyang, China

Meng Chen
Affiliated Hospital of Hebei University, Baoding, China

Ying Yu and Sisi Pan
Pfizer Investment Co.,Ltd, Shanghai, China

A. E. Kates
Division of Infectious Disease, Department of Medicine, School of Medicine and Public Health, University of Wisconsin-Madison, Madison, WI, USA

D. Thapaliya and T. C. Smith
Department of Biostatistics, Epidemiology and Environmental Health Services, College of Public Health, Kent State University, Kent, OH, USA

M. L. Chorazy
Department of Epidemiology, College of Public Health, University of Iowa, Iowa City, IA, USA

Stefan Erb and Andreas Widmer
Division of Infectious Diseases and Hospital Epidemiology, University Hospital Basel, University of Basel, Basel, Switzerland

Reno Frei
Division of Infectious Diseases and Hospital Epidemiology, University Hospital Basel, University of Basel, Basel, Switzerland
Division of Clinical Microbiology, University Hospital Basel, University of Basel, Basel, Switzerland

Jeroen Ensink
Environmental Health Group, Faculty of Infectious and Tropical Diseases, London School of Hygiene and Tropical Medicine, London, UK

Lauren D'Mello-Guyett
Environmental Health Group, Faculty of Infectious and Tropical Diseases, London School of Hygiene and Tropical Medicine, London, UK
Maji Safi kwa Afya Bora Ifakara (MSABI), Morogoro, Tanzania

Fatuma Matwewe
Maji Safi kwa Afya Bora Ifakara (MSABI), Morogoro, Tanzania

Hamisi M. Malebo
National Institute for Medical Research, Dar es Salaam, Tanzania

Robert M. Njee
National Institute for Medical Research, Dar es Salaam, Tanzania
Ministry of Health, Community Development, Gender, Elderly and Children, Dar es Salaam, Tanzania

Vladimira Hinic
Division of Clinical Microbiology, University Hospital Basel, University of Basel, Basel, Switzerland

Index

www.ingramcontent.com/pod-product-compliance
Lightning Source LLC
LaVergne TN
LVHW080737210926
848485LV00003B/571